WORLD COTTON GERMPLASM RESOURCES

Edited by **Ibrokhim Y. Abdurakhmonov**

World Cotton Germplasm Resources
http://dx.doi.org/10.5772/56978
Edited by Ibrokhim Y. Abdurakhmonov

Contributors

Marina Sanamyan, Richard Percy, Lori Hinze, James Frelichowski, Ibrokhim Y. Abdurakhmonov, Warwick Stiller, Iain Wilson, Mauricio Ulloa, Linghe Zeng, Mehboob-Ur- Rahman, Zainab Rahmat, Abid Mahmood, Khalid Abdullah, Yusuf Zafar, Tianzhen Zhang, Narayanan Srinivasan Srirangam, Parchuri Vidyasagar, K. Srinivasu Babu, Yinghua Jia, Junling Sun, Xiongming Du, Manikanda Boopathi

Published by InTech

Janeza Trdine 9, 51000 Rijeka, Croatia

Publishing Process Manager Iva Lipovic

Technical Editor InTech DTP team

Cover InTech Design team

First published July, 2014

Printed in Croatia

Additional hard copies can be obtained from orders@intechopen.com

World Cotton Germplasm Resources, Edited by Ibrokhim Y. Abdurakhmonov

p. cm.

ISBN 978-953-51-1622-6

For EU product safety concerns:
IN TECH d.o.o., Prolaz Marije Krucifikse Kozulić 3, 51000 Rijeka, Croatia,
info@intechopen.com or visit our website at intechopen.com.

Meet the editor

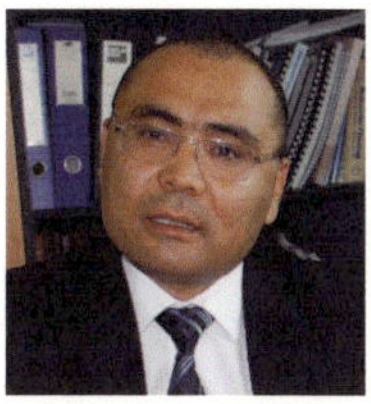

Ibrokhim Y. Abdurakhmonov received his B.S. Degree (1997) in biotechnology from the National University of Uzbekistan, and received M.S. Degree in plant breeding (2001) from Texas A&M University, Texas, USA. He received his PhD degree (2002) in molecular genetics, Doctor of Science degree (2009) in genetics and full professorship (2011) in molecular genetics and molecular biotechnology area from the Institute of Genetics and Plant Experimental Biology, Academy of Uzbek Sciences, Tashkent, Uzbekistan. He is a founder and director of the Center of Genomics and Bioinformatics, Uzbekistan. His research areas include plant genomics, marker-assisted selection, transgenomics, proteomics and bioinformatics. Prof. Abdurakhmonov currently serves as associate editor in several international scientific journals on plant sciences. He is a member of executive board of International Cotton Researchers Association (ICRA), USA. He has received 2010 TWAS prize in agriculture, Uzbekistan government award "Mark of Uzbekistan" in 2010, and ICAC Cotton Researcher of the Year 2013.

Contents

Preface

Being a golden reservoir and fulcrum for biodiversity of useful genes, plant germplasm resources, already conserved *in situ* at the centers of origin and *ex situ* in worldwide plant germplasm collections, are the vital natural resources of earth to provide growing human population with enough food and nutrients, feed, medicinal compounds, clothes, etc. Plant germplasm resources are the basic foundation of plant research to safeguard agriculture from biotic (phytopathogens, pests, and invasive species) and deteriorating abiotic threats (drought and salinity including global climate change) in the globalization and technological advances of the 21st century.

Therefore, understanding the importance of exploration, collection, preservation, storage, maintenance, and propagation of plant germplasm resources are the key tasks and obligations of mankind in the front of future generations. Further, evaluation, characterization, description, exploitation and sharing of available germplasm resources and collections are the stepping stones to provide sustainable agriculture for food and product security. Understanding this, mankind historically paid a great attention and has collected and preserved a wealth of available genetic resources of many plant species worldwide. One of such worldwide plant germplasm resources is available for cotton, which we addressed in this book.

The cultivated *Gossypium spp* . (cotton) is a unique natural fiber producing cash crop for mankind. Besides its fiber, cotton plants provide human livelihoods and animal livestock with the oil and protein portion of the cottonseed – a potential raw material source for alternative bioenergy. The worldwide economic impact of the cotton industry is estimated to ~$500 billion/yr with an annual utilization of ~115-million bales or ~27-million metric tons of cotton fiber. Such economically valuable cotton crop (*Gossypium* genus) includes approximately 45 diploid and 5 allotetraploid species that are largely spread in tropical and subtropical regions of the world. Diploid cottons, referred as Old World cottons, are classified into eight cytogenetically defined genome groups that have African/Asian, American, and Australian origin. Hybridization between diploid Asian cottons (A-genome) and diploid American cottons (D-genome) and subsequent polyploidization about 1.5 million years ago in American continent created the five AD allotetraploid lineages that include the commercially important widely grown coarse fibered (also called Acala or Upland, short stapled, Mocó, and Cambodia cotton) and silk fibered (also called long staple fibered Pima, Sea Island or Egyptian cotton) cotton species.

To protect above-mentioned significant economic value, byproducts and biodiversity of *Gossypium* genus, cotton growing countries worldwide put significant efforts to collect and preserve the cotton genetic resources for the last century period. Such major collections, including breeding materials and wild-species germplasm, genetic and cytogenetic stocks for cotton gene pools exist in Australia, Brazil, China, India, France, Pakistan, Turkey, Russia, United States of America, and Uzbekistan. However, there is evidence that not all collections in an adequate maintenance and shape, having numerous challenges to maintain the collections that make vulnerable some important germplasm and species to extinction.

Here we invited key leaders of worldwide cotton germplasm resources to describe their collections in order to provide readers with updated information on existing cotton germplasm resources. Although some existing collections in Brazil, France, and Russia as well as a leading cytogenetic collection from the United States of America are missing in this book, we successfully compiled key chapters from several leading cotton growing countries including Australia, China, India, Pakistan, United States of America, and Uzbekistan. These 11 peer-reviewed chapters written by 61 distinguished authors, describing the cotton germplasm collections of six countries and germplasm resources of D-genome New World cotton species, provided updated information on the current status and detailed inventory of available cotton germplasm. All chapters also targeted to address past and current progress; enrichment of collections with novel germplasm resources including Bt-cotton, RNA interference and markers assisted selection lines; new trends and molecular tools in germplasm evaluations, development of database, understanding genetic diversity and its exploitation in cotton breeding; future perspectives of existing collections; critical challenges and opportunities in preserving the cotton genetic resources; and the ongoing multi-national communication and collaboration to enhance the germplasm protection, preservation, and evaluation. As an additional literature to published reports, this book should be a comprehensive encyclopedic reading source for plant research community and students to readily gather important information on worldwide cotton genetic resources.

Working with chapter manuscripts and compiling this book has been a great pleasure. I sincerely thank the authors of the book chapters for their response to our invitation, the great efforts putting valuable information together, and their patience with editorial process of chapter manuscripts. I thank following peer-reviewers for their critical reviews of manuscript contents, time, efforts and constructive suggestions on improvement for chapters of the book: **Anna Blenda** , Department of Genetics and Biochemistry, Clemson University, Clemson, South Carolina, USA; **Rafiq Chaudhry**, Technical Information Section, International Cotton Advisory Committee, Washington D.C., USA; **Greg Constable** , CSIRO Plant Industry, Narrabri, Australia; **Vinita Gotmare** , Central Institute for Cotton Research, Nagpur, India; **Johnie N. Jenkins** , United States Department of Agriculture (USDA), Strakville, Mississippi USA; Siva P. Kumpatla, Department of Trait Genetics and Technologies, Dow Agrosciences, Iowa, USA; **Jean-Marc Lacape** , Department of System Biology, CIRAD, Montpellier, France; **Alan E. Pepper** , Department of Biology, Texas A&M University, College Station, Texas, USA; **Richard G. Percy** , United States Department of Agriculture (USDA), College Station, Texas, USA;

Sukumar Saha , United States Department of Agriculture (USDA), Strakville, Mississippi, USA; Mauricio Ulloa, United States Department of Agriculture (USDA), Lubbock,Texas, USA; and **Jonathan F. Wendel** , Department of Ecology, Evolution, & Organismal Biology, Iowa State University, Iowa, USA.

I greatly acknowledge the Intech Editorial Board for considering this book project and its publication. I thank Ms. **Ivana Lorković** and Ms. **Iva Lipović** , InTech Publishing Process Managers, for coordination of the entire book editing and publication process.

Ibrokhim Y. Abdurakhmonov
Center of Genomics and Bioinformatics,
Academy of Sciences of Uzbekistan,
Ministry of Agriculture and Water Resource,
"Uzcottonindustry" association,
Tashkent,
Uzbekistan

Chapter 1

Australian Cotton Germplasm Resources

Warwick N. Stiller and Iain W. Wilson

Additional information is available at the end of the chapter

http://dx.doi.org/10.5772/58414

1. Introduction

1.1. History

Cotton has been sporadically cultivated in Australia since the late 1700s with varying degrees of success until the advent of the modern intensively managed and mechanised industry in the latter half of the Twentieth Century. There were initial attempts to establish an industry during the mid 1800s to fill the demand in Britain for lint caused by declining production during the US Civil War, but with the return of US production after the war this new incarnation of an Australian industry was relatively short lived. In the early 1900s, financial incentives were introduced by the Queensland State Government to promote production in that State and by 1934 around 4000 tonnes of cotton lint, primarily from imported cultivars, were being produced. However, by the mid 1900s production was again virtually non-existent because of the prohibitively high cost of labour [1]. By the 1960s, the development of proper infrastructure for irrigation and mechanised pickers led to a rapid increase in area and production in northern NSW and southern and central Qld which was aided by the development of locally adapted cultivars in the 1980s and 1990s. An industry was also attempted in the Ord River Irrigation Area in the tropical region of Western Australia. However, this had collapsed by 1973 predominantly due to insect resistance to pesticides, but the crop continued to flourish in the Eastern part of Australia where the insect pressure was lower. Genetically modified cotton (Ingard®-Monsanto's MON531 *Cry1Ac* Bt) was first commercialised in 1996 and by 2005 over 90% of the area was grown to GM cultivars (Monsanto's Bollgard II® and Roundup Ready Flex®). In the 2011/12 season, the cotton area exceeded 700,000 ha, was >99% GM and produced over one million tonnes of lint.

The Australian cotton industry covers a wide north-south geographical range of 13° latitude (Figure 1); is based on a combination of heavy clay soils; and is challenged by a range of pests and diseases. The industry is predominantly upland cotton (*Gossypium hirsutum*), with up to

2% of pima cotton (*Gossypium barbadense*). Since 2010, as a result of a long drought and eventually loss of infrastructure to support its processing, there has been no Pima cotton grown in this country. The Commonwealth Scientific and Industrial Research Organisation (CSIRO) cotton breeding program has developed and released over 100 very successful cultivars adapted to local conditions with a high yield and quality. By 2000, these had displaced all imported cultivars and any other local competition and currently all cotton grown commercially in Australia stems from that program. Between 1995 and 2009, yield progress from the CSIRO program was an impressive 18.3 kg ha^{-1} $year^{-1}$, with 48% of that yield improvement directly attributed to cultivar, 28% to improved management and 24% to the interaction between cultivar and management [2], making Australia one of the highest yielding cotton producers per hectare globally.

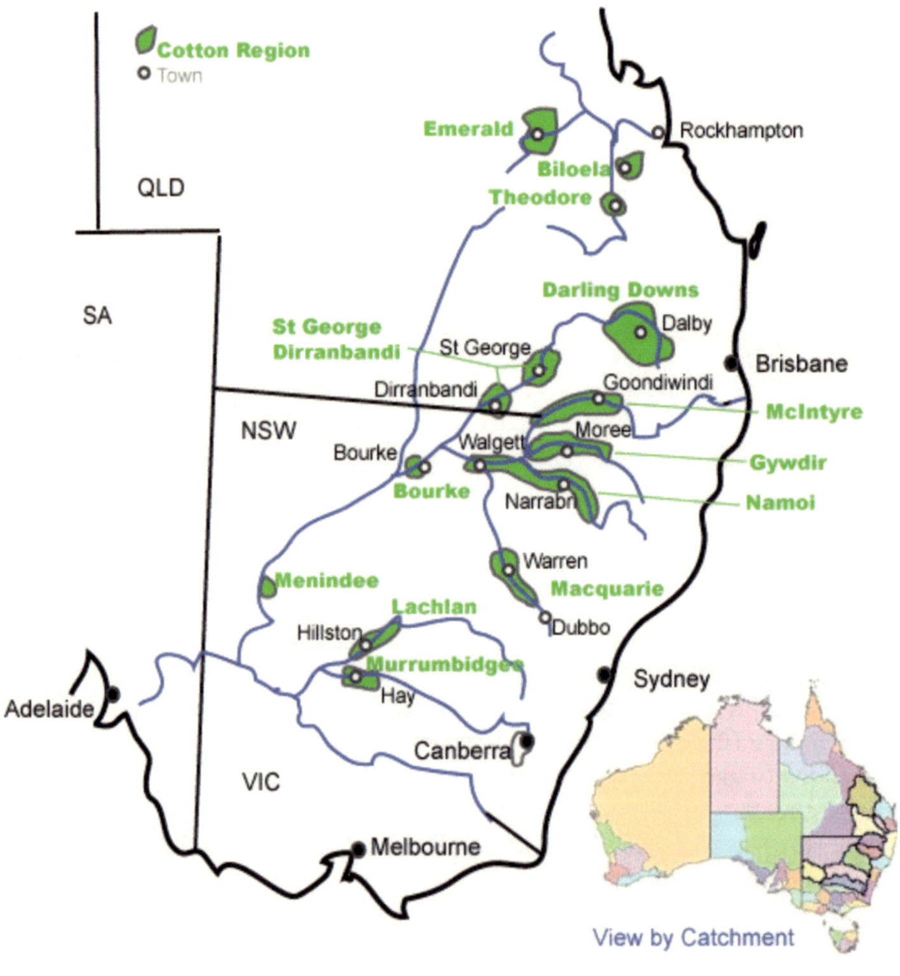

Figure 1. Australian cotton production regions

1.1.1. History of cotton breeding programs in Australia

Cotton breeding in Australia began in a very piecemeal manner with most early growers relying on unimproved and imported US cultivars. The first concerted effort to breed locally adapted cultivars came when a cotton research station was established in Central Queensland in 1923 and a Queensland DPI breeding program eventually released local cultivars to replace some of the imported cultivars. The first locally selected cultivar was Miller 43-9-0. This program also worked on insect host-plant resistance, producing a jassid-resistant hairy cultivar that was discontinued with the advent of widespread mechanical harvesting that was less tolerant of hairy leaf trash adhering to the cotton. This breeding program closed in 1990.

With bounties to encourage production and construction of dams to facilitate irrigation, cotton expanded into more temperate areas in the 1960s and particularly through the 1980s. In 1972, breeding programs in southern NSW (CSIRO) and in northern Western Australia (CSIRO) were all consolidated at one location at Narrabri in northern New South Wales (NSW), where NSW Agriculture had established a breeding program in 1960. The NSW Agriculture program initially screened overseas cultivars for suitability to the unique combination of soils and climate in northern NSW, but evolved to study resistance to Verticillium wilt. This program closed in 1980. The CSIRO breeding program in southern NSW had a particular emphasis on earliness and suitability for ultra narrow row systems. This program used a wide range of germplasm for breeding, including from USSR and US Texas material to produce a number of early-maturing cultivars such as Riverina Poplar and Riverina Gold [3]. This program closed in 1972 with the move to Narrabri.

Until the mid-1980s, the majority of cultivars grown in Australia were still imported from the US, principally Deltapine Smoothleaf, DP16, DP61 and DP90. The Delta and Pineland Company established a breeding program in 1990 and marketed a number of cultivars, particularly GM, over the next decade. This US company changed hands and withdrew from marketing cultivars in 2010 as CSIRO developed cultivars had displaced the majority of even their locally bred offerings, but it still retains a breeding station in Australia.

The CSIRO breeding program in northern Western Australia originally concentrated on adaptation to a system of sowing before the tropical wet season, then relying on fruit set during the dry season before harvest in winter [4]. This system and regional production collapsed due to heavy insect pressure and resistance by *Helicoverpa armigera* to insecticides. This program moved to northern NSW in 1972 and initially had strong emphasis on host plant resistance, with success in releasing okra leaf cultivars with tolerance to mites and *Helicoverpa* [5, 6] that set the foundations for future cultivar development by CSIRO. This program has grown rapidly since 1972 and has released many cultivars which now dominate the Australian cotton production system [7].

2. Challenges faced in breeding of Australian cultivars

Breeding challenges have largely been dictated by unique biotic and abiotic limitations on production and the need for Australia to remain competitive with other producing countries that have lower labour costs. There has therefore always been a high focus on improving yield potential as a first priority and incremental increases in fibre quality to meet changing spinning requirements that might restrict the marketability of Australian cotton. Overlaid on these efforts has been targeted breeding for yield protection from losses caused from individual biotic and abiotic factors. Some of the early emphasis on breeding for host-plant resistance to insects has changed with the advent of genetically modified traits, but this has just moved the priorities to other challenges. A key asset to the breeding has been access to a diverse collection of germplasm from around the world, building on a quite diverse suite of base cultivars developed in the early 1970s and 1980s that have allowed CSIRO to tackle challenging insect, disease and weed issues.

2.1. Insects

A number of important pests of cotton are found in Australia that have necessitated the establishment of intensive pest management programs [8]. Cotton breeders have initiated programs to address host plant resistance and eventually released local cultivars containing *Bt* traits to confer resistance to the most important *Lepidopteron* pests.

The key pests of cotton in Australia are the larvae of two lepidopteron species, *Helicoverpa armigera* and *H. punctigera*, together with cotton aphid (*Aphis gossypii*), green mirid (*Creontiades dilutus*), spider mites (*Tetranychus urticae*) and silverleaf whitefly (*Bemisia tabaci* B-Biotype). From the 1960's to early 2000's, pest management was highly reliant on use of insecticides, mostly broad spectrum organophosphates, carbamates and pyrethroids as well as endosulfan. Crops were sprayed around 12-16 times per season [9]. This has brought with it predictable problems of pesticide resistance, destruction of natural enemy populations resulting in pest resurgence and outbreaks of secondary pests such as aphids [10] and spider mites [11], health concerns and off-farm movement into sensitive riverine environments [9].

Deployment of Ingard® (Monsanto's Bollgard) cotton in 1996 reduced insecticide use on those crops by about 50%, but efficacy was limited due to declining expression of *Cry1Ac* through the growing season. Ingard® cotton was always seen as an interim technology and during this period its area was capped at 30% to reduce the risk that *Helicoverpa spp.* would develop resistance to this critical insecticidal protein. This regulation limited the influence of the technology on the industry. The strong reliance on insecticides continued on the remaining 70% of conventional cotton and led to ongoing selection for resistance to insecticides in *H. armigera,* secondary pest problems and selection of pesticide resistance in these secondary pests. For instance, by the early 2000's spider mites were resistant to organophosphates, the pyrethroid bifenthrin and chlorfenapyr, and cotton aphids were resistant to organophosphates, the carbamate pirimicarb and pyrethroids [12].

The deployment of Bollgard II® in 2003/04, for improved resistance management and removal of the 30% area cap, resulted in a dramatic uptake of this technology. It also led to a massive decline in pesticide use (by about 85% [13]), especially relative to earlier years but also in comparison with contemporary conventional cotton that had also significantly reduced its reliance on pesticides. This technology essentially saved the cotton industry from insecticide resistance in *H. armigera,* although a pre-emptive *Bt* resistance management strategy was initiated [12].

Over the past 10 years, silverleaf whitefly has occasionally reached pest status in some regions of the Australian cotton industry. It was first reported in cotton regions in 1994 [14], and the first major outbreak occurred in the Emerald production region in 2001/02. There are limited effective chemical control options for whitefly and they are also very expensive, so there is large emphasis on sampling protocols, thresholds and cultural control of this pest [15].

A range of other minor pests have occurred since 2000, many of which are related to the introduction and use of Bollgard II®. Reduced spraying for *Helicoverpa* has allowed survival of pale cotton stainers (*Dysdercus sidae*), jassids (*Austroasca viridigrisea*) and thrips (*Frankliniella schultzei* and *F. occidentalis*) late in the season and in some years these species have all caused damage and sporadically required control [12].

2.2. Weeds

In Australia, weeds are generally less of a problem in cotton than insects such as *Helicoverpa,* but many areas do have a reasonably high incidence of problematic weeds particularly on former grazing and/or flood-prone land [16]. Some of the problem weeds are *Ipomea spp., Cyperus rotundas, Polymeria spp., Conyze bonariensis,* and *Datura spp.* Weed control systems have changed in the last decade: production has changed from a cultivation-based system with residual herbicides and hand hoeing, to a system of minimal cultivation, with the use of herbicide tolerant cultivars (glyphosate and glufosinate) and few if any residual herbicides [17]. This has caused weed composition to shift to glyphosate tolerant species (particularly *Conyze sp.*) and has the real risk of developing glyphosate resistant weed populations.

2.3. Diseases

Many diseases of cotton are present in Australia and have necessitated the establishment of breeding projects to confer host resistance.

Bacterial blight of cotton caused by *Xanthomonas axonopodis* pv. *malvacearum* was historically the most important and widespread disease in Australian cotton. This disease was present in all crops and averaged around 20% of bolls affected though the mid-to late-1980s. The use of standard differential cultivars showed that Race 18 of the pathogen was predominant [18] and that infected seed was the major factor in the epidemiology of the disease. The disease was partially controlled through the production of blight-free planting seed. The CSIRO breeding program has released cultivars with immunity to blight and this disease is no longer found in Australian production systems due to 100% uptake of blight-resistant cultivars.

Verticillium wilt caused by *Verticillium dahliae* has been an important disease in Australia for many years, especially in the older growing regions of the Namoi, Gwydir and McIntyre. It is assumed that this pathogen is endemic to Australia. To date, all the Australian Verticillium isolates that have been tested are categorised as 'non-defoliating' strains [19]. Despite not having the more severe 'defoliating' strains that occur in other countries, yield reductions of up to 20% have been recorded [20]. The majority of cultivars now grown commercially have relatively strong resistance to Verticillium wilt, but in seasonal conditions that favour the disease (temperature between 22-27°C [21]) and high number of rain days during the boll filling period [Allen S.J, pers comm.], significant productions losses still occur in some regions so improving resistance remains a breeding focus at a somewhat lower priority than other diseases.

Fusarium wilt caused by *Fusarium oxysporum* f sp. *vasinfectum*, was first recognised in Australia in 1993 [22] and is characterised by causing plant mortality at any time throughout the season, from seedling emergence through to harvest. By the end of 1999, the disease was present in six of the ten cotton production areas in Eastern Australia, but only widespread in two of those areas [23]. Subsequently, it has been shown that this is a unique strain of Fusarium and is substantially different to strains that are pathogenic to cotton in other countries [24]. This new Australian strain is identified as race 6 and is associated with alkaline clays, absence of nematodes [25], seedling death and an optimum temperature of 18 to 23°C [26]. Fusarium in the USA are races 1 and 2 and are associated with acid sands and nematodes [25], symptoms occur in mid-season with no plant mortality and an optimum temperature of 30 to 32°C [27]. It is assumed that the Australian pathogen evolved locally on weeds within our production system [28]. The extreme virulence and persistence of this pathogen and its ability to be readily transported in soil, water or trash raised concern within the industry when it was first discovered [29], particularly because most commercially grown cultivars in 1994 were highly susceptible. Production losses of virtually 100% have been reported for some fields. Substantial progress has been made in developing more resistant cultivars. However, for fields that have a high level of inoculum, the most resistant cultivar may still only have 10% survival in seasons that favour the disease so it remains a significant breeding challenge.

Cotton bunchy top disease (CBT) was first recorded in the late 1990s when a severe outbreak occurred in several Australian growing regions. Economic losses in that season alone were estimated at AUD$70 million [30], with nearly all Australian cotton cultivars being susceptible to the disease. The cotton aphid (*Aphis gossypii*) was identified as the vector and since then, there have only been sporadic outbreaks as the vector has generally been well controlled but its incidence is now very widespread across the industry. The causal agent has subsequently been identified as a Polerovirus and has some similarities to cotton blue disease found in Africa, Asia and the Americas [30]. Currently no commercial cultivars in Australia have resistance to this disease, although a readily accessible source of resistance has been identified in Australian material and cultivars are due for release around 2017.

Black root rot caused by *Thielaviopsis basicola* was first reported on cotton in Australia in 1990 [31]. It is now present in almost all cotton fields in NSW, as well as many in Qld. Diseased plants show stunted growth early in the season when the cooler temperatures favour the pathogen. While the pathogen does not kill plants, it can cause significant yield loss in cooler and shorter season regions due to the delay in crop maturation. The wide host range of the pathogen and persistence of the chlamydospores makes effective control through crop rotation very difficult. No *G. hirsutum* or *G. barbadense* cotton cultivars have been shown to have any significant resistance to this pathogen, so breeders must look to primary, secondary or tertiary germplasm or to GM approaches for control of this disease.

Alternaria leaf spot caused by *Alternaria macrospora* has caused severe defoliation of cotton grown on less fertile soils when the crop is exposed to extended periods of wet weather. These conditions occasionally occur in some Queensland growing regions. All upland cultivars currently grown have some degree of resistance, so the disease is considered of minor importance [20].

Reniform nematodes, *Rotylenchulus reniformis*, associated with stunting of cotton plants have only recently been identified in Australia [32] and are yet to be considered of economic importance. There was an isolated detection in 2003 in central Qld, but a more widespread identification was made in 2012, so it may become more important with time and pre-emptive breeding for resistance may be desirable.

2.4. Other industry challenges

A range of other industry challenges are also being, or need to be, addressed through breeding. There is a constant awareness of the dangers of having a narrow genetic base from which cultivars are developed. However, it is also acknowledged that broadening the genetic base through the introduction of exotic germplasm can often have a detrimental effect on yield [33]. In Australia, there is clear evidence of continuing yield improvement through selection within a 'narrowing' germplasm pool. In a high input, high yield industry such as Australia, there is a requirement for continued yield improvement to counter the ever increasing cost of production. While some of these improvements can come from improved management, historical data indicates that new cultivars are expected to provide at least 50% of the increase [2].

Many of the new challenges are related to the introduction of new technology or new environmental standards. The introduction of GM insect resistance traits into Australia in the mid 1990s simplified many aspects of pest management. However, it was soon discovered that the combination of high fruit retention of insect-protected crops together with early-maturity genotypes resulted in crops that had a fruiting cycle shorter than the available growing season and thus were not capitalising on the inherent yield potential of the cultivars. This had a detrimental effect on yield, so longer season, more indeterminate germplasm was subsequently used to deploy the GM traits. This remains a challenge as the industry expands into the southern (shorter season) regions of Australia where yield expectations of growers are similar to the fuller season traditional regions and may require a different approach to breeding.

Most Australian cotton is exported to Asia and spun on ring-spinning frames. Although this spinning technology has been used for around 100 years, modern machines continue to run faster and spinning companies demand greater throughput. This places greater stresses on the fibre, so there is a continual demand for higher quality fibre. There are well documented negative associations between yield and quality [34] which makes the simultaneous improvement of both yield and fibre quality difficult. In addition, breeders are also expected to address changing future fibre quality requirements due to changes in spinning technology or the yarn that is required by the textile industry.

At a time of increased awareness of the potential for climate change, greater scrutiny is also being placed on climate-related aspects of agricultural production [35]. Australia already has a limited water supply, so increases in water-use efficiency (WUE) are being sought through management and breeding. In addition, the energy consumed and the emissions produced by a cotton crop are also being closely examined. Due to the heavy influence that yield has in the WUE calculation, this must continue to be the major focus of breeding programs. The efficient use of other resources, such as nitrogen fertiliser, will significantly influence the emissions from a crop [36, 37], so breeding programs also have responsibilities to continue research in this area.

3. Content and description of Australian cotton germplasm collections

Initially, Australian plant breeders acquired and maintained their own germplasm collections. However, in the early 1980s the Commonwealth and State governments established a series of genetic resource centres to conserve national germplasm collections. The Australian Tropical Crops and Forages Genetic Resource Centre (ATCF) Biloela, Qld is the centre that included cotton. Currently, the only other two cotton collections in Australia reside at CSIRO Plant Industry in Narrabri, NSW and Canberra, ACT.

Unfortunately, the ATCF cotton collection is, at present, only funded to maintain germplasm under long-term storage, so the collection is not actively maintained or expanded. However, germplasm can still be requested from this collection. The CSIRO collection at Narrabri is maintained and funded by the dedicated breeding program. The CSIRO collection in Canberra is largely dedicated to the long-term storage of indigenous Australian species that have been collected through germplasm explorations [38] over the last few decades. Table 1 describes the number of cultivated tetraploid accessions amalgamated across the ATCF and CSIRO Narrabri collections. This includes both cultivars as well as locally developed and introduced germplasm. Table 2 describes the wild accessions held in all three collections.

Species	Description	Number of accessions
G. hirsutum	Germplasm	952
	Cultivars	611
	Landraces	10
	Total	*1573*
G. barbadense	Germplasm	51
	Cultivars	45
	Landraces	3
	Total	*99*
Other hybrids/genetic stocks		12

Table 1. Number of cultivated tetraploid accessions in Australian collections.

http://dx.doi.org/10.5772/58414

Species	Number of accessions	Genome*
Primary gene pool		
G. tomentosum	6	AD3
G. mustelinum	1	AD4
G.darwinii	1	AD5
Secondary gene pool		
G. herbaceum	39	A1
G. arboreum	211	A2
G. anomalum	4	B1
G. logicalyx	1	F1
G. thurberi	5	D1
G. trilobum	1	D8
G. davidsonii	2	D3-d
G. klotzschianum	1	D3-k
G. armourianum	1	D2-1
G. harknessii	1	D2-2
G. aridum	1	D4
G. raimondii	1	D5
Tertiary gene pool		
G.sturtianum	64	C1
G.robinsonii	3	C2
G. stocksii	3	E1
G. somalense	2	E2
G.australe	159	G
G.nelsonii	39	G
G.bickii	28	G1
G.costulatum	1	K
G.cunninghamii	2	K
G.enthyle	1	K
G.exiguum	3	K
G.nobile	1	K
G.pilosum	1	K
G.populifolium	1	K
G.pulchellum	1	K
G.rotundifolium	3	K
unclassified	8	

* As per [39]

Table 2. Number of wild primary, secondary and tertiary tetraploid and diploid accessions in Australian collections.

3.1. Australian native *Gossypium*

Australia is home to 17 native *Gossypium* species that are found exclusively in Australia and are distantly related to cultivated cotton. These contain the C, G and K genome species. The distribution and characterisation of these diploid species has been reasonably well documented [40-43]. The potential for transferring traits from these species, together with techniques for the production of fertile hybrids has also been reported [44, 45]. There is interest in a number of traits from these species, however, research has largely focused on disease resistance [46, 47], glandless, and seed-glanded plants [45, 48]. Despite this research, there are no documented cases of successfully transferring economically important traits from the wild Australian *Gossypium* species to cultivated cotton. There still remains interest in this area and improvements in molecular techniques may facilitate the successful introgression of traits.

3.2. Plant quarantine requirements

Australia has strict plant quarantine regulations which aim to safeguard Australia's plant health status to maintain overseas markets and protect the economy from the impact of exotic pests and diseases. This is administered by the Commonwealth (Federal) Department of Agriculture, Fisheries and Forestry (DAFF) Biosecurity based on policy determined in consultation with industry stakeholders (http://www.daff.gov.au/bsg) [verified December 2013]. For cotton, these requirements are quite onerous and costly, which restricts capacity for importing cotton seed into Australia.

3.3. Focus of the collections

Both the ATCF and the CSIRO Canberra collections have actively collected wild *Gossypium* accessions. As can be seen in Table 2, this has largely focused on *G. sturtianum, G. australe, G. nelsonii* and *G. bickii.* However, the major focus of the CSIRO Narrabri and ATCF collections have been the collecting of overseas cultivars, predominantly *G. hirsutum*, for use in the Australian cotton breeding programs. Over time, these programs have had a range of objectives as mentioned previously which is reflected in the material accumulated. Major areas of interest have been general genetic diversity, targeted host-plant resistance to insects and diseases, crop maturity, fibre quality and yield.

3.4. Key contributors to collections

Over time, germplasm representing most cotton producing countries has been sourced. This has either come directly from breeders (through exchange), acquisition of commercially released cultivars, or requests to centralised cotton collections. Initially, germplasm was sourced in larger numbers to rapidly develop the collections, however, as time has gone on, the requests for germplasm have been much more focused, as for example when Fusarium wilt was discovered in the early 1990s in Australia. Although this is a locally evolved strain that is unique to Australia, significant efforts went into searching for germplasm that had improved levels of resistance. Extensive literature searches were undertaken to identify potential germplasm from other countries to evaluate for resistance. Once a genotype had been identified, various databases were searched and institutions contacted in an attempt to find a source for the material. Although germplasm was sourced from a number of countries, the USDA collection in TX proved to be an extremely valuable resource for resistance to Australian isolates of Fusarium. This example highlights the need to be aware of what is available, to seek out that germplasm and request it under as favourable terms as possible.

3.5. Current status of collections

Although the ATCF collection is acknowledged as a valuable national resource, funding of this collection remains uncertain. On the other hand, the CSIRO collection at Narrabri is a live collection associated with an active breeding program. Although not an extensive collection by world standards, containing around 1000 introduced cultivars and germplasm, it is nonetheless a critical component of the CSIRO breeding program. The collection is continually being added to when new material is identified which may contain diversity for traits of interest. Many of these relate to insect and disease resistance, but yield, fibre quality and maturity are also targeted.

3.6. Storage and renewal of germplasm collections

The ATCF collection is maintained under long-term conditions in which germplasm is preserved as fuzzy seed that is dried to 6% moisture content at 15°C. Once the seed is dry, it is sealed in laminated aluminium bags and stored at -20°C. Under these conditions, it is expected that viability will be maintained for at least 50 years. Previously, when funding was available, all accessions were routinely monitored for germination every 10 years and regenerated if germination fell below 60% of the starting germination. Seed was either regenerated in the field or greenhouse with controlled pollination. Germplasm was extensively characterised in the past, but this is no longer undertaken. The collection maintains an in-house seed management database that manages germplasm passport, collection, characterization, inventory, seed health, regeneration and distribution data. The passport and characterisation data are freely available via the Australian Plant Genetic Resources Information System Web site (http://www2.dpi.qld.gov.au/extra/asp/auspgris) [verified December 2013]. A national review of Plant Genetic Resource Centres in Australia has determined that this website will be replaced with GRIN-Global. However, a deadline for this transition has not been finalised.

The CSIRO Narrabri collection is maintained in short-term storage as delinted seed at 7°C and 50% relative humidity. Around 1 kg of each accession are stored in cotton bags. A 10g backup collection is also maintained in sealed laminated aluminium bags at 4°C in an additional facility on the same site. Each accession is regenerated in the field every 10 years, or when stocks have been depleted to less than 200g. During regeneration, accessions are inspected and compared to known visual characteristics and off types are removed. Accessions that are photoperiod sensitive are grown in the greenhouse during the winter when the short days promote flowering. In addition, those accessions in which purity is considered vital to maintain are also grown in the greenhouse. The CSIRO breeding program maintains an internal database where accession data is recorded. This database is not publicly available.

The CSIRO Canberra collection is in long-term storage at -20°C. This collection provides a resource, but is not currently funded or maintained. Many of its accessions are also available from major US germplasm collections, as US researchers were often involved in the initial exploration. As the majority of these lines have been collected during genetic explorations, an internal database contains details of the collector, location and date. This database is not publicly available. There has been a decline in funding in CSIRO over the last few decades for extending germplasm collections for native *Gossypium* and other crop relatives like *Glycine*, as more and more biodiversity research shifts to consolidation of national collections, electronic archiving of data and making them more broadly accessible on-line.

There are increasing challenges associated with maintenance and regeneration of these collections. Ensuring genetic purity of accessions has always been difficult when regeneration is conducted in the field. However, the GM era has added another level of complexity to the problem. Even though Australia does not have large numbers of insects that will cause cross pollination in cotton (only the European honey bee), measurable out-crossing can occur in some seasons and some locations [49, 50]. Care must be taken to locate regeneration blocks away from known sources of bee activity as well as isolated from commercial GM cotton crops. CSIRO also has substantial activities in areas of biotech research in addition to the traits sourced from third parties and some of these activities are discussed in a later section. This research is geographically isolated (in Canberra) from the breeding program and only traits that have reached the advanced field evaluation stage are grown at Narrabri. As CSIRO is developing cultivars for release commercially, stewardship of germplasm and GM traits is extremely important and internal quality assurance protocols are rigorously adhered to. These protocols dictate that all material needs to be tested via protein or DNA analysis prior to handover to commercial partners for seed increase and sale.

3.7. Germplasm passport data

The current status of the accession descriptions varies depending on when and who imported them, as well as the donor. As many characteristics are either invisible or not able to be determined except in specific environments (e.g., disease resistance), the data provided by the donor is often critical. However, in many cases, particularly for older material, this information is simply not available for many accessions that may have been obtained via an intermediary collection or supplier. When it was actively funded, the ATCF collection generated substantial passport data on all lines including morphological characteristics, boll size, lint percent and fibre quality parameters. This is invaluable information for a breeder searching for specific characteristics. Descriptions in the CSIRO collection are more *ad-hoc*. This is largely a function of the collection not being 'public', and simply a resource for the breeding program that operates it. The data that does exist largely relate to the traits that were initially identified as being of interest *i.e.*, HPR to insects and disease or fibre quality.

3.8. Sharing and exchange

The ATCF collection is based on a national collection model with small quantities (20-30 seeds) of germplasm freely available to researchers worldwide. The CSIRO collection is not publicly available, but historically, genuine exchange with other breeding programs has been practised. In recent years however, commercial agreements and patents have made this exchange difficult. This has restricted the amount of new material added to the collection. However, it is imperative that exchange of germplasm continues. Many of the patent and commercial 'in confidence' issues can be addressed with specific (though often restrictive) material transfer agreements. This can allow new germplasm to be evaluated prior to negotiating further freedoms to utilise germplasm in a breeding program.

4. Other cotton germplasm resources beyond seed collections

4.1. Mapping populations

Improving disease resistance against indigenous Australian strains of Fusarium has been a high priority in the Australian breeding program and a number of new sources of resistance have been identified through the screening of introductions (mostly) from the US, China and India where Fusarium is also endemic. To investigate the genetic basis of the Fusarium wilt resistance in the Indian *G. hirsutum* cultivar MCU-5, a bi-parental cross was made between MCU-5 and Siokra 1-4; a *Fusarium* susceptible Australian okra leaf *G. hirsutum* cultivar [51]. An F_3 population consisting of 244 lines was developed from this cross, and from single seed decent from each F_3 line, 244 F_4 lines subsequently produced. The F_3 and F_4 populations were assayed for Fusarium wilt resistance using a glasshouse bioassay [52] and genotyped with 151 markers (95 SSR and 56 AFLP). QTL analysis revealed the presence of multiple regions that were associated with resistance that provide targets for introgression into elite cultivars to improve Fusarium wilt resistance [51]. Subsequently, it was found that MCU-5 which was derived from a multi-line cross between Indian Cambodia-type cultivars (MCU-1 and MCU-2) and cultivars from East Africa, the West Indies and the US, including some contribution from *G. barbadense,* also possesses significant resistance to non-defoliating strains of *Verticillium dahliae,* as well as possessing significantly longer fibre than Siokra 1-4.

In an international collaboration with CIRAD (France), CSIRO obtained a 140 RIL inter-specific population ranging from the F_6 to F_9 stages of selfing through single seed descent. The two parents; Guazuncho 2 (*G. hirsutum*), and VH8-4602 (*G. barbadense*), were chosen for their agronomic performance (Guazuncho 2) and superior fibre quality parameters (VH8-4602) [53]. This population was grown in several countries including Australia in the glasshouse and field and analysed for many different traits (including fibre, leaf shape hairiness, boll size and number and earliness) and genotypes consisting of 1,745 loci derived from 597 SSR and 763 ALFP markers [54-56]. Not all of the lines performed well under Australian conditions with only about 55 flowering within an acceptable timeframe for harvesting and thus seed stocks are severely restricted for most of the RILs. The QTLs associated with fibre traits identified in Australia may help generate markers for selection for these traits in breeding populations. The population also represents a resource for linking markers with mite resistance, as the parent lines show differentiation in resistance.

4.2. Near isogenic lines of host plant resistance traits

Cotton mutants can be of interest to cotton breeders for their agronomic or host plant resistance possibilities. Near Isogenic lines (NIL) are plants that mostly genetically identical except in DNA regions associated with a specific trait or gene mutation. They are usually created by the repeated backcrossing of a mutant plant to a recurring parent, and are useful for quantifying the effect of the mutation or phenotype on agronomic performance, by reducing genetic background differences between the mutant and the normal plant type. Although very important for defining the agronomic value of an altered phenotype, NILs require a large investment of time to produce. Thomson [57] developed NILs for glabrousness (T_2^{arm}), frego bract (fg), okra leaf (L_2^0), and nectariless (ne_1,ne_2). These mutations are known to affect resistance to specific insects and diseases, and in the case of glabrous also reduces lint trash [57]. All 16 NIL combinations of the four mutants were developed in the Deltapine 61 background. The 16 NIL were derived from an initial crossing of a Deltapine-related experimental line homozygous for all four mutant characters and Deltapine 61. Four backcrosses were then made with Deltapine 61. A final backcross was made and from a large F_2 population homozygous genotypes were selected and maintained. Subsequent hybridizations were done using lines from this original population as parents and a total of nine cultivars were released up until 1999 including the original Siokra and Sicot cultivars.

4.3. Mutant populations

Mutation and mutation breeding is a tool for producing novel variation that potentially cannot be found in existing cotton species, for genetic improvement and in aiding the study of gene function. Mutations are nucleotide base changes within the genome of an organism that are not brought on by normal recombination and segregation, and occur naturally at a low frequency. Many naturally derived mutant cotton plants have been isolated that contain no fibre, which has aided our molecular understanding of fibre formation [58]. The rate of mutation can be greatly increased or induced in plants using chemical mutagens, ionizing radiation or transposable elements. Induced mutants have been generated and used to create valuable traits in many major crops, but have only occasionally been used in improving cotton. Mutagenesis of cotton has resulted in 'naked and tufted' seeds, herbicide resistance and plants with longer fibre [59-62] that have direct application within the cotton industry. Other mutants, such as those possessing inferior fibre traits, provide powerful tools for understanding what genes are associated with fibre formation [58].

CSIRO is investigating the general usefulness of mutagenised cotton populations for conventional plant breeding. Populations of *G. hirsutum*, *G. barbadense* and *G. arboreum* have been mutagenised with the chemical mutagens sodium azide and ethyl methanesulfonate, as well as heavy-ion mutagenesis using the Riken Ring Cyclotron at the RI Beam facility in Japan in collaboration with Dr Tomoko Abe. The mutagenised populations are currently being screened for a number of traits including: herbicide resistance, fibre traits, boll size, plant architecture and flowering.

http://dx.doi.org/10.5772/58414

4.4. Transgenics

A transgenic cotton plant contains gene/s that have been artificially inserted. The inserted gene (known as a transgene) may come from another cotton plant, or from a completely different species, such as *Bt* cotton; which possesses the *Bt* toxin from the bacterium *Bacillus thuringiensis*. Transgenic technology enables plant breeders to bring together in one plant traits from potentially any organism, not just from within Upland cotton or sexually compatible species. Potentially this technology could be a quicker and cleaner method of bringing in traits from poor agronomic sources compared to backcrossing, but regulatory costs makes this currently unfeasible. Transgenic technology also provides the means for studying specific genes in cotton and enables the definitive assignment of genes to specific functions through either overexpression or silencing of individual genes or gene families.

It is difficult and time consuming to generate transgenic cotton, as it requires *Agrobacterium tumefaciens* mediated gene insertion via callus, generated via tissue culture. It was found in the 1980s that Coker cultivars were generally superior for gene transfer using tissue culture, although a small number of Australian cultivars could be transformed with relatively low efficiency [63]. Coker 315 is the cultivar used for all transformation events in Australia as it was thought to possess better agronomic traits under Australian conditions compared to other transformable Coker cultivars, such as Coker 312 that have been used by international biotech companies. Currently, all transgenic traits present in Australian commercial cultivars were obtained internationally under License from either Monsanto or Bayer CropScience. The focus of Australian transgenic R&D work has been on developing potential traits of more specific relevance to the Australian Industry and on basic research to understand gene function, particularly the functions of genes involved in fibre initiation and formation, plant defence and seed oil formation. Such work has demonstrated the importance of GhMyb 25 [64], GhMyb25-like [65] and GhHD-1 [66] for fibre initiation and for controlling fibre initial numbers. As part of CSIRO research, transgenic cotton plants that are altered in the expression of GhMYB109 were imported under a Material Transfer Agreement for research use [67]. CSIRO transgenic research has demonstrated through altering the expression of a cotton sucrose synthase [68] or overexpressing a potato sucrose synthase [69] the essential role of the different sucrose synthases in cotton fibre and seed formation. Expression of the *Talaromyces flavus* glucose oxidase gene in cotton demonstrated increased resistance against Verticillium wilt [70], and plants with suppressed Cadinene synthase gene expression revealed its role in bacterial blight infection [71]. Although cotton is principally a crop grown for fibre, its seeds are also a valuable source of oil. Transgenic silencing of key fatty acid desaturase genes altered the cottonseed oil composition to improve its nutritional profile, making it more competitive with other oilseed crops has also been achieved, although commercialisation of this trait is still under discussion [72]. Currently none of these CSIRO transgenic derived traits have been incorporated into commercial cultivars.

Successful expression of transgenes in cotton also requires the ability to precisely express genes at high levels. Experiments with transgenic plants have demonstrated the value of the soybean lectin gene promoter to drive transgenes in the embryo of cotton seeds [73], and subterranean clover stunt virus promoters and terminators [74] for general and high level expression in cotton. The CSIRO derived sub-clover duplicated stunt7 viral promoter was deregulated in 2008 as a commercial event in cotton (T304-40) driving the *Cry1Ab* insect resistance gene and forms part of Bayer CropScience's TwinLink product. A cotton rubisco small subunit promoter has also been shown to be expressed at high levels in green photosynthetic tissues throughout the development of cotton in the field and hence a useful promoter for expressing transgenes in leaves [75].

5. Molecular markers for germplasm characterisation

Molecular markers are DNA tags or sequence differences (polymorphisms) that provide the ability to quickly track the presence of specific DNA regions associated with a trait, through a segregating population. They are widely used for basic research in plant biology and genetics and are now essential to the CSIRO cotton breeding program for selecting homozygous transgenic lines on a large scale, monitoring the purity of transgenic breeding lines, and stacking traits by marker assisted selection. Upland cotton has limited intra-specific genetic polymorphism compared to other crops as revealed by a number of molecular marker and genetic diversity analyses [76-78], due to the relatively recent polyploidisation (estimated 1-2 mya) [79, 80] that created the species as well as domestication and selection. This has hindered application of molecular markers to breeding, as to obtain large numbers of polymorphic markers for detailed mapping required crossing *G. hirsutum* to *G. barbadense* (inter-specific), which are largely unsuitable for cultivar improvement in breeding programs.

Two major technological breakthroughs have occurred in the marker field since ~2010 that have removed many limitations associated with marker technology and its application in cotton.

1. Next-generation sequencing (NGS) can sequence DNA millions of more times than previous methods [81]. This has opened up the possibility to discover a larger number of single nucleotide polymorphisms (SNP, single DNA base changes) in cotton that are the most common form of difference between individuals or cultivars, and should be sufficiently abundant to discriminate between any two *G. hirsutum* lines. NGS has also enabled the completion of the genome sequence of the diploid cotton *Gossypium raimondii* [82] that is related to the D-genome present in Upland cotton. The genome sequence of a diploid A-genome containing cotton species is likely to be publicly available in the near future, and will make it easy to compare and align any short sequence reads from NGS to find large numbers of widely distributed nucleotide differences between cultivars that can be used for mapping and breeding.

2. New high-throughput genotyping (HTG) platforms based on SNPs have been developed that can accurately call millions of SNPs in large populations [83, 84]. These technologies enable complete genome coverage of markers between *G. hirsutum* cultivars in a fraction of the time required by conventional marker approaches.

5.1. SNP discovery in germplasm important for Australia

To ensure that SNPs are informative to the breeding populations being developed in Australia, it is essential to find SNPs among cotton cultivars that constitute the major germplasm sources of the elite cultivars we are developing. The most straightforward method to identifying SNPs, in the absence of the Upland cotton genome sequence, is to sequence expressed gene transcripts (RNA-seq) by isolating mRNA and converting it into cDNA for sequencing. This method has been used successfully for many other plants such as maize and wheat [85]. RNA-seq targets SNP discovery to genes that are actively transcribed and therefore more likely to be associated with conferring trait differences. The disadvantage is that cDNA is likely to have lower SNP frequencies than non-expressed regions as they are constrained by the genes function. CSIRO RNA-seq data was generated on a set of 18 cultivars that represented significant genetic variation present within current Australian commercial cultivars were selected; containing old Australian and US cultivars, as well as cultivars from China and India. Over 50 million reads (of ~90 bp) for each Upland cotton sample was obtained. We found the key to identifications of varietal SNPs confidently was when a sub-genome-specific SNP was also found in close proximity to the varietal SNP (Figure 2). This enabled representative sequences from both genomes in each cultivar to be identified and compared. From the 18 cultivars ~38,000 varietal SNPs were identified. A selected subset of >1,500 of these putative SNPs were analysed using a combination of SNP platforms (GoldenGate and Sequenom) and it was found that these SNP could be validated at a rate >90% [Zhu, Q-H, pers comm.].

```
Cultivar-1A   ......AGCGTAGTCAGATTAAGTGGAATCCCTGATG......
Cultivar-1D   ......AGCCTAGTCAGATTGAGTGGAATCCCTGATG......
Cultivar-2A   ......AGCGTAGTCAGATTGAGTGGAATCCCTGATG......
Cultivar-2D   ......AGCCTAGTCAGATTGAGTGGAATCCCTGATG......
```

Figure 2. Stretch of DNA sequence from two cultivars showing the sequences for both the A and D genomes. SNPs with the best validation rates are where a varietal SNP (in red) is in close proximity to a sub-genome-specific SNP (in blue) that allows determination of which genome the specific short reads sequences are derived from.

Although RNASeq data has allowed us to progress towards being able to effectively use SNPs for genotyping in breeding projects, the protein coding regions of genomes have been found to have a significantly lower level of DNA polymorphism than non-coding regions, so polymorphisms within genes between closely related cultivars are going to be less frequent and hence less useful. With the availability of the assembled *G. raimondii* genome and possibly of the *G. arboreum* genome soon, to serve as a framework for short read sequence alignment, our SNP identification will in future be performed using genomic DNA sources.

5.2. International cotton SNP consortium

SNP Chips enable high throughput parallel analysis (millions at a time) whereas older markers like SSR markers tend to be performed only one or a few at a time. Therefore SNP Chips represent a significant improvement over older technologies for large-scale genotyping.

Recently an international cotton consortium was formed to create a 70,000 public Illumina Infinium SNP array for cotton. This array was made available for purchase in late 2013 and contains ~ 50,000 intra-specific *G. hirsutum* SNPs, ~16,000 inter-specific SNPs predominantly from *G. barbadense* but also *G. tomentosum* and *G. mustelinum*, and small numbers (~4,000) of SNPs from two diploids *G. longicalyx* and *G. armourianum*. The publicly available SNPs were provided by a number of international groups including; CSIRO, Texas A&M, University of California-Davis, Cotton Incorporated, Brigham Young University and United States Department of Agriculture-Agricultural Research Service, Centre de Coopération Internationale en Recherche Agronomique pour le Développement (CIRAD), Council of Scientific and Industrial Research-National Botanical Research Institute (CSIR-NBRI), and Dow AgroSciences. These arrays will provide unprecedented numbers of makers to be screened across cotton germplasm and will likely be the genotyping method of choice for a number of years.

5.3. Genotype-by-sequencing

SNP Chips represent a major advance in genotyping of cotton. However, SNP Chip platforms still possess limitations. Since cultivated cotton is an allotetraploid it is often difficult for these platforms to differentiate between the two cotton sub-genomes, and from our experience only ~34% of the polymorphic SNP markers act as co-dominant markers (can discriminate between both homozygous alleles and their heterozygote class, see Figure 3A) on a GoldenGate or Fluidigm platform, whereas the majority act as dominant markers (can only differentiate accurately between both homozygote classes but the heterozygote class cannot be differentiated from one of the homozygote classes, see Figure 3B). Dominant markers reduce the amount of information that can be obtained from an individual, but they are still very useful for mapping (eg., commonly used AFLP markers are all dominant markers). In addition SNP platforms can only interrogate the SNPs that have already been indentified and placed on the chip, and once manufactured, new SNP Chips are unlikely to be remade for several years, so any newly discovered SNPs will be unable to be included and assayed.

We are investigating genotyping using NGS alone, which is called Genotype-by-Sequencing (GBS). GBS uses an amplified subset of genome from individual lines or plants to identify base differences between them [86, 87]. Using bioinformatic analyses the SNPs are found on-the-go when comparing the two sets of sequences, so no prior information about the genotypes is required. The SNPs found are then analysed as separate markers. The advantage of GBS is that SNPs are found in the analysis of the DNA fragments compared, and so informative SNPs linked to a trait are more likely to be identified. Also SNPs from different genomes can be easily separated based on the presence/absence of specific sub-genome related SNPs (which are much more common than varietal SNPs) and so most markers can be selected to be co-dominant (i.e., heterozygous alleles can be scored). This makes this genotyping technology especially suitable for polyploids such as cotton, and is becoming the genotyping method of choice in, for example, wheat which has three similar genomes (A, B and D) [86].

http://dx.doi.org/10.5772/58414

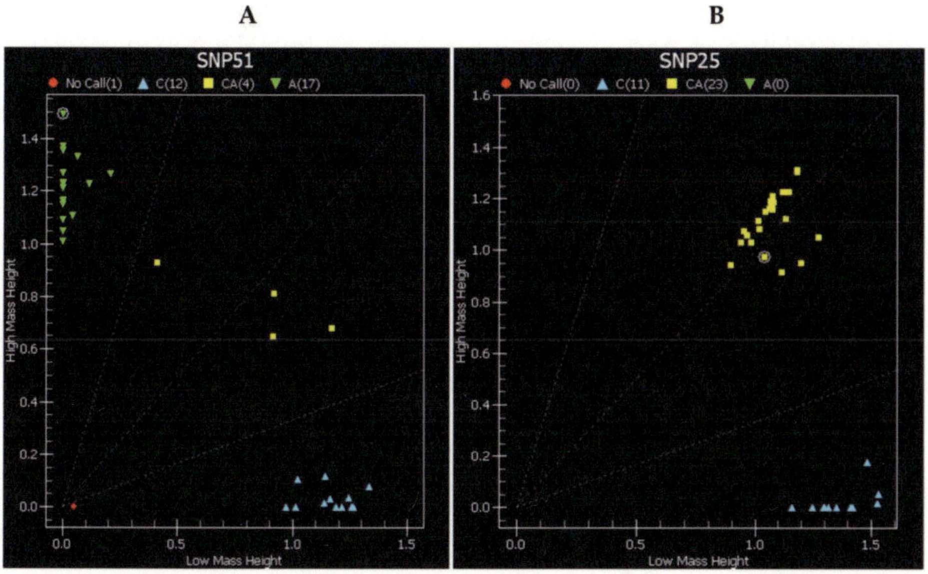

Figure 3. Typical *G. hirsutum* varietal SNP profiles using the Sequenom platform. Each spot represents a different cultivar being assessed for the presence of a specific SNP. A) Co-dominant example, a particular polymorphic nucleotide is scored either as homozygous A (Green) or C (Blue) or heterozygous for C and A (Yellow). B) Dominant example, a particular polymorphic nucleotide can only be scored either as homozygous A (Blue) or heterozygous CA (Yellow), homozygous C (blue) cannot be scored due to tetraploid nature [Zhu, Q-H, pers comm.].

5.4. Genetic diversity analysis

Possessing significant genetic diversity within a breeding program is extremely important for future crop improvement. Where detailed pedigree information is known, breeders can specifically select parents for crossing based on their trait package and degree of relatedness. However, it is often the case that detailed knowledge about the pedigrees of cultivars is lacking, especially for imported cultivars, and this may hamper their use in cotton improvement. Molecular markers provide an alternative means of determining levels of relatedness and ancestry between cultivars. Many studies have used markers to determine the diversity levels with cotton populations [88], however most have suffered from insufficient numbers of marker required to generate accurate estimates. The first major use of a large public cotton SNP chip and other high throughput genotyping technologies by CSIRO will be to enable more accurate diversity estimates within breeding populations and seed repositories. Breeders should be quickly able to determine diversity estimates and phylogenies between cultivars, as well as identify shared genetic regions between members of the same pedigree. This data will enable the use of more diverse germplasm which may contain unique traits to be effectively integrated into the breeding program.

5.5. Linking SNPs to traits

With improvements in SNP identification and the availability of large scale public cotton SNP chip, the availability of molecular makers will no longer be a limiting issue in cotton research and the main task will be linking markers to important traits that will aid in their introgression into elite varieties. Most of our initial focus will be to link SNPs to disease resistance traits, as increased disease resistance has been responsible for a significant amount of our variety based yield improvements. Common methods for linking markers to traits involve the creation of bi-parental crosses that segregate for the trait of interest, followed by selfing, genotyping and trait assessment in the F_2 or F_3 populations. Where possible immortal genetic populations, in which each line is inbred and can be propagated simply by self-pollination, such as recombinant inbred populations or inbred backcross (IBC) populations are used as phenotyping is much simpler (only looking at homozygote classes) and repeatable. These immortals lines have been very helpful when assaying for disease resistance (Verticillium wilt, Fusarium wilt and black root rot) as disease phenotypes are often environmentally affected and difficult to score. The new high-throughput marker technology should greatly accelerate these traditional genetic studies in cotton. However, such populations require significant amounts of time and labor invested in their creation. With the availability of high throughput SNP genotyping between *G. hirsutum* cultivars, other approaches consistent with conventional breeding strategies can now be routinely performed. One such method involves locating chromosomal segment substitutions derived by repeated backcrossing of the trait into an elite cultivar. Backcrossing is used by breeders to transfer a limited number of desirable traits from one parent (possibly poor agronomically) to an elite parent, and involves multiple rounds of crossing back to a recurring elite line; with each backcross reducing the amount of donor DNA present in the offspring. This methodology can be used to find markers linked to the trait(s) after as little as 3 cycles of backcrossing and then selfing, as individuals with the desired trait can now be compared using whole genome SNP analysis to reveal which genomic regions are associated with the donor parent. The markers in the donor regions can be confirmed as being linked to the trait in a further cycle of backcrossing, selfing and selection. Once the marker linkage has been verified, marker-assisted backcrossing can then eliminate the need for further trait phenotyping until the desired elite cultivar is obtained. We are using this system to find linked markers for disease and fibre traits and for introgression of traits from other cotton species.

The ability to scan the whole genome quickly and identify regions from the donor plant makes this strategy practical in cotton and is limited only by reliability and robustness of the trait and the time it takes to cycle through multiple generations. An added advantage of this method to find markers is that the germplasm produced at the end of the process is already partly introgressed into an elite cultivar and can be a parent for more advanced crosses with other elite material. A SNP Chip can also be used to identify backcrossed individuals with the lowest levels of donor DNA at each backcrossing step, reducing the number of backcrosses required to produce an elite cultivar with the trait of interest. This is especially useful to separate the trait of interest from regions nearby that may carry genes that result in poor yield (linkage drag), such as Okra leaf trait.

5.6. Genome wide association mapping

Large scale genotyping of cotton at an economical price enables genotyping large diverse collections of *G. hirsutum* lines. To link SNP markers to important traits in cotton the most manageable route is to perform genome wide association studies on elite cultivars and their pedigrees, avoiding the time and energy required in the creation of specialised genetic populations examining small numbers of traits. Association genetic analysis is a method for linking specific markers with phenotypes using established populations of individuals, and has been extensively used in human/animal genetic analyses where defined genetic crosses are often difficult to generate [89]. The extent of genome-wide allelic association (linkage disequilibrium: LD) is the key starting point for association mapping. The extent of LD has been quantified and association mapping has been successfully applied for many plant species (e.g., [90]) including cotton [91, 92]. The application of LD-based association mapping for cotton will facilitate comprehensive utilization of existing genetic diversity conserved within cotton germplasm cultivars.

CSIRO is interested in using association analysis on a large number of well defined cotton varieties to find markers linked to disease resistance, fibre quality and yield component traits. The bottleneck for this type of research is the difficulty in adequately phenotyping a large number of cultivars for agronomically important traits. To obtain an accurate measurement of the most important trait, yield, requires significant replication both within a field, across geographical regions and over multiple seasons. This restricts the numbers of varieties that can be tested lowering the power of the analyses. It is also possible to model genetic/environmental (GxE) interactions for specific traits using association analysis, but that requires a magnitude larger level of replication under different management conditions, as well as significant knowledge about the environmental conditions in which the traits were measured (and therefore is unlikely to be undertaken by our research teams in the near future).

5.7. Mining diversity in other cotton species

The cotton genus (*Gossypium*) contains ~50 species that are widely geographically distributed from arid to tropical regions and morphologically diverse ranging from herbaceous perennials to small trees. These species are usually divided into three gene pools with regard to their use for genetic improvement of Upland cotton though only a few sources have been extensively used. The primary gene pool consists of *G. barbadense, G. tomentosum, G. mustelinum* and *G. darwinii* which are tetraploid species with the same A and D genome complement that are sexually compatible with Upland cotton. The secondary gene pool is represented by diploids with A, D, B or F genomes that require synthetic tetraploid formation or a synthetic hexaploid bridging species for traits to be introgressed into Upland cotton [39, 44]. The tertiary gene pool consists of other diploid species with a completely different genome type such as C, E, G or K that show relatively poor or no recombination with the A or D-genome and thus traits from these species are likely to require isolation of the causal genes and transfer into cultivated Upland cotton by genetic modification.

Once a representative A-genome diploid sequence is completed, and its information added to the already published D genome, it will be possible to use this information as a scaffold to determine the gene coding regions for different *Gossypium* species. The coding sequences from these genomes will identify new diversity within genes already associated with disease and stress that could be targets for introgression. Traditionally the work required to introgress traits from anything other than *G. hirsutum* or *G. barbadense* has been prohibitive. However the ability to identify important genes via re-sequencing of other *Gossypium* species means that markers for these traits can be found rapidly and used in marker assisted backcrossing strategies as mentioned above. Therefore, in future we will be able to access much more diverse germplasm for unique traits with potential targets for introgression including glandless seeds (in a glanded plant) and Fusarium wilt resistance that are present in indigenous Australian *Gossypium* species [47, 48].

5.8. Exploiting mutant collections of cotton

As previously mentioned, induced mutations can produce novel variation that can be directly used for crop improvement and aid in identifying which genes are important for specific traits. Now that a genome sequence is available for cotton, the major basic research challenge is to uncover the genes responsible for major agronomic traits from the more than 50,000 genes present in this species. The advent of NGS technology and the completed *G. raimondii* genome sequence has opened up practical ways of achieving this via a reverse genetics approach; where a mutation in a specific gene sequence is first identified in a plant by sequencing and the phenotype of this plant is then compared against the not mutated or wild-type plant to identify the physiological, morphological or agronomic consequences of the disruption of that gene and hence its possible function. Traditionally mutated plants with interesting phenotypes are selected from large populations of mutagenised plants, and researchers work back to find where the mutation that caused the novel trait is located within the genome (forward genetic approach). However the space/land required in order to select for interesting mutants is substantial for a large plant like cotton, and the tetraploid nature of Upland cotton, potentially makes finding valuable mutants more difficult (as for some traits both the A and D genome genes would need to be simultaneously mutated to result in a phenotype). The reverse genetics approach, is to first obtain a large collection of plants carrying chemically or radiation induced mutations spread throughout the genome that are identified through NGS. Since NGS can rapidly re-sequence a genome as long as an existing reference genome is known, sequencing the randomly mutated plants will identify single base changes in gene sequences caused by chemical mutagenesis similar to how SNPs are already identified between cultivars. Using specialised DNA capture technologies that only isolate DNA from expressed regions of the genome to reduce the sequence complexity [93, 94], this procedure would be cost effective. A large library of plants harbouring these known mutations, would be made by subjecting cotton seeds to induced mutagenesis and plants (M1 generation) grown and allowed to self seed. The M2 seeds would then be planted, leaf material isolated and the gene sequences of these plants sequenced and the multiple mutations in each plant identified. By collecting seeds from the M2 plants, a database of the sequence changes would be identified and associated with specific seed lots and mutations causing loss of gene function of any selected gene could be identified. The M3 seeds from that plant would be planted and using markers specific for the mutation (a type of SNP marker), plants selected that were homozygous for the mutation [95]. The phenotype of these plants would then be compared to homozygous wild-type plants at this location from the same seed lot.

The availability of mutant lines in most or all of the cotton genes would provide the cotton community with the means of testing gene function in a large number of genes at an unprecedented rate. Lines with mutations in a particular gene would need to be found in both subgenomes, then crossed and progeny selected that were mutated for both copies of the genes in order to categorically define its function. Once a gene has been confirmed as being associated with an important trait, the sequence of this gene could be sequenced from many different cotton cultivars and related species to identify variants that may possess superior qualities for targeted introgression. Currently, large mutagenic populations of *G. arboreum* and *G. hirsutum* are being established at CSIRO in order to locate genes involved in fibre formation and disease and insect resistance.

5.9. Seed genotyping

NGS and high throughput genotyping will enable large numbers of specific traits to be linked to specific markers, thus increasing the importance of marker assisted selection in the breeding of cotton. However the ability to easily stack a moderate number of traits becomes quickly impractical in the field, where extremely large population would need to be grown to identify plants carrying all the correct combination of markers. To overcome this problem a number of companies have developed non-destructive seed based screening methodologies to screen markers. 'Seed chippers' [96] use complicated robotics and liquid handling equipment to remove small portions of embryo, extracting DNA and performing genotyping. This technology was first demonstrated in maize and then soybean but is beginning to be adapted to work in cotton. Seed-based screening will play an essential role in future transgenic trait stacking and marker-assisted breeding of disease and fibre traits in cotton as it will allow the very small proportion of plants with the favorable allele combination to be identified. Seeds selected that contain the correct marker combinations will be planted in the field and selections for fibre and yield traits performed normally, with the knowledge that other desired traits are already present.

6. Success stories of germplasm utilization in Australian cotton improvement

6.1. Disease resistance

As mentioned previously, bacterial blight was the most important disease in Australian cotton when the modern Industry first started with estimated yield losses up to 20%. Bacterial blight resistance was introduced to the CSIRO breeding program from Tamcot SP37, which supplied the B_2, B_3 and B_7 genes [97]. The first blight resistant cultivar was released in 1985 and had rapid adoption. Importantly, this cultivar also had high yield, high gin turnout, wide adaptation and the okra leaf trait. This cultivar was selected from a large breeding population that was initially developed in 1974, which demonstrates the considerable lag from introduction of a trait to commercial release.

Verticillium wilt continues to be an import disease for the Australian industry. However, there have been major successes in developing cultivars with good resistance to this disease. A major breakthrough was the release of Sicala V-1 in 1991, the first CSIRO cultivar with significant resistance, and its higher yielding replacement, Sicala V-2 in 1994. These cultivars show greatly reduced levels of infection, less severe symptoms and higher yields compared to their predecessors and have transformed those regions where Verticillium wilt severely limited yields. None of the parents of the population these cultivars were developed from had significant resistance to Verticillium wilt and would generally have been considered susceptible. The source of resistance has therefore been considered to be the result of additive effect of alleles at multiple loci. Molecular techniques may one day be able to determine the source and composition of this resistance.

After Fusarium wilt was first identified in Australian cotton in the early 1990s, new cultivars were required to allow viable production in the regions where the disease was present. It was quickly established that there was cultivar variability for resistance and a few cultivars did show some degree of resistance (Sicot 189, Delta Emerald). Most other commercial cultivars were very susceptible to the disease and had survival rate of close to zero in some situations. An initial screen from the CSIRO germplasm collection in 1994 tested 36 *G. hirsutum* genotypes from the USA, South America, Africa, Asia and Europe. As with the local cultivars, most were susceptible, but a few genotypes showed field survival up to 50% higher than the best Australian cultivars. Over the next few years over 200 genotypes from the collection were evaluated, with material from countries/regions/programs that showed promise in the early evaluations targeted. In 2004 a new cultivar, Sicot F-1, was released from the CSIRO breeding program which had at least twice the resistance of the best cultivar in 1994. Progress in breeding for improved Fusarium resistance continues, with the initial sources of resistance being derived from Indian and Chinese *G. hirsutum* parents and more recently, improved resistance from *G. hirsutum* and *G. barbadense* landrace cottons.

The key to the breeding success of soil borne fungal diseases has been the availability of screening sites with high levels of inoculum and therefore the opportunity for selection of reduced disease incidence and symptoms, together with high yield. The germplasm collections have been invaluable in accessing material for evaluation of resistance.

6.2. Commercial utilisation of the okra leaf mutant

The okra leaf (OL) mutant of upland cotton is characterised by deep lobing and some reduction in leaf area. This L_2^o allele is partially dominant over the normal leaf (l_2) shape. Although considerable research has been done on the effects of this leaf shape, only in Australia have OL cottons been grown on a major scale, accounting for between 40-60% of Australian seed sales between 1987 and 1993. As reviewed by Thomson [6] the published benefits of OL include host plant resistance to a range of insect and mite pests (boll weevil *Anthonomus grandis*, whitefly *Bemisia tabaci*, spider mites *Tetranychus spp.* and bollworms *Heliothis* and *Helicoverpa spp.*), earlier maturity, increased water-use efficiency and reduced boll rot. However, the OL trait has been associated with increased numbers of plant bugs (*Lygus spp.*), mirids (*Creontiades spp.*) and cotton flea hoppers (*Pseudatomoscelis seriatas*). The yield effect of OL has been reported as being anywhere from negative to positive and is thus far from clear cut.

In the 1970s, the CSIRO breeding program at Narrabri was focused on increasing yield, quality and disease resistance, but also had a strong commitment to increasing resistance to insects. To this end, significant effort was allocated to the OL trait, with large breeding populations developed as well as considerable research into the effect on yield. It was concluded that while there was a small (5%) reduction in yield potential, under commercial production systems with normal levels of insect damage there was no significant yield difference between OL and normal leaf (NL) near-isogenic lines. In addition, in situations where some insect damage was permitted, OL out-yielded NL by up to 10% [6]. A similar observation was reported by Brook *et al.* [98] who stated that OL was infested with fewer pests than NL and suffered less damage from a given density of pests and the reduction in yield caused by pest damage at high yield levels was less in OL than NL.

Thomson [6] reported the reasons why OL has been so successful in Australia when it has either largely failed or been ignored in other countries. As mentioned at the beginning of this chapter, the modern cotton industry is relatively new in Australia, only being a significant industry since the early 1960s. Because growers did not have a long tradition of growing cotton, they had no fixation on what a cotton plant should look like – their concern being solely on performance. The absence of a yield penalty in commercial production systems as mentioned above was also a significant factor in the adoption of OL cottons. Importantly, the Australian OL cottons were not developed by backcross as most other studies have reported (e.g. [99-101]. Rather, as reported by [6], they were developed by hybridisation using wide crosses and large populations with heavy selection pressure for yield performance. Research, together with commercial experience demonstrated the host plant resistance of OL to spider mites and *Helicoverpa* as well as improved insecticide efficacy probably due to better spray penetration in the crop canopy. Lastly and of significant importance, the first OL cotton released for commercial sale (Siokra 1-1) was also the first cultivar in Australia to be completely resistant to bacterial blight. This was undoubtedly a significant factor in its rapid acceptance by growers.

7. Conclusions

The challenge of maintaining genetic diversity in this era of fierce intellectual property protection and commercial reality is significant. One of the ways this is being addressed in the CSIRO breeding program is by developing diversity through utilisation of the genetic resources outside the cultivated tetraploids. This can mean using landrace cottons, but more importantly evaluating traits in the secondary germplasm pool (A and D genomes) and accessing those traits by developing synthetic tetraploids. This approach to diversity requires considerable effort and a long-term vision; however, it does have the potential to pay substantial dividends in unlocking traits previously unavailable from within elite cultivars. To justify this approach, there generally must be present a crucial trait of commercial importance not available in existing germplasm and/or forward-looking funding.

Access to a broad germplasm pool and the ability to import material from other breeding programs combined with rigorous selection regimes for yield and quality under the unique Australian climate has meant that the CSIRO cotton breeding program has maintained yield progress while many other programs are plateauing in yield. Australian cultivars have had considerable success in the US, particularly Texas where there are some similarities in climatic challenges and are now being marketed worldwide under the FiberMax™ brand.

New DNA sequencing technologies will accelerate the identification of genes involved in important agronomic traits, and via marker assisted seed selection, new and novel traits will be introgressed into elite cultivars that should further improve Australian cotton yield and quality.

Author details

Warwick N. Stiller[1*] and Iain W. Wilson[2]

*Address all correspondence to: warwick.stiller@csiro.au

1 CSIRO Plant Industry, Narrabri, NSW, Australia

2 CSIRO Plant Industry, Canberra, ACT, Australia

References

[1] Basinski JJ. The cotton growing industry in Australia. Journal of the Australian Institute of Agricultural Science 1965;31:206-22.

[2] Liu SM, Constable GA, Reid PE, Stiller WN, Cullis BR. The interaction between breeding and crop management in improved cotton yield. Field Crops Research 2013;148:49-60.

[3] Low A. Cotton cultivars in Australia. Cotton Growing Review 1974;51:26-34.

[4] Thomson NJ, Basinski JJ. Cotton in the Ord Valley of northern Australia. Cotton Growing Review 1962;34:81-92.

[5] Thomson NJ. Host plant resistance for cotton. Journal of the Australian Institute of Agricultural Science 1987;53:262-70.

[6] Thomson NJ, editor. Commercial utilisation of the okra leaf mutant of cotton-the Australian experience. Proc World Cotton Research Conf-1, Feb 14-17 1994, Brisbane, Australia: CSIRO; 1994

[7] Constable GA, Reid PE, Thomson NJ. Approaches utilized in breeding and development of cotton cultivars in Australia. In: Jenkins J, Saha S, editors. Genetic Improve-

ment of Cotton: emerging technologies. Enfield, New Hampshire: Science Publishers, Inc.; 2001. p1-15.

[8] Fitt GP, Wilson LJ, Kelly D, Mensah R. Advances in integrated pest management as a component of sustainable agriculture: The case study of the Australian Cotton Industry. In: Peshin R, Dhawan AK, editors. Integrated Pest Management: Innovation-Development Process: Springer Science and Bussiness Media BV; 2009. p507-24.

[9] Wilson LJ, Mensah RK, Fitt GP. Implementing IPM in Australian cotton. In: Horowitz AR, Ishaaya I, editors. Novel approaches to insect pest management in field and protected crops. Netherlands: Springer Press; 2004. p97-118.

[10] Wilson LJ, Bauer LR, Lally DA. Insecticide-induced increases in aphid abundance in cotton. Australian Journal of Entomology 1999;30;38:242-3.

[11] Wilson LJ, Bauer LR, Lally DA. Effect of early season insecticide use on predators and outbreaks of spider mites (Acari : Tetranychidae) in cotton. Bulletin of Entomology Research 1998;88(4):477-88.

[12] Wilson L, Downes S, Khan M, Whitehouse M, Baker G, GRundy P, et al. IPM in the transgenic era: A review of the challenges from emerging pests in Australian cotton systems. Crop and Pasture Science 2013;64:737-49.

[13] Constable G, Llewellyn D, Wilson L, Stiller W. An industry transformed" The impact of GM technology on Australian cotton production. Farm Policy Journal 2011;8(1): 23-41.

[14] Gunning RV, Byrne FJ, Conde BD, Connelly MI, Hergstrom K, Devonshire AL. First Report of B-Biotype *Bemisia-Tabaci* (Gennadius) (Hemiptera, Aleyrodidae) in Australia. Journal of the Australian Entomological Society 1995;34:116-20.

[15] Sequeira RV, Naranjo SE. Sampling and management of *Bemisia tabaci* (Genn.) biotype B in Australian cotton. Crop Protection 2008;27(9):1262-8.

[16] Werth JA, Preston C, Roberts GN, Taylor IN. Weed management practices in glyphosate-tolerant and conventional cotton fields in Australia. Aust Journal of Experimental Agriculture 2006;46(9):1177-83.

[17] Charles GW, Taylor IN. Herbicide resistance and species shift in cotton: the need for an integrated weed management (IWM) approach. In: Swanepoel A, editor. World Cotton Research Conference-3; Cape Town, South Africa: Agricultural Research Council-Institute for Industrial Crops; 2003. p818-28.

[18] Allen SJ. Predominance of race 18 of *Xanthomonas campestris* pv. *malvacearum* on cotton in Australia. Plant Disease 1991;75:43-4.

[19] Schnathorst W, Evans G. Comparative Virulence of American and Australian Isolates of *Verticillium-albo-atrum* in *Gossypium hirsutum*. Plant Disease Reporter 1971;55(11): 977-80.

[20] Allen SJ, editor. The distribution, importance and control of diseases of cotton in Australia. Beltwide Cotton Conference; 1992; Nashville TN: National Cotton Council of America.

[21] Bell AA. Verticillium wilt. In: Hillocks RJ, editor. Cotton Diseases. Wallingford, UK: CAB International; 1992. p87-126.

[22] Kochman JK. Fusarium wilt in cotton-a new record in Australia. Australasian Plant Pathology 1995;24(1):74.

[23] Allen SJ, Lonergan PA. Control strategies for Fusarium wilt of cotton in Australia. In: Dugger P, Richter D, editors. Beltwide Cotton Conference; San Antonio, TX: National Cotton Council of America, Memphis, TN.; 2000.

[24] Kim Y, Hutmacher RB, Davis RM. Characterisation of California isolates of *Fusarium oxysporum* f.sp. *vasinfectum*. Plant Disease 2005;89:366-72.

[25] Colyer PD. A comparison of Fusarium wilt in Australia and the United States. In: Dugger P, Richter D, editors. Beltwide Cotton Conference; Nashville, TN: National Cotton Council of America, Memphis, TN; 2003.

[26] Wang B, Dale ML, Kochman JK. Studies on a pathogenicity assay for screening cotton genrmplasm for resistance to *Fusarium oxysporum* f. sp. *vasinfectum* in the glasshouse. Australian Journal of Experimental Agriculture. 1999;39(8):967-74.

[27] Hillocks RJ. Fusarium wilt. In: Hillocks RJ, editor. Cotton Diseases. Wallingford, UK: CAB International; 1992. p127-60.

[28] Wang B, Brubaker CL, Summerell BA, Thrall PH, Burdon JJ. Local origin of two vegetative compatibility groups of *Fusarium oxysporum* f. sp *vasinfectum* in Australia. Evolutionary Applications 2010;3(5-6):505-24.

[29] Allen SJ. The Australian cotton industry response to the Fusarium wilt problem. In: Dugger P, Richter D, editors. Beltwide Cotton Conferences; Altanta, GA: National Cotton Council of America, Memphis, TN; 2002.

[30] Ellis MH, Silva TF, Stiller WN, Wilson LJ, Vaslin MFS, Sharman M, et al. Identification of a new Polerovirus (family Luteoviridae) associated with cotton bunchy top disease in Australia. Australasian Plant Pathology 2013;42(3):261-9.

[31] Allen SJ. *Thielaviopsis basicola*, a new record on cotton in Australia. Australasian Plant Pathology 1990;19:24-5.

[32] Bauer B, Smith L, Scheikowski L, Lehane J, Cobon J, O'Neil W. Reniform nematode: A new pest of Australian cotton and it's distribution in the Dawson Valley. The Australian Cotton Grower 2013;34(5):28-32.

[33] Bowman DT. Public cotton breeders-do we need them? Journal of Cotton Science 1999;3:139-52.

[34] Clement JD, Constable GA, Stiller WN, Liu SM. Negative associations still exist between yield and fibre quality in cotton breeding programs in Australia and USA. Field Crops Research 2012;128:1-7.

[35] Stokes C, Howden M. Adapting agriculture to climate change. In: Cleugh H, Smith MS, Battaglia M, Graham P, editors. Climate change: science and solutions for Australia. Collingwood, VIC, Australia: CSIRO; 2011. p85-96.

[36] Rochester IJ. Assessing internal crop nitrogen use efficiency in high-yielding irrigated cotton. Nutrient Cycling in Agroecosystems 2011;90(1):147-56.

[37] Rochester IJ. Using seed nitrogen concentration to estimate crop N use-efficiency in high-yielding irrigated cotton. Field Crops Research 2012;127:140-5.

[38] Craven LA, Stewart JM, Brown AHD, Grace JP. The Australian wild species of *Gossypium*. In: Constable GA, Forrester NW, editors. World Cotton Research Conference-1; February 14-17, 1994; Brisbane, Australia: CSIRO, Melbourne; 1994. p278-81.

[39] Stewart JM. Potential for crop improvement with exotic germplasm and genetic engineering. In: Constable G, Forrester N, editors. Challenging the future: Proceedings of the World Cotton Research Conference-1; February 14-17; Brisbane, Australia: CSIRO, Melbourne; 1994. p313-27.

[40] Anon. The biology and ecology of cotton (*Gossypium hirsutum*) in Australia. 2002. August 2002. http://www.ogtr.gov.au/internet/ogtr/publishing.nsf/content/cotton-3/$FILE/biologycotton.pdf

[41] Brown AHD, Brubaker CL. Genetics and the conservation and use of Australian wild relatives of crops. Australian Journal of Botany 2000;48(3):297-303.

[42] Brubaker CL, Brown AHD. The use of multiple alien chromosome addition aneuploids facilitates genetic linkage mapping of the Gossypium G genome. Genome 2003;46(5):774-91.

[43] Lopez-Lavalle LAB, Matheson B, Brubaker CL. A genetic map of an Australian wild Gossypium C genome and assignment of homoeologies with tetraploid cultivated cotton. Genome. 2011;54(9):779-94.

[44] Brubaker CL, Brown AHD, Stewart JM, Kilby MJ, Grace JP. Production of fertile hybrid germplasm with diploid Australian Gossypium species for cotton improvement. Euphytica 1999;108(3):199-213.

[45] Mergeai G. Forty years of genetic improvement of cotton through interspecific hybridisation at Gembloux Agricultural University: Achievements and prospects. In: Swanepoel A, editor. World Cotton Research Conference-3; Cape Town, South Africa: Agricultural Research Council-Institute for Industrial Crops; 2003. p119-33.

[46] Lopez-Lavalle LAB, McFadden H, Brubaker CL. The effect of Gossypium C-genome chromosomes on resistance to Fusarium wilt in allotetraploid cotton. Theoretical Applied Genetics 2007;115(4):477-88.

[47] McFadden H, Beasley D, Brubaker CL. Assessment of Gossypium sturtianum and G-australe as potential sources of Fusarium wilt resistance to cotton. Euphytica 2004;138(1):61-72.

[48] Brubaker CL, Benson CG, Miller C, Leach DN. Occurrence of terpenoid aldehydes and lysigenous cavities in the 'glandless' seeds of Australian Gossypium species. Australian Journal of Botany 1996;44(5):601-12.

[49] Llewellyn D, Fitt G. Pollen dispersal from two field trials of transgenic cotton in the Namoi Valley, Australia. Molecular Breeding 1996;2(2):157-66.

[50] Llewellyn D, Tyson C, Constable G, Duggan B, Beale S, Steel P. Containment of regulated genetically modified cotton in the field. Agriculture, Ecosystems & Environment 2007;121(4):419-29.

[51] Lopez-Lavalle LAB, Gillespie VJ, Tate WA, Ellis MH, Stiller WN, Llewellyn DL, et al. Molecular mapping of a new source of Fusarium wilt resistance in tetraploid cotton (*Gossypium hirsutum* L.). Molecular Breeding 2012;30(2):1181-91.

[52] Lopez-Lavalle LAB, Potter N, Brubaker CL. Development of a rapid, accurate glasshouse bioassay for assessing Fusarium wilt disease responses in cultivated Gossypium species. Plant Pathology 2012;61(6):1112-20.

[53] Lacape JM, Jacobs J, Arioli T, Derijcker R, Forestier-Chiron N, Llewellyn D, et al. A new interspecific, *Gossypium hirsutum* x *G. barbadense,* RIL population: towards a unified consensus linkage map of tetraploid cotton. Theoretical Applied Genetics 2009;119(2):281-92.

[54] Lacape JM, Llewellyn D, Jacobs J, Arioli T, Becker D, Calhoun S, et al. Meta-analysis of cotton fiber quality QTLs across diverse environments in a *Gossypium hirsutum* x *G. barbadense* RIL population. BMC Plant Biology 2010;28;10.

[55] Lacape JM, Gawrysiak G, Cao TV, Viot C, Llewellyn D, Liu SM, et al. Mapping QTLs for traits related to phenology, morphology and yield components in an inter-specific *Gossypium hirsutum* x *G. barbadense* cotton RIL population. Field Crops Research 2013;144:256-67.

[56] Liu SM, Llewellyn DJ, Stiller WN, Jacobs J, Lacape JM, Constable GA. Heritability and predicted selection response of yield components and fibre properties in an inter-specific derived RIL population of cotton. Euphytica 2011;178(3):309-20.

[57] Thomson NJ, Reid PE, Williams ER. Effects of the Okra Leaf, Nectariless, Frego Bract and Glabrous Conditions on Yield and Quality of Cotton Lines. Euphytica 1987;36(2): 545-53.

[58] Wu YR, Machado AC, White RG, Llewellyn DJ, Dennis ES. Expression profiling identifies genes expressed early during lint fibre initiation in cotton. Plant Cell Physiology 2006;47(1):107-27.

[59] Brown N, Smith CW, Auld D, Hequet EF. Improvement of Upland Cotton Fiber Quality through Mutation of TAM 94L-25. Crop Science 2013;53(2):452-9.

[60] Bechere E, Auld DL, Dotray PA, Gilbert LV, Kebede H. Imazamox Tolerance in Mutation-Derived Lines of Upland Cotton. Crop Science 2009;49(5):1586-92.

[61] Bechere E, Auld DL, Hequet E. Development of 'naked-tufted' seed coat mutants for potential use in cotton production. Euphytica 2009;167(3):333-9.

[62] Herring AD, Auld DL, Ethridge MD, Hequet EF, Bechere E, Green CJ, et al. Inheritance of fiber quality and lint yield in a chemically mutated population of cotton. Euphytica 2004;136(3):333-9.

[63] Cousins YL, Lyon BR, Llewellyn DJ. Transformation of an Australian Cotton Cultivar-Prospects for Cotton Improvement through Genetic-Engineering. Australian Journal of Plant Physiology 1991;18(5):481-94.

[64] Machado A, Wu YR, Yang YM, Llewellyn DJ, Dennis ES. The MYB transcription factor GhMYB25 regulates early fibre and trichome development. Plant Journal 2009;59(1):52-62.

[65] Walford SA, Wu YR, Llewellyn DJ, Dennis ES. GhMYB25-like: a key factor in early cotton fibre development. Plant Journal 2011;65(5):785-97.

[66] Walford SA, Wu YR, Llewellyn DJ, Dennis ES. Epidermal cell differentiation in cotton mediated by the homeodomain leucine zipper gene, GhHD-1. Plant Journal 2012;71(3):464-78.

[67] Pu L, Li Q, Fan XP, Yang WC, Xue YB. The R2R3 MYB Transcription Factor GhMYB109 Is Required for Cotton Fiber Development. Genetics 2008180(2):811-20.

[68] Ruan YL, Llewellyn DJ, Furbank RT. Suppression of sucrose synthase gene expression represses cotton fiber cell initiation, elongation, and seed development. Plant Cell 2003;15(4):952-64.

[69] Xu SM, Brill E, Llewellyn DJ, Furbank RT, Ruan YL. Overexpression of a Potato Sucrose Synthase Gene in Cotton Accelerates Leaf Expansion, Reduces Seed Abortion, and Enhances Fiber Production. Molecular Plant 2012;5(2):430-41.

[70] Murray F, Llewellyn D, McFadden H, Last D, Dennis ES, Peacock WJ. Expression of the *Talaromyces flavus* glucose oxidase gene in cotton and tobacco reduces fungal infection, but is also phytotoxic. Molecular Breeding 1999;5(3):219-32.

[71] Townsend BJ, Poole A, Blake CJ, Llewellyn DJ. Antisense suppression of a (+)-delta-cadinene synthase gene in cotton prevents the induction of this defense response

gene during bacterial blight infection but not its constitutive expression. Plant Physiology 2005;138(1):516-28.

[72] Liu Q, Singh SP, Green AG. High-stearic and high-oleic cottonseed oils produced by hairpin RNA-mediated post-transcriptional gene silencing. Plant Physiology 2002;129(4):1732-43.

[73] Townsend BJ, Llewellyn DJ. Spatial and temporal regulation of a soybean (Glycine max) lectin promoter in transgenic cotton (*Gossypium hirsutum*). Functional Plant Biology. 2002;29(7):835-43.

[74] Schunmann PHD, Llewellyn DJ, Surin B, Boevink P, De Feyter RC, Waterhouse PM. A suite of novel promoters and terminators for plant biotechnology. Functional Plant Biology. 2003;30(4):443-52.

[75] Amarasinghe B, Faivre N, Wu, Udall J, Dennis E, Constable G, et al. Genomic approaches to the discovery of promoters for sustained expression in cotton (*Gossypium hirsutum* L.) under field conditions: expression analysis in transgenic cotton and Arabidopsis of a Rubisco small subunit promoter identified using EST sequence analysis and cDNA microarrays. Plant Biotechnology 2006;23:437-50.

[76] Abdalla AM, Reddy OUK, El-Zik KM, Pepper AE. Genetic diversity and relationships of diploid and tetraploid cottons revealed using AFLP. Theoretical Applied Genetics 2001;102(2-3):222-9.

[77] Wendel JF, Brubaker CL, Percival AE. Genetic Diversity in *Gossypium hirsutum* and the Origin of Upland Cotton. American Journal of Botany 1992;79(11):1291-310.

[78] Iqbal MJ, Aziz N, Saeed NA, Zafar Y, Malik KA. Genetic diversity evaluation of some elite cotton varieties by RAPD analysis. Theoretical Applied Genetics 1997;94(1): 139-44.

[79] Wendel JF, Olson PD, Stewart JM. Genetic Diversity, Introgression, and Independent Domestication of Old-World Cultivated Cottons. American Journal of Botany 1989;76(12):1795-806.

[80] Wendel JF, Cronn RC. Polyploidy and the evolutionary history of cotton. Advances in Agronomy, Vol 78. 2003;78:139-86.

[81] Schuster SC. Next-generation sequencing transforms today's biology. Nature Methods 2008;5(1):16-8.

[82] Paterson AH, Wendel JF, Gundlach H, Guo H, Jenkins J, Jin DC, et al. Repeated polyploidization of Gossypium genomes and the evolution of spinnable cotton fibres. Nature 2012;492(7429):423-+.

[83] Huang XH, Wei XH, Sang T, Zhao QA, Feng Q, Zhao Y, et al. Genome-wide association studies of 14 agronomic traits in rice landraces. Nature Genetics 2010;42(11):961-U76.

[84] Cavanagh CR, Chao SM, Wang SC, Huang BE, Stephen S, Kiani S, et al. Genome-wide comparative diversity uncovers multiple targets of selection for improvement in hexaploid wheat landraces and cultivars. Proceeding of the National Academy of Science U.S.A. 2013;110(20):8057-62.

[85] Barbazuk WB, Emrich SJ, Chen HD, Li L, Schnable PS. SNP discovery via 454 transcriptome sequencing. Plant Journal 2007;51(5):910-8.

[86] Deschamps S, Llaca V, May GD. Genotyping-by-Sequencing in Plants. Biology 2012;1(3):460-83.

[87] Gore MA, Chia JM, Elshire RJ, Sun Q, Ersoz ES, Hurwitz BL, et al. A First-Generation Haplotype Map of Maize. Science 2009;326(5956):1115-7.

[88] Fang DD, Hinze LL, Percy RG, Li P, Deng D, Thyssen G. A microsatellite-based genome-wide analysis of genetic diversity and linkage disequilibrium in Upland cotton (*Gossypium hirsutum* L.) cultivars from major cotton-growing countries. Euphytica 2013;191(3):391-401.

[89] de Bakker PIW, Yelensky R, Pe'er I, Gabriel SB, Daly MJ, Altshuler D. Efficiency and power in genetic association studies. Nature Genetics 2005;37(11):1217-23.

[90] Gupta PK, Rustgi S, Kulwal PL. Linkage disequilibrium and association studies in higher plants: Present status and future prospects. Plant Molecular Biology 2005;57(4):461-85.

[91] Abdurakhmonov IY, Kohel RJ, Yu JZ, Pepper AE, Abdullaev AA, Kushanov FN, et al. Molecular diversity and association mapping of fiber quality traits in exotic *G. hirsutum* L. germplasm. Genomics 2008;92(6):478-87.

[92] Abdurakhmonov IY, Saha S, Jenkins JN, Buriev ZT, Shermatov SE, Scheffler BE, et al. Linkage disequilibrium based association mapping of fiber quality traits in *G. hirsutum* L. variety germplasm. Genetica 2009;136(3):401-17.

[93] Neves LG, Davis JM, Barbazuk WB, Kirst M. Whole-exome targeted sequencing of the uncharacterized pine genome. Plant Journal 2013;75(1):146-56.

[94] Hodges E, Xuan Z, Balija V, Kramer M, Molla MN, Smith SW, et al. Genome-wide in situ exon capture for selective resequencing. Nature Genetics 2007;39(12):1522-7.

[95] Wang TL, Uauy C, Robson F, Till B. TILLING in extremis. Plant Biotechnology Journal 2012;10(7):761-72.

[96] Gao SB, Martinez C, Skinner DJ, Krivanek AF, Crouch JH, Xu YB. Development of a seed DNA-based genotyping system for marker-assisted selection in maize. Molecular Breeding 2008;22(3):477-94.

[97] Bird LS. Registration of Tamcot SP37H cotton. Crop Science 1979;19:412.

[98] Brook KD, Hearn AB, Kelly CF. Response of Cotton to Damage by Insect Pests in Australia-Compensation for Early Season Fruit Damage. Journal of Economic Entomology 1992;85(4):1378-86.

[99] Andries JA, Jones JE, Sloane LW, Marshall JG. Effects of okra leaf shape on boll rot, yield, and other important characters of upland cotton, *Gossypium hirsutum* l. Crop Science 1969;9:705-10.

[100] Meredith WR. Effect of environments and genetic backgrounds on evaluation of cotton isolines. Crop Science 1983;23:51-4.

[101] Meredith WR, Wells R. Normal vs. Okra leaf yield interactions in cotton. I.Performance of near isogenic lines from bulk populations. Crop Science 1986;26:219-22.

Chapter 2

Cotton Germplasm Resources in China

Yinghua Jia, Junling Sun and Xiongming Du

Additional information is available at the end of the chapter

http://dx.doi.org/10.5772/58595

1. Introduction

1.1. History of cotton germplasm research in China

China is one of the oldest countries that was found to have a long history of growing cotton. The remotest record was searched in one of the Chinese historic literature book *Shang Shu.Yu Gong* (about 300 BC), which described that cotton named *Jibei* was used to weave colorful cloth by the native people in the island of South China [1-2,4]. The primary species of cotton were two diploids including *G. arboreum* L. in South China and *G. herbaceum* L. in West China, but *G. arboreum* L. was only kept growing in the south of the Five Ridges area, Hainan Island and Yunan until Huang Daopo (about 1245—1330AD) improved the technology of waving cotton fiber and brought it to Songjiang in Shanghai from Yazhou in Hainan. Then, *G. arboreum* L. was widely cultivated in the mid and lower reaches of the Yangtze River and was spread to North China in Ming Dynasty. *G. herbaceum* L. was firstly found to be planted in Xinjiang, but it was not popularized across the country, and was only cultivated in Xinjiang and Gansu Provinces in the past years. *G. hirsutum* L. was firstly imported to China by Zhang Zhidong in 1892-1893 and was cultivated in Hubei. *G. barbadense* L. was imported to China earlier than *G. hirsutum* L. and was mainly in Yunan province as perennial cultivars [3-5]. Now China is the largest producer and consumer of cotton in the world. According to the World Bank, from 2005-2007, China produced 28.4 to 37 million bales of cotton and consumed 45 to 51.5 million bales in the country's domestic textile mill industry. On average, cotton was produced on ~5.6 million ha in China within three predominant growing areas including Xinjiang area, the Yellow River area, and the Yangtze River area. Similar to India, China's adoption of Bt-hybrids and cultivars have resulted in marked yield increases in recent years [6-7].

The Chinese cotton germplasm collection located at the Institute of Cotton Research of Chinese Academy of Agricultural Sciences in Anyang. A medium-term working collection located at Anyang, and a long-term collection located at Beijing, which was established in 1958. An *in vivo* collection of wild species was housed at Hainan Island. The earliest medium-term germplasm bank for cotton was built in Baibi town in 1959-1960, and the seeds must be reproduce every three years, which could preserve the cotton seeds for 4-5 years because of the primitive condition. Then a semi-automatic temperature controlling medium-term germplasm bank was rebuilt in 1979-1982, which was enlarged for the storage area and was constituted of two rooms. This semi-automatic germplasm bank could kept the seeds for more than ten years at 0℃. An automatic temperature controlling medium-term grmplasm bank was built in Anyang city in 2000-2002, which could prolong the preservation of the seeds for fifteen years at 0+2℃ below 50% relative humidity. Now a new germplasm bank has been rebuilt based on the old building in Baibi town in 2011-2012, which is larger and can hold more than 30000 cotton germplasm lines at the temperature 0C and 50% relative humidity. The *in vivo* collection garden was built in Yachen, Shanya, Hannan in 1979 due to the warm and moist weather in the winter. Till now, more than 36 wild species were nursed in that place.

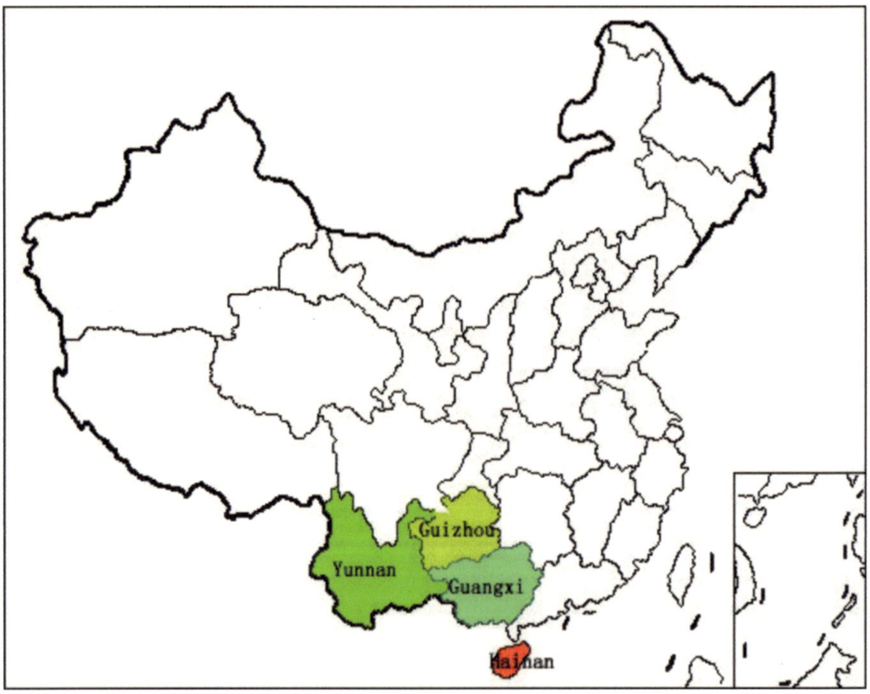

Figure 1. Map of exploration of *G. arboreum* L. in south-west china

Six professors have been in charge of the germplasm bank and *in vivo* garden from 1958 to 2013, and made important contributions to the development of cotton germplasm in China. Prof. Meng Shiheng was the first researcher in charge of cotton germpasm work during 1957-1960, and he established the early system of preservation of cotton, including information collection of pedigree and specimens. Xiang Xianlin continued the work and built seven ecological conservation sites from 1958-1989. Xiang edited and published the first two

http://dx.doi.org/10.5772/58595

catalogues of cotton germplasm in China [8-9]. She organized the collection, conducted evaluation and exploration of *G. arboreum* L. in the south-west China. Later Prof. Liu Guoqiang was in charge and kept on the work of cotton germplasm. He arranged to classify and evaluate all the cultivars in the germplasm bank from 1981 to 2001. Prof. Liu edited and published the latest catalogue books of cotton germplasm in China [10-12]. Prof. Du Xiongming added molecular method in the evaluation of the diversity of cotton germplasm, and identification the genes related to elite agronomic traits in recent years [13]. Prof. Wang Kunbo was in charge of the preservation of wild species of cotton. He built the nursery station for *in vivo* preservation, and evaluated the characters of species with FISH and molecular method [14].

2. Collection of cotton germplasm in China, exploration, exchange with other countries

From last century, collection in homeland has gone through three stages of development. The first stage was the years before the 1949. Wang Shanquan and Feng Zhefang firstly started to collect the *G. arboreum* L., from thirteen provinces in the country including Jiangsu, Zhejiang, Liaoning, Shangdong (in 1922-1923) etc., and acquired 112 lines with diversity phenotypes [1]. Later, Central Agricultural Research Institute continued the work and collected 1200 *G. arboreum* L. But most of these lines were lost during World War Two. The second stage was the middle of the last century. In 1956-1957, the Ministry of Agriculture announced to support for collection of the landraces across the country assisted by the local government. Until 1961, almost 1007 cotton lines were received from all over the country, including 697 *G. hirsutum* L., 25 *G. barbadense* L., 256 *G. arboreum* L., one *G. herbaceum* L. and five wild cottons. Regular collection expeditions were also organized at this stage. The crop explorations have covered most of South-west China. In 1975, Xiang Xianlin, Ma Xijing and Wang Biying explored Luxi, Yinjiang, Longchuan, Jinghong, Mengla in South–west of Yunnan Province. In 1980, Xiang Xianlin explored Yaxian, Linshui, Baoting, Yuedong, Baisa, Danxian, Dongfang, Wenchang in Hainan province with the help of local government. In 1983, Xiang Xianlin, Zhang Zhujie, Yang Shiquan explored the south of Guizhou Province, and in the same time Liu Guoqiang and Shen Duanzhuang explored the north of Guangxi Province. In this stage, the agricultural institutes in the main provinces also kept their cultivars genetic stocks and sent to the long-term germplasm bank in Beijing after evaluation till 1995. The third stage was years after 2000. In 2002-2013, lines preserved in local agricultural institutes of Xianyang, Tangshan, Xiaoshan, Jiuquan, Bazhou, Binchuan, were sent to Institute of Cotton Research of Chinese Academy of Agricultural Sciences for long-term preservation. Explorations of landrace cotton were also carried out in this stage. Profs. Wang Kunbo and Du Xiongming organized the explorations in Yunan, Guizhou, Guangxi Province separately from 2002 to 2013 (Table 1).

Years	Locations	Acquirement	Explorer and institute
1922-1933	Thirteen provinces in china, including Shangdong, Jiangsu, Zhejiang, Liaoning	112 *G. arboreum* L. were collected	Wang Shanquan, Feng Zhefang
1939-1949	All over the country, including Sichuan, Yunanan	1200 *G. arboreum* L. were collected	Wang Shanquan, Feng Zhefang, Xi Yuanling, Chenren et al in Central Agricultural Institute
1952		73 *G. arboreum* L. were collected	Huabei Agriculture Research Institute
1956-1961	All over the country		Agriculture Ministry and Xiang Xianlin
1980	Hainan Province, including Yaxian, Baoting, Linshui, Yuedong, Baisha, Danxian, Dongfang, Wenchang	78 accessions including *G. arboreum* L., and *G. hirsutum* L.	Xiang Xianlin in Institute of Cotton Research of Chinese Academy of Agricultural Sciences, science and technology department in Hiannan province.
1983	Guizhou province, including Kaili, Chongjiang, Rongjiang, Sandou, Luodian, Wangmo, Guanling, Zhenning	36 *G. arboreum* L. and 16 *G. hirsutum* L.	Xiang Xianlin, Zhang Zhuxian in Institute of Cotton Research of Chinese Academy of Agricultural Sciences, and Yang Shiquan in Guizhou
1983	Guangxi province, including Donglan, Bama, Nandan, Sanjiang, Fuchuan, Guiping, Debao, Jingxi, Pingguo	18 *G. arboreum* L. and 22 *G. hirsutum* L.	Liu Guoqiang, Fu Huaiqin in Institute of Cotton Research of Chinese Academy of Agricultural Sciences, Sheng Duanzhuang in Jiangsu Academy of Agricultural Sciences
2002	Guangxi, Guizhou, Yunan province	89 *G. arboreum* L., 43 *G. hirsutum* L.and 18 *G. barbadense* L.	Wang Kunbo, Liu Fang et al in Institute of Cotton Research of Chinese Academy of Agricultural Sciences
2005	Yunnan, Guangxi province, including Mojiang, Jiangcheng, Kaiyuan, Maguan, Funing, Napo, Leye, Longlin, Tiandong, Pingguo, Daxin, Debao, Shangsi	Six *G. arboreum* L., two *G. barbadense* L.	Liu Guoqiang, Jia Yinhua in Institute of Cotton Research of Chinese Academy of Agricultural Sciences
2009	Guizhou, Guangxi province	16 *G. arboreum* L.	Du Xiongming, Zhou Zhongli, Jia Yinhua, Sun Junling, He Shoupu in Institute of Cotton Research of Chinese Academy of Agricultural Sciences
2012-2013	Guangxi, Guizhou, Yunnan province	26 *G. arboreum* L. and 105 *G. barbadense* L.	Sun Junlin, Jia Yinhua, He Shoupu, Pan Zaoe et al in Institute of Cotton Research of Chinese Academy of Agricultural Sciences

Table 1. Cotton germplasm exploration in China during the past years

http://dx.doi.org/10.5772/58595

Years	Locations	Acquirement	Explorer and institute
1984	Mexico		Hu Shaoan in Institute of Cotton Research of Chinese Academy of Agricultural Sciences, Chen Zhongfang in Institute of industrial Crops, Jiangsu Academy of Agricultural Sciences
1979-1993	Mexico, including Sonora, Sinoloba, Baja California Sur, Colima, Yucatan, Michoacan, Colima	243 wild species and Landraces, including race *punctatum*, race mexicanum, race *richmondii*, race *latifolium*, race *morilli*, race *mariegalante*, race *parmeri*	Shen Duanzhuang, Huang Junqi, Xiao Songhua, Zhou Baoliang et al in Institute of industrial Crops, Jiangsu Academy of Agricultural Sciences
2011-2013	Hawaii, USA	20 *G. tomentosum* Nuttall ex Seemann	Wang Kunbo, Liu Fang, Zhou Zhongli in Institute of Cotton Research of Chinese Academy of Agricultural Sciences
2013	Brazil		Wang Kunbo, Liu Fang in Institute of Cotton Research of Chinese Academy of Agricultural Sciences
2013	Australia		Wang Kunbo Liu Fang in Institute of Cotton Research of Chinese Academy of Agricultural Sciences

Table 2. Cotton germplasm exploration in cotton origination place during the past years

Collections obtained from foreign countries are showed in Table 2 and Table 3. The earlier introduction of germplasm of Upland cotton were Deltapine lines imported from USA which were the main varieties grown in China in 1950s [15-17]. Following, Acala and Stonville lines were also introduced to China which helped to enhance new cultivars by the native breeders based on these materials. From 1980 to 1997, Ma Jiazhang, Xiang Shikang, and Liu Guoqiang imported genetic stocks, PD lines and *G.barbadense* separately. The Soviet Union was also one of the countries that provided their varieties and lines including the early mature and resistant Upland cottons, short branch Sea island cottons and various hybrid lines. Recently, many accessions were exchanged between China and other countries, including Russia and Uzbekistan. The expeditions to the origin sites were mainly made in Mexico, Brazil and Australia. Till now, 2,236 cotton accessions including 2,024 *G. hirsutum* L., 198 *G. barbadense* L. and 14 G. arboretum L were introduced from 53 foreign countries in the last 100 years. The top five countries with a large number of introductions were United States of America, Russia, Australia, Pakistan and Egypt.

Years	Collection Issues
1977	Import 9 wild species from Czechoslovakia Prague tropical subtropical Agricultural Research Institute of Kasetsart University, including *G. australe Mueller, G. trilobum (DC.) Skovsted, G. tomentosum, G. bickii, G. sturtianum, G. davidsonii, G. klotzschianum, G. davidsonii, G. herbaceum var africanum*
1980	Import 50 genetic stocks from USA, and 7 *G.hirsutum* landraces from Mexico
1982	Import 21 wild species from USA, including *G. nandewarense* Derera, *G. capitis-viridis* Mauer, *G. armourianum* Kearn, *G. gossypioides* (Ulbr) Standl, *G. longicalyx* J.B.Hutch & Lee, *G. triphyllum* (Harv, Sond) Hochr, *G. incanum* (Schwartz) Hillc, *G. aridum* (Rose&Standley) Skovsted, 3 wild species from French including *G. turneri* Fryx, *G. laxum* Phillips, *G. nelsonii* Fryx.
1983	Import 27 PD lines from USA, and 33 lines from French
1984	Import 6 wild species from Mexico, including *G. aridum* and *G. laxum*
1986	Import 38 lines from Pakistan, including 6 wild species and 7 *G. arboreum* L.
1986	Import 6 wild species from The Commonwealth Scientific and Industrial Research Organisation in Australia, including *G. cunninghamii* Todaro, *G. costulatum* Todaro, *G. populifolium* (Bentham) Mueller ex Todaro
1987	Import 79 GP lines and 3 wild species including *G. bickii*, *G. triphyllum*, *G. anomalum*, and 11 lines from Pakistan
1989	Import 3 wild species from Cote d'Ivoire, including *G. incanum* (Schwartz) Hillc, *G. turneri* Fryx, *G. mustelinum* Miers &Watt
1990	Import 52 lines, including 3 wild species
1991	Import 55 lines from USA, 8 lines from French, 5 line from Egypt, 1 line from Burma, 1 line from Barbados
1992	Import 94 lines from Australia, including 16 wild species
1990-1995	Import 8 *G. hirsutum* landraces and 4 wild species from Mexico including *G. schw endimanii* Fryxell)
1999	Import 35 lines from Mexico
2001	Import 36 MAR lines from USA
2006	Import 418 *G. hirsutum* landraces from USA
2008	Import 100 lines from Uzbekistan
2009-2013	Import 990 lines from Russia

Table 3. Cotton germplasm importing and collection from foreign country

3. Status of cotton germplasm preservation in China

Funding for maintenance of the collections was provided by the Chinese government under the National Key Technology Research and Development Program, and the National Key Basic Research and Development Program, Funds primarily provided by the National Science Foundation of China, the Ministry of Science and Technology, and the Ministry of Agriculture. There are five full-time staff members assigned to the maintenance and conservation of the germplasm collection. The total collection consists of 8,868 accessions that represent cultivated species (*G. arboreum, G. herbaceum, G. hirsutum, G. barbadense*) and 32 wild species (Table 4 and

Table 5). In these collections, most of the accessions were originated from all China, and the other accessions were imported from 52 countries (Table 6).

Species	Total	Catalogued	Cataloguing
G. hirsutum L.	7402	6305	1057
G. barbadence L.	633	532	101
G. arbareum L.	433	350	83
G. herbaceum L.	18	15	3
G. hirsutum lanraces	350	350	
Wild species	32	15	17
Total	8868	7567	1261

Table 4. Cotton germplasm in the medium-term germplasm bank

7,221 accessions were preserved for long-term in Beijing at-18°C under 57% relative humidity. The collection in Anyang, considered the working collection, contains 8,868 accessions and is maintained at 0°C under 50% relative humidity. The Hainan Island nursery site maintained an *in vivo* collection of 391 wild species and *G. hirsutum* landrace stock accessions in a garden under natural field conditions [18-19]. Over time, the Chinese collection has grown through international germplasm exchange and expeditions. The germplasm expeditions covered most of southern China (Hainan Island, Guangxi, and Guangzhou) and the mountainous areas of Yunnan and west Sichuan provinces. *G. hirsutum* landrace germplasm has also been collected from southern Mexico.

The seeds of germplasm accessions in the working collection were renewed according to individual accession germination rates. When germination rates fell under 65%, or the weight of individual accession was no more than 150g, these accessions would be increased and renewed for the maintaining of the viability, genetic integrity and releasing for the research. 50-100 seedlings of each individual should been kept in the field for the harvest of enough healthy seeds. The field was chose according to the environments of origins of the accessions for propagation. The *G. hirsutum* L. has been propagated in Anyang, Nanjing, Kuche, and Liaoyang, in the past years. The *G.barbadence* L. has been grown in Kuche or Turpan of Xinjiang because of low rainfall and high temperature weather. The lines sensitive to the Verticillium wilt and Fusarium wilt were grown in disease free field. Some lines that were photoperiod and temperature sensitive were grown in Sanya of Hainan province. The main agronomic traits were checked according to the database descriptors in the germplasm bank, and the mixed seedlings were weeded out for keeping the purity of the accessions and the true accuracy of the database. Cotton germplasm preserved in the local institutes last century were renewed for enough seeds with purity and vitality. Every year more than 300 accessions were renewed for better seed vitality (Table 7).

Species	Origin
G. nandewarense Derera	Nandeware, New South Wales, Australia
G. sturtianum Willis	Centre and South Australia
G. robinsonii Muell	West Australia
G. costulatum Tod	Kimberley, Australia
G. cunninghamii Tod	North Australia
G. populifolium (Benth) Muell ex Tod	Kimberley, Australia
G. australe Muell	Centre and North Australia
G. bickii Prokhanov	Centre Australia
G. nelsonii Fryx	Centre Australia
G. thurberi Tod	Arizona, USA; Sonora and Warburg, Mexico
G. trilobum Skov	Mexico
G. davidsonii Kell	Baja California, Mexico
G. klotzschianum Anderss	Galapagos islands
G. armourianum Kearn	San Marcos and Baja California, Mexico
G. harknessii Brandg	Baja California, Mexico
G. turneri Fryx	Sonora, Mexico
G. gossypioides (Ulbr) Standl	Warburg, Mexico
G. aridum (Rose & Standley) Skov	Mexico
G. schwendimanii Fryx	Mexico
G. lobatum Gentry	Mexico
G. laxum Phillips	Guerrero, Mexico
G. raimondii Ulbr	Centre and West Peru
G. anomalum subsp.*senarense* (Wawra & Peyr) Vollesen	Niger, Chad, Sudan, Ethiopia
G. capitis-viridis Mauer	cape verde islands
G. incanum (Schwartz) Hillc	Yemen
G. somalense (Gürke) J.B.Hutch	Sudan, Ethiopia, Somalia, Kenya
G. stocksii Mast in Hook	Somalia, Oman, Pakistan
G. longicalyx J.B.Hutch & Lee	Sudan, Uganda, Tanzania
G. triphyllum (Harv, Sond) Hochr	Angola, Botswana, Namibia
G. tomentosum Nutt & Seem	Hawaii
G. mustelinum Miers &Watt	Brazil
G. darwinii Watt	Galapagos islands

Table 5. Wild species in the germplasm bank in China

Origin	G. hirsutum L.	G. barbadence L.	G. arbareum L.	G. herbaceum L.	Origin	G. hirsutum L.	G. barbadence L.	G. arbareum L.	G. herbaceum L.
Afghanistan	1				Kenya	5			
Albania	1	3			Mali	2			
Angola	1				Mexico	17	1		
Argentina	7				Nepal	5			
Australia	154				Nicaragua	1			
Brazil	4				Nigeria	3			
Bulgarian	14				North Korea	3			
Burkina Faso	2				Pakistan	99		1	
Burma	1				Peru	1			
Burundi	1				Portuguesa	1			
Cambodia	1				Somalia	2			
Cote d'Ivoire	10				Soviet Union	355	135		
Canada		1			Spain	3			
Chad	1				Sudan	8	1		
Cameroon	2				Sweden	1			
Cuba	4				Syria	7	3		
Czech	1				Tanzania	5			
Egypt	1	41			Turkey	6			
France	29				Uganda	11			
Ghana	1				USA	1200	13	11	
Greece	6				Uzbekistan	11			
Hungary	1				Vietnam	5			
India	15		1		Yemen	1			
Indonesia	2				Yugoslavia	2			
Iran	1				Zambia	1			
Japan	4		1		Other	4			

Table 6. The Collections from different countries in the medium-term germplasm bank

Years	2001	2002	2003	2004	2005	2006	2007	2008
Accession Number	997	1058	574	700	586	1336	404	400

Table 7. Seed propagation of cotton germplasm in recent years

4. Evaluation of cotton germplasm in China

For the utilization of the cotton germpasm, all the accessions in the germplasm bank were evaluated with different method, including the main agronomic traits and mutant beneficial genes. We took charge of some national projects such as *"Propagation, Identification, evaluation and utilization of cotton germplasm", "Construction molecular map of cotton germplasm and molecular marker for the genes with important traits", "Germplasm enhancement and utilization of cotton"* etc., for elite germplasm evaluation. All these projects were in cooperative with provincial cotton research institutes and national universities. We are seeking to have some chances to make international cooperation on collection and evaluation.

4.1. Evaluation of agronomic traits

Germplasm accessions were evaluated by field investigation according to *"Descriptors and Data Standards for Cotton Germplasm"* utilizing the IPGRI description standards for cotton [20]. Sixty-six agro-economic characters were evaluated, including 41 morphological and agronomic characters, 13 fiber quality, 4 seed quality, 8 disease, insect, multi-adversity resistance characters among 6372 accessions. The main characters were early maturity, mid-maturity, late maturity, clustering of bolls, dwarfness, pubesence, naked seeds, big boll, high lint percentage, long fiber, strong fiber, high oil content, high protein content, low gossypol content, high gossypol content, high Fusanrium wilt resistance, high Verticillium wilt resistance, root disease resistance, aphids resistance, bollworm resistance, red pink boll worm resistance, spider resistance, draught resistance, salinity resistance, humidity resistance, cold resistance, color of fiber, male sterility, and genetic markers (Table 8). The Chinese Crop Germplasm Information System (CGRIS) served as a central repository for all germplasm accession characterization and evaluation information for China and was freely available at http:// icgr.caas.net.cn/ cgrisintroduction.html (verified on July 17th 2009). Cotton germplasm evaluation and characterization data was first stored on an offline, internal database and then periodically deposited onto the CGRIS online database.

The evaluation of environment adaptation was also carried out in the past years. All germplasms from the foreign origins were divided into three types based on the latitude, including tropical type, subtropical type and temperate zone type, and were grown in Lujiang in Yunan province, Nanjing in Jiangsu province, Yuncheng in Shanxi province, Kuerle in Xinjiang province. It was found that the germplasm from USA were adaptable in Yellow River area and Yangtze River area because of the similar latitude and weather, and the germplasms from

Years	Fiber quality	Fusarium wilt	Verticillium wilt	Drought	Salt	Boll -worm	Aphid	Pink worm	Tetranychid mite
1957-1990	2943	2344	2345	2844	2888	365	364	359	1
1991-2000	1242	888	897	1053	1064	337	356	337	346
2001-2005	491	470	485	477	484	198	202	208	207
2006-2009	501	416	500	487	500	284	499	500	498

Table 8. Evaluation of the main traits in cotton during the past years

Central Asia grew very well in Xinjiang province, but these from Brazil and Africa produce only in Yunan. This provided a guidance for the further introduction germplasm in different area. Some better fiber quality lines were screened after the evaluation in different environments, such as Chuan77-1, Acala1517-70, Acala1517-77, LineF, upland, FJA, Zaoshuchangrong7, ITMA96497, Hopical. Now Nanjing, Anyang, Kuerle, Kuche and Shijiazhuang were chosen as the appointed locations for the environment adaption evaluation of the cotton germplasm in China.

The *G.arboreum* L in China was selected to evaluate for special agronomy traits, such the fiber quality, abiotic resistance, specific follower color and leaf. Some important traits were classified into different types including oil and protein contents in the seeds, fiber fineness, and boll maturity based on the evaluation of all the germplasm.

4.2. Evaluation with molecular method

The genetic diversity of main sources germplasm of Upland cotton were studied on the basis of simple sequence repeat (SSR) markers. These germplasm of Upland cotton included the cultivars bred in different periods and grown in different ecological areas, the lines transferred with genes and exotic DNA, and the introgression lines from interspecific hybridization [13]. Meanwhile, SSR fingerprinting analysis were set up to indentify the elite germplasm with high yield and good fiber quality, and QTLs mapping were carried out to screen the markers linked or associated with the beneficial genes [21-24]. Those studies presented an overview of the genetic diversity of the cotton germplasm in China, and provided a guideline for breeders to develop new cultivars efficiently.

4.2.1. Evaluation of introgression G.hirsutum lines

The introgression *G.hirsutum* lines were created by different institutes and collected in the germplasm bank in the past years, which possessed some important beneficial genes from the wild species. Our research showed that there were specific SSR loci among the different exotic *G.hisutum*. Around 45.2% of 155 interspecific lines possessed specific SSR loci [13]. The percentage of the lines with exotic specific SSR loci among the exotic *G.hirsutum* which may be transferred from *G. barbadense* and *G. thurberi* was highest, reached 62.1% and 71.1% respectively. The second was those with the specific SSR loci of *G. anomalum* and *G. bickii* etc., reached 57.1% and 42.9% respectively (Table 9). Because the numbers of exotic gene transformation were different, the specific SSR loci detected were very different. The *G. hirsutum* with exotic *G. barbadense* genes possessed 1-4 specific SSR loci, and those with *G. thurberi* had 1-5 specific loci. Through analysis of the agricultural traits of the introgression lines with specific SSR loci, the correlation between specific SSR loci and the main elite traits of the introgression lines was found. The results showed that the more specific SSR loci of exotic species, the better the fiber length and strength, the more tolerance of drought stress etc., and the elite strains with resistance to Verticillium wilt maybe selected from the germplasm with specific SSR loci (Table 10). This indicated that there were desirable markers and genes related to high fiber quality, tolerance to draught, resistance to Verticillium wilt etc. among these exotic *G. hirsutum* lines. For example, the variety Shenmian 5 in *G.hirsutum* with exotic genes of *G. barbadense* had 5 specific SSR loci. This caused its high fiber quality with length 34.1 mm and strength 24.3 Cn/tex, which indicated the high fiber quality of *G. barbadense* may be transferred into Shenmian 5. Similarly, the character of resistance to Verticillium wilt of *G. hirsutum* variety Shenmian 718 maybe resulted from *G. barbadense* since it had 2 specific SSR loci of *G. barbadense.* The high fiber quality traits of *G. hirsutum* variety Acala SJC-1, FJA and J line with consanguinity of *G. thurberi* maybe also resulted from potential high quality genes of *G. thurberi.* Moreover, the similar molecular and agronomic characters of exotic *G. hirsutum* of *G. barbadense* and *G. thurberi* indicated *G. barbadense* may be originated from *G. thurberi* [13].

Exotic species	No. of accessions	No. of specific loci	Percentage of lines with specific loci(%)	Average specific loci	Range of specific loci
G. barbadense	29	8	62.1	2.6	1-4
G. arboreum	21	2	4.8	2.0	2
G. thurberi	45	15	71.1	1.7	1-5
G. sturtianum	12	2	25.0	2.0	2
G. bickii	7	1	42.9	1.0	1
G. anomalum	7	3	57.1	1.8	1-3
G. hirsutum race mexicanum	5	1	20.0	1.0	1
G. raimondii	5	2	40.0	1.0	1
Total introgression lines	155	25	45.2	1.8	1-5

Table 9. The specific SSR loci of introgression genes among some exotic *G. hirsutum*

For confirming the detail information of each accession, the database of fingerprints was set up to describe and distinguish some lines. "Decimal string code" was given to each individual based on the fingerprints after running gel with SSR markers, and then the information of the code as an identification number was integrated with the existent database. This helped to keep the uniformity of the accessions in the germplasm bank and the releasing lines. Till now

	Drought tolerance (%)	Salt tolerance (%)	Verticillium Wilt tolerance (%)	Fusarium Wilt Resistance (%)	Bollworm resistance (%)
Specific SSR loci	0.521**	-0.051	-0.100	-0.068	0.026
Lines with specific loci(%)	-0.029	-0.439*	0.475*	-0.288	-0.494**
	Length (mm)	Uniformity (%)	Strength (cN/tex)	Elongation (%)	Micronaire
Specific SSR loci	0.185	0.020	0.085	-0.009	-0.139
Lines with specific loci(%)	0.215	0.192	0.438*	0.319	0.100

* showed significance at 5%, ** showed significance at 1%

Table 10. Correlation coefficient between SSR loci and fiber traits and stress resistant traits

330 cultivars have been assigned with the "Decimal string code", and more lines will be done in the future [25].

4.2.2. Identification of the genes or QTLs in the specific germplasm

For further finding and using the potential beneficial genes, QTLs mapping and cloning of genes were carried out using the mutant lines that were developed through physical and biologic methods or/and collected from other institutes. A new fiber developmental mutant *G. hirsutum* line GZnn with fuzzless-seed was analyzed by traditional genetics methods and SSR marker analysis. It was found that GZnn possessed a qualitative trait of naked seed that was controlled by one recessive gene. Using SSR marker technology, we located this fuzzless-gene on chromosome 10 and named it n_4, which was different from N_1 (on chromosome 12), n_2 (on chromosome 26) and n_3 (found in USA in recent years). This gene was closely linked with SSR marker S1495-120. Some other novel fiber quality QTLs were also detected using genetic population of the interspecific crossed line J02-508 which was segregated for fiber length and fiber strength. The fiber length of line Su7235 was found to be controlled by one major gene and many minor genes. A dwarf gene which was thought to be caused by the absence of gibberellin (GA) and recovered by spraying GA in the seedling stage, was also found and mapped[22]. Other genes about the big boll, high lint percent, brown fiber, resistance to *Verti*cillium wilt, and glandless in the seedling [21-24]. Some important genes controlling the drought and salt tolerance, yield, fiber quality and boll opening stage, were screened with the method of association mapping using a germplasm resources.

5. Germplasm release and utilization

The purpose of the collection and evaluation of cotton germplasm is to release and utilization for the improvement of breeding based on the screening of the beneficial genes. The procedures were made to fit for the normal release and utilization for the research. Since recorded files, a large number accessions have been released and helped to promote the yield, quality and resistance in the development of cotton breeding in China.

5.1. Germplasm release

Formal germplasm seed requests within China are needed to provide to the Cotton Research Institute of the Chinese Academy of Agricultural Sciences. A Material Transfer Agreement is required to distribute seeds of requested germplasm. Seed requests from outside of China require a complex procedure for approval. Cotton characterization and evaluation database is linked with Chinese Germplasm Resource System (CGRIS: http://icgr.caas.net.cn). More than 11241 accessions cotton germplasm have been released for the customers in China and a few foreign counties till 2006 (Table 11). Since 2007, different accessions have been grown in the field every year and have been arranged for demonstration in the boll opening stage for the selection and utilization of the researchers. Through this way, the researchers could visually recognize and know the lines in the germplasm bank, and decide what they want to choose for the breeding and other research. Therefore, the numbers of accessions released in recent years which were selected by the researchers themselves increased dramatically every year.

Province/ Country	Accession number	Number of organizations	Province/ Country	Accession number	Number of organizations
Henan	2525	27	Shanghai	20	4
Xinjiang	1803	21	Tianjin	11	3
Jiangsu	981	22	Jilin	4	1
Hebei	863	24	Xizang	3	1
Beijing	862	15	Guangdong	1	1
Shandong	573	18	Yunnan	1	1
Hubei	542	15	USA	204	
Jiangxi	422	9	Brazil	52	
Hunan	356	11	Russia	50	
Sichuan	330	5	Vietnam	18	
Shanxi	314	8	Australia	12	
Zhejiang	257	4	Ethiopia	10	
Liaoning	256	6	Pakistan	15	
Anhui	122	16	Marcello	6	
Shanxi	101	5	Kazakhstan	3	
Gansu	52	5	India	1	
Hainan	28	4	Others	190	
Chongqin	25	2	Total	11241	

Table 11. The accessions released in the different areas during the past years

5.2. Germplasm utilization

5.2.1. Utilization of basic germplasm

All these accessions shared with the researchers have helped to develop some import cultivars. Some basic accessions have made important contribution to the improvement of cotton breeding, which could be summarized in three stages in the development of cotton germplasm. In the first stage, the germplasm imported from USA, such as TX 53, Stoneville 4, Stoneville 4B, Stoneville 2B, Coker 100, D.P.L 14, D.P.L 15, and Empire, were the main basic lines to promote the breeding level in China [15-17,26-27]. More than one thousand new lines were bred based on these basic lines. Guannong No.1 is the typical cultivar that was bred using the basic line King, and also was used as new basic line for the new cultivar breeding. In the second stage, the cultivars and germplasm selected by the Chinese breeders, such as Yishuhong, Jingmian 1, Ganmian 1, Xuzhou 209, Xuzhou 1818, Dongting 1, Zhongmiansuo 2, Zhongmiansuo 3, Zhongmiansuo 4, Zhongmiansuo 7, Jiangsumian 1, Jiangsumian 2 and Jiangsumian 3, became the new basic lines, which were commercialized and grown in larger areas. Some lines with resistant genes also were used as the basic lines, such as Liaomian 1, Liaomian 3, Shanmian 3, Shanmian 4, Shanmian 5, 52-128, 57-681, and D.P.L 16 from USA, as well as 24-21 and KK1543 from the Soviet Union. New cultivars that were created using these basic lines, replaced the varieties imported from foreign countries in commercialization. In the third stage, the basic lines with the resistant to the disease, early maturity, high lint percentage and male sterility, were used that resulted in the resistant lines 86-1 and Zhongmiansuo 12, early mature lines Heishan mian 1 and Zhongmiansuo 10, high lint percent and heterotic line Jimian 1, and male sterile line Dong A. The glandless lines such as Lambright GL-5 and Mcnair 210 introduced from USA, helped to create new type of cultivars in China. The basic germplasm lines of *G. barbadense* were fewer than the *G.hirsutum*. Only seven lines were most frequently-used in the breeding of *G. barbadense*, such as C6022, 8763 I and 9122 i from the Soviet Union, Menoufi from Egypt, Xinhaimian, Junhai and Changrong 3 from China.

Some important cultivars have been bred after the basic lines were introduced to the breeders in China. Zhongmiansuo 12 was from the crossing of Uganda 3 and Xingtai 6871, which was the first high yielding cultivars that was resistant to Fusarium wilt and was ever grown in nearly 50% cotton area in China during 1992-1996. Lines 52-128, 57-681-52-128 and 57-681 were selected from D.P.L 15 and Texas 531 bred by Sichuan cotton institute, and became the important lines that provided the gene source of resistance to Fusarium wilt. In China, Liaomian 1 and Liaomian 2 were the pioneer varieties with Verticillium wilt. Resistance. Two varieties of Zhong 8004 and Zhong 8010 resistant to Verticillium wilt were produced. Lines Shan 1155 and Zhong 3474 with resistance to Fusarium and Verticillium wilt provided resistant genes for seven varieties. In the 1990s, almost 111 varieties had the resistant genes of Verticillium wilt from the lines 86-6, Chuan 737, Chuan 2802, Shan 2234, Shan 6192, Chuanmian 239, Huai 910 and Chuanmian 243.

5.2.2. *Utilization of germplasm with beneficial traits and genes*

Germplasm with beneficial agronomic traits were utilized in the past year for purpose of the good quality, high yield, and multiple resistance in the cotton breeding. Nine PD lines with good fiber quality, such as PD 4548 and PD 2164, have been the origin of eleven new cultivars including Emian 21, Lumian 14, and Wanmian 10. The new varieties Xinluzao 6, Xinluzao9 and Xiangzamian 9 came from the contribution of line Bellsiro with good fiber quality [24, 26]. Lumian 9 had the pedigree of Acala. In the field of resistant research, Simian 3 that was important and popular in commercialization, was devoloped by importing the Fusarium wilt resistant genes from the line Yankang 76-75. Also Liaomian 5 was the origin of Verticillium wilt resistant gene and contributed to the breeding of six new varieties including Zhongmiansuo 20 and Lumian 7. Chuanmian 109 that possessed the gene of resistance to aphid, helped to create the cultivars Chuanmian 109-1 and Jingmian 1 with the resistant to the aphid. In recent years, more and more varieties were bred through composing different kinds of powerful genes from the special germplasm lines. For example, Chuang 075 was from the lines Zhongmiansuo 12, Yumian 19 and Zhnongmiansuo 21 with Verticillium wilt resistance. Zhongmiansuo 44 developed from the line Zhong 2369 with Fusarium wilt resitance, the line Tamcot CD3Hal with drought tolerance and the line Zhongmiansuo 17 with high yield. Zhongmiansuo 49 derived from the early mature line Jing 444 and the line Zhongmiansuo 35 with salt tolerance and high yield. Zhongmiansuo 48 with good fiber quality, big boll and high yield, was from the big boll line Su9108.

5.2.3. *Utilization of special germplasm with specific traits*

Some special cotton germplasm showed different characteristics to the standard lines in the traits of leaf shape, flower color, bract shape, absence of nectarines, fiber color etc. The first special trait used in the breeding was okra leaf, which reduced the vegetative growth for keeping well light ventilation, and was resistant to *Syllepte derogata Fabricius*. The varieties with okra leaf were very popular in the cotton growing areas. The oldest cultivar with okra leaf used in china was Okra leaf TX 8207 selected from normal leaf TX 8207, which was the important variety before 1958. The second famous cultivar with okra leaf was Biaoza A1, a hybrid commercialized in Xinjiang. The virescent trait was also used in the breeding for indentifying the false hybrid in the seedling stage. Frego-bract providing the resistance to the bollworm, pink bollworm and boll weevil through the narrow and twisted bract, helped to create the new cultivar Zhongmiansuo 33. The absence of nectary in the leaf and bract could reduce the attraction to insects, and was used in the breeding of morphological resistance to insects such as Zhong 5909 and Ji U82-3[28]. The glandless trait attracted the researchers when it was found to be lower poisonous to the health of people for the oil and protein consumption. Many varieties with glandless such as Zhong 13 and Yumian 6 have been selected in the past years and were grown in some special areas. The cultivars with brown and green fiber were also created. The first two colored cotton cultivars in China were Zhongxu 1 and Lvxu 1, which genes were transferred from the wild cotton. In recent years, more and more colored cotton cultivars were bred by different researchers, such as the brown fiber cultivars Zhong 263,

Zhong 163, Zhongmiansuo 51, Xincai 3, Xiangcaimian and Zhongmiansuo 81, and green fiber cultivars Lv 4560 and Zhongmiansuo 82.

5.2.4. Utilization of wild species

Wild species possess many beneficial genes that have been swept in the domestication of cotton. Researchers in China started to study and untilize the wild species very early. The most famous variety was Shiyuan 321 from the hybridization of *G.thurberi*, *G.barbadense* and *G.hirsutum* by the institute of Genetic and Developmental Biology, Chinese Academy of Sciences(CAS) and Shijiazhuang Academy of Agricultural Sciences. Jinmian 2 was the second commercialized variety from the *G.thurberi*, *G.anomalum* and *G.hirsutum*, which possessed the traits such as resistance to Verticillium wilt, Fusarium wilt and bollworm, early maturity, high yield, and good fiber quality. Qinyuan 4 was commercialized with the multiple cross of *G. sturtianum* and two *G. hirsutum* (Zhongmiansuo 12 and Acala SJ-1), which is resistant to Fusarium wilt and tolerant to drought. Other lines were also created by different institutes in China, such as the line HST2 from the hybridization of *G. sturtianum* and *G. hirsutum* with the resistant to Verticillium wilt, Fusarium wilt, pinkworm and drought, line HAS from *G. sturtianum*, *G. hirsutum*, and *G. arboretum*, line 92-26-2 from *G. hirsutum* and *G. anomalum*, line 92-48-1 from *G. thurberi*, *G. barbadense* and *G. hirsutum*, line BZ201 from *G. thurberi*, *G. hirsutum* and *G. hirsutum* landrace, line BZ401 from *G. hirsutum* and *G. anomalum*, line JSCG7235 from *G. hirsutum* and *G. anomalum* with long fiber length and strong fiber strength.

6. Future perspectives and suggestions

In future, further research need to be carried out based on the current result of cotton germplasm in China for providing the development of cotton breeding. First, expeditions to the origin sites should be emphasized in the following stage of collection, especially expeditions in the origin sites of wild species and landraces. Exchange with the countries that had special and more diversity germplasm should be continued for enriching the diversity of cotton in China. Second, the method of evaluation should be renewed, and new methods such as the association analysis with new generation sequencing technology should be used in the procedure of screening of important germplasm carrying beneficial genes. The genes with drought and salt tolerance that are required urgently in North-west China cotton production suffering from water deficiency and salinity, should be identified accurately with high throughput methods. Third, new lines should be created through comprehensive techniques using the current germplasm resources. One novel line could significantly change the reputation of cotton breeding. Forth, high efficient database should be set up for recording all the information of the cotton germplasm, including the agronomic traits and molecular data.

Author details

Yinghua Jia*, Junling Sun and Xiongming Du

State Key Laboratory of Cotton Biology/ Institute of Cotton Research of Chinese Academy of Agricultural Sciences (ICR, CAAS),Anyang, Henan, China

References

[1] Xianlin, X., Duanzhuang, S., Guoqiang, L., Zhongfang, C., Qinfang, X., Ruohai, W., Siyin, Q., Huaiqin, F. *G. arboreum* L in China. ISBN 7-109-01295-6/S.927; 1989

[2] Shuchun, M., Yabin, L., Hezhong, D., Shu, B., Yongzeng, L., Helin, D. Cotton cultivation. ISBN 978-7-54781-516-8; 2013

[3] Shankang, S., Xianlin, X., Jianhua, C., Siyin, Q., Lianqin, L., Guanglan, X., Guochun, Z., Shubi, C., Rui, Y. Cotton Breeds in China. 16144.2314; 1981

[4] Xiongmin, D., Guoqiang, L., Junlin, S., Zhongli, Z., Yinhua, J., Zaoe, P. Cotton Breeds in China (1978-2007). ISBN 978-7-80233-727-5; 2009

[5] Ruohai, W., Xiulan, L. Historical Account of Cotton in China. ISBN 978-7-80233-244-7; 2007

[6] Leslie, M., Stephen, M., Robert, S. Cotton and Wool Situation and Outlook Yearbook. Market and Trade Economics Division, Economic Research Service, U.S. Department of Agriculture 2007.

[7] Campbell, BT., Saha, S., Percy, R. Status of the Global Cotton Germplasm Resources. Crop Science 2010 ; 50 1161–1179.

[8] Catalogues of cotton germplasm in China. Institute of Cotton Research of Chinese Academy of Agricultural Sciences; 1975

[9] Catalogues of cotton germplasm in China. Institute of Cotton Research of Chinese Academy of Agricultural Sciences; 1978

[10] Catalogues of cotton germplasm in China. Institute of Cotton Research of Chinese Academy of Agricultural Sciences; 1990

[11] Catalogues of cotton germplasm in China. Institute of Cotton Research of Chinese Academy of Agricultural Sciences; 1995

[12] Catalogues of cotton germplasm in China. Institute of Cotton Research of Chinese Academy of Agricultural Sciences; 2000

[13] Chaoyou, P., Xiongming, Du., Zhiying, Ma. Evalution of the introgressed lines and screening for elite germplasm in Gossypium. Chinese Science Bulletin 2006 ; 51(3) 304-312.

[14] Renhai, P., Tao, Z., Fang, L., Jian, L., Chunying, W., Shaohui, Li., Xiangdi, Z., Yuhong, W., Kunbo, W. Preparations of Meiotic Pachytene Chromosomes and Extended DNA Fibers from Cotton Suitable for Fluorescence *In Situ* Hybridization. PLoS ONE 2012; 7(3) e33847

[15] Zikang, H., Daofan, J., Jiaju, P. Cotton Genetics and Breeding in China. ISBN 978-7-53313-324-5; 2013

[16] Zikang, H. Cotton Breeds and Pedigree in China. ISBN 978-7-10911-378-7; 2007

[17] Zikang, H., Youlu, Y., Fuxin, Y. Cotton Heterosis and Hybrid in China. ISBN 978-7-10912-646-6; 2008

[18] Guoqiang, L., Huaiqin, F., Jinding, L., Kunbo, W. Cotton Genetic Resources and Traits in China. ISBN 7-109-05373-3/S. 3421; 1998

[19] Yongwen, J., Yongzhong, Q., Jiahe, F., Yongxing, Z. Inventory of germplasm in the Field Gene Bank in China. ISBN 7-80167-802-8/S. 617; 2005

[20] Xiongming, D., Zhongli, Z. Descriptors and Data Standard for Cotton (Gossypium spp). ISBN 7-109-10427-3; 2005

[21] FuguangL, YouluY. Cotton Molecular Breeding. ISBN 978-7-5655-0678-9; 2013

[22] Cao, Z., Junling, S., Yinhua, J.et al. Morphological Character, Inheritance and Exogenous Hormone Response of a Cotton Super Dwarf Mutant in G.hirsutum. Plant Breeding 2010; 130 67-72

[23] Hongjie, F., Junling, S., Jie, W. et al. Genetic effects and heterosis of the fibre colour and quality of brown cotton (Gossypium hirsutum). Plant Breeding 2011; 130 450-456

[24] Sheng, W., Guohong, Z., Yinhua, J., Xipongmin, D. Molecular Cloning and Characterization of an Adenylyl Cyclase-Associated Protein from Gossypium arboreum L. Agricultural Sciences in China 2009; 8 (7) 777-783

[25] Xiwen, W. Genetic Diversity Evaluation and Establishment of SSR Digital Fingerprint of the Elite Germplasm Resources in Cotton. Post-Graduate thesis. Sichuan Agricultural University; 2009

[26] Jizhong, Sun. Cotton. ISBN 978-7-10905-758-6; 1999

[27] Shenghan, Z. Pedigree of Cotton Breeds in China. ISBN 978-7-53644-516-0-9; 2000

[28] Yingfan, C., Xiaohong, H., Jianchuan, M., Quan, S., Jianping, Y., Jinggao L. Molecular research and genetic engineering of resistance to Verticillium wilt in cotton: A review. African Journal of Biotechnology 2009; ISSN 1684–5315 pp. 7363-7372

Chapter 3

Exploitation of Chinese Upland Cotton Cultivar Germplasm Resources to Mine Favorable QTL Alleles Using Association Mapping

Hongxian Mei, Xiefei Zhu, Wangzhen Guo,
Caiping Cai and Tianzhen Zhang

Additional information is available at the end of the chapter

http://dx.doi.org/10.5772/58587

1. Introduction

Cotton (*Gossypium* spp.) is the most important natural textile fiber source globally. The worldwide economic impact of the cotton industry is estimated at approximately $500 billion per year with an annual utilization of about 27 million metric tons of cotton fiber [1].The tetraploid species *Gossypium hirsutum* L. (n=26, AD genome), commonly referred to as Upland cotton, accounts for 95% of the world's cotton production [2]. Most of the objectives in cotton breeding, such as yield, fiber quality, biotic-and abiotic-stress tolerance, are all complex traits, which are controlled by a large number of quantitative trait loci (QTLs). It is becoming progressively more difficult to improve these traits using conventional breeding methods due to their complex architecture and inheritance [3]. Fortunately, the development in applied genomics research has provided alternative tools to improve efficiency in plant breeding programs. Molecular markers tightly linked to the target genes or QTLs can be used for marker-assisted selection (MAS) and/or genomic selection (GS) [4-5]. In the past two decades, the availability of abundant molecular markers has made tagging QTL harboring functional genes through family-based linkage mapping a routine process, and a large number of QTLs for fiber quality properties [6-40], yield and its components [6, 8, 10-11, 14, 18-19, 27, 30-32, 36, 40-45], nematode resistance [46-49], Verticillium wilt resistance [50-53] as well as Fusarium wilt resistance [54-60] have been identified in cotton.

However, approximately 80% of the previously reported QTLs could not be confirmed in subsequent studies, and few have actually been applied in breeding programs [61-62]. This may be because most QTLs were population-specific, and the genetic variations detected in a unique bi-parental population were not shared with other genetic populations, or shared but fixed in the parental lines. In addition, limited genetic recombination events in most populations used for linkage mapping make it difficult to map QTL with a high resolution, which severely limits their application in breeding programs. With the potential to exploit all recombination events that occurred in the evolutionary history of natural populations, linkage disequilibrium (LD) based association mapping (AM) has become a powerful approach for the dissection of complex traits and identification of causal variation with modest effects for target traits in many plant species [3, 63] including cotton [64-73]. Furthermore, although AM has been successfully used to detect the QTLs underlying quantitative traits in some crops, from a breeding standpoint, detecting associated loci is just the first step; analyzing the genetic effects of alleles and identifying favorable alleles will be more beneficial for target trait improvement. For example, Breseghello and Sorrells identified several potentially beneficial alleles for kernel size and milling quality by comparing the average phenotypic value with specific alleles and null alleles in a soft winter wheat population [74]; Jia et al. identified some putative resistant alleles for Sheath Blight resistance in a rice panel composed of 217 accessions from the USDA core collection, and found that the number of putative resistant alleles presented in an entry was highly and significantly correlated with the decrease of ShB rating [75].

China is the world's largest cotton-growing nation, but not a cotton domestication region. Most Upland cotton cultivars developed in China were derived from a few germplasm resources such as Deltapine (DPL), Stoneville (STV), Foster, King and Uganda, all of which were introduced from abroad [76]. More than 8800 accessions have been collected, developed, and maintained in Chinese cotton germplasm collection [77]. Among these collections, *G. hirsutum* varieties and breeding lines comprise about 83% of the total. Current and obsolete cultivars have been and continue to be the main resources for cotton breeding programs in China. Dissecting the genetic basis of main breeding objective traits will be of great benefits to germplasm evaluation and future molecular breeding. In this chapter, we reviewed QTLs underlying yield and its components, fiber quality properties and Fusarium wilt resistance detected by association mapping and their favorable alleles identified in 2 Chinese Upland cotton AM panels [71-73]. We hope that these results should provide useful information for further understanding the genetic basis of these traits, and would facilitate future breeding process by MAS in Upland cotton.

2. Favorable QTL alleles for yield and its components

In recent years, demand for cotton fiber in the world market has dramatically increased. While cotton acreage has declined worldwide in the past few years, mainly it was due to strong competition from other crops as well as production costs [1]. To improve lint yield of Upland cotton cultivars will remain critical for meeting worldwide demand and maintaining profitability for cotton growers. A total of 356 representative Upland cotton cultivars and breeding lines were selected from the cotton germplasm collection in Cotton Research Institute, Chinese Academy of Agricultural Sciences (CRI-CAAS), and from the collection in our laboratory, and assembled to construct an AM panel. The population consisted of 348 cultivars developed in China, seven introduced from the U.S. including the genetic standard line TM-1, and one introduced from Uganda. According to their release year, the 348 Chinese cultivars could be divided into the following six groups: I (1930–1960, 26 lines); II (1961–1970, 26 lines); III (1971–1980, 39 lines), IV (1981–1990, 83 lines); V (1991–2000, 125 lines); and VI (2000–2005, 49 lines). The cultivars introduced from abroad, DPL 15, DPL 16, STV 2B, King, Foster 6 and Uganda 3, were used as a check group for genetic diversity and allele transmission evaluation, because they had been used as the main founder parents in China's Upland cotton breeding programs [71]. Yield and its components of the accessions were evaluated in three diverse environments, including lint yield per plant (LP), seed cotton yield per plant (SY), bolls per plant (BN), boll weight (BW), lint percentage (LP), lint index (LI) and seed index (SI). Three hundred and eighty-one pairs of SSR primers that amplify loci evenly covering the tetraploid cotton genome [78] were selected to genotype the 356 accessions.

The Bayesian model-based program STRUCTURE 2.3 was used to infer the population structure using 66 unlinked or weakly linked SSR markers as described in reference [79]. The length of the burn-in period and the number of Markov Chain Monte Carlo replications after burn-in were all assigned at 100,000 with an admixture and allele frequencies correlated model. Five independent run iterations were performed with the hypothetical number of subpopulations (k) ranging from 1 to 10. However, the result showed that the LnP(D) value corresponding to each hypothetical k kept increasing with k value and did not show any peak (Figure 1). Thus an ad hoc statistic Δk [80] was joined to correctly estimate the population structure. The Δk value showed a much higher likelihood at k=2 than at k=3-10 (Figure 1), suggesting that the total panel could be divided into 2 major subpopulations. Based on the correct k, all accessions were assigned to each of the two subpopulations (P1 and P2), for which the membership value (Q value) was >0.5, and the population structure matrix (Q) was generated for further association mapping. The P1 group contained 115 accessions including 63 cultivars from Yellow River cotton growing region, 46 lines from North and Northwest China regions, and 6 cultivars from Yangtze River region. The P2 group consisted of 241 accessions including 116 lines from Yellow River region, 107 lines from Yangtze River region, 10 lines from the North and Northwest China regions, and 8 lines introduced from abroad (see reference [71] for details). The software SPAGeDi was used to calculate the pair-wise relatedness [81]. For the kinship coefficient values, 86.85% was less than 0.05, 8.56% had a range of 0.05–0.10, and the remaining 4.59% showed various degrees of genetic relatedness. Based on the results of the relatedness analysis, a K matrix was constructed for further association mapping.

Marker-trait association analysis were performed with the MLM model, considering both kinship (K) and population structure (Q), implemented in TASSEL software [82]. At the α=0.01 (-log$P$=2) level, a total of 195 significant associations were detected between 82 SSR markers and 7 lint yield traits. Among these, most of the associations (125 of 195) were detected in only one environment, and the proportion of phenotypic variation explained by markers ranged from 1.52% to 9.40%, with an average of 3.70% (see reference [71] for details). After Bonferroni correction [83], 55 associations were found to be significant ($P \leq 0.05/145$,-log$P \geq 3.46$) between 26 SSR markers and 7 lint yield traits (Table 1). Most of the associations could be detected in

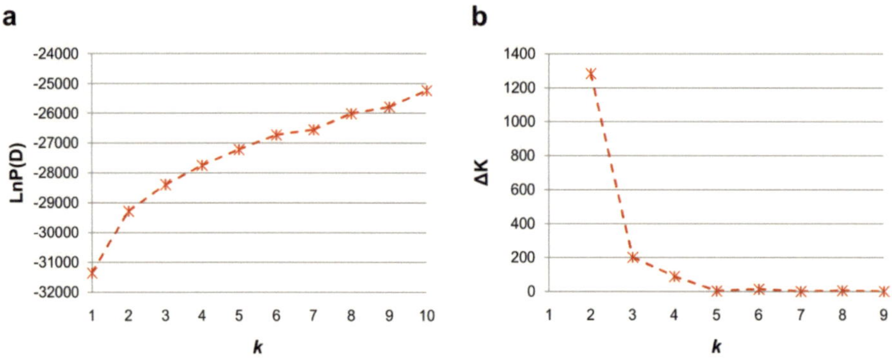

Figure 1. Estimated LnP(D) and Δ*k* over five repeats of STRUCTURE analysis (a) LnP(D) for *k* from 1 to 10 for 356 accessions. Note that Ln*P*(D) value of each hypothetical *k* kept increasing with *k* value. (b) Δ*k* for *k* from 2 to 9 for 356 accessions. The Δ*k* value showed a much higher likelihood at *k*=2 than at *k*=3–10, suggesting that the total panel should be divided into two major subpopulations

more than one environment, and the proportion of phenotypic variation explained by markers ranged from 1.63% to 9.40%, with an average of 4.51%. The number of SSR markers associated with LY, SY, BN, BW, LP, LI and SI were 9, 4, 6, 4, 14, 17 and 1, respectively. Seventeen loci were co-associated with two or more different traits (Table 1), for example, NAU3269 (Chr. 5) and NAU3100 (Chr. 23) were simultaneously associated with FY, SY, BN, LP, and LI, and most of the lint yield-associated loci were associated with at least one of its components. These associations coincided with phenotypic correlations among these traits [71]. This might result from pleiotropy of a single causal gene or tight linkage of multiple causal genes. We found that 10 of 14 markers associated with LP were detected in all three environments, which was consistent with the results in phenotypic evaluation that LP possessed the highest broad-sense heritability (h_B^2=75.77%) [71]. The phenotype of complex traits often result from the combined actions of multiple genes and environmental factors [3]; only those traits with high heritability can be stably detected. The resulting stably associated markers should be useful for cotton breeding with broad adaptability to different environments.

Traits	Marker loci	Chr.	Position	-LogP			*R*²(%)		
				E1	E2	E3	E1	E2	E3
LY	NAU3269	A05(Chr.05)	182.215	3.43	4.42	3.33	2.83	4.60	3.05
	NAU5166	A10(Chr.10)	23.423	ns	5.49	ns		5.40	
	NAU2935	A10(Chr.10)	51.592	ns	4.00	ns		4.72	
	JESPR204	A13(Chr.13)	59.714	4.12	3.00	ns	4.60	4.08	
	CIR246	D02(Chr.14)	112.473	ns	ns	3.55			4.44
	BNL3594	D06(Chr.25)	7.66	ns	4.51	ns		7.65	
	TMK19	D06(Chr.25)	70.38	4.30	2.77	3.97	4.21	3.21	4.28

Traits	Marker loci	Chr.	Position	-LogP			R^2(%)		
				E1	E2	E3	E1	E2	E3
	NAU3100	D09(Chr.23)	25.262	3.67	5.38	4.31	4.08	7.08	5.41
	NAU2776	D10(Chr.20)	9.452	ns	3.81	2.54		4.41	2.76
SY	NAU3269	A05(Chr.05)	182.215	2.25	4.16	2.43	1.85	4.41	2.19
	CIR246	D02(Chr.14)	112.473	ns	ns	4.23			5.36
	BNL3594	D06(Chr.25)	7.66	ns	4.61	ns		7.97	
	NAU3100	D09(Chr.23)	25.262	ns	4.03	2.82		5.61	3.84
BN	NAU6584	A03(Chr.03)	74.975	3.53	2.29	ns	3.93	2.91	
	NAU3269	A05(Chr.05)	182.215	2.08	3.52	3.45	1.74	3.64	3.44
	BNL3594	D06(Chr.25)	7.66	ns	3.62	ns		6.67	
	TMK19	D06(Chr.25)	70.38	3.58	ns	2.41	3.71		2.84
	NAU493	D07(Chr.16)	113.413	3.91	ns	ns	3.38		
	NAU3100	D09(Chr.23)	25.262	ns	3.48	ns		4.92	
BW	BNL1414	A09(Chr.09)	95.911	ns	3.26	3.72		4.18	4.45
	NAU4047	A12(Chr.12)	11.118	3.29	4.17	ns	3.32	4.61	
	NAU3398	A13(Chr.13)	3.311	3.47	3.46	ns	5.65	6.03	
	JESPR208	D09(Chr.23)	118.225	ns	4.01	3.69		5.15	4.45
LP	NAU3269	A05(Chr.05)	182.215	3.54	2.21	2.72	3.18	2.02	2.59
	NAU5166	A10(Chr.10)	23.423	2.33	4.36	2.74	1.80	4.10	2.44
	NAU2508	A10(Chr.10)	128.028	4.45	3.62	4.68	5.23	4.81	6.09
	NAU980	A11(Chr.11)	0	3.40	ns	3.75	5.65		6.72
	JESPR135	A11(Chr.11)	55.787	3.79	6.64	3.80	3.16	6.45	3.54
	NAU3398	A13(Chr.13)	3.311	3.50	ns	ns	4.99		
	JESPR204	A13(Chr.13)	59.714	3.73	2.96	2.22	4.41	3.96	3.11
	BNL3590	D03(Chr.17)	39.284	4.70	ns	2.89	4.91		338
	TMK19	D06(Chr.25)	70.38	5.97	4.58	3.67	6.04	5.18	4.19
	NAU3100	D09(Chr.23)	25.262	4.50	3.35	2.89	5.35	4.58	4.00
	NAU3917	D10(Chr.20)	31.125	ns	3.57	ns		4.03	
	BNL1404	D11(Chr.21)	33.571	4.48	6.20	3.51	3.81	6.01	3.23
	Gh508	D11(Chr.21)	54.48	2.15	3.37	3.81	1.63	3.06	3.54
	NAU2361	D11(Chr.21)	101.215	4.05	4.30	4.03	6.37	7.34	7.03
LI	NAU3269	A05(Chr.05)	182.215	4.98	2.77	2.38	4.92	2.63	2.32
	NAU980	A11(Chr.11)	0	8.85	2.34	2.80	8.96	4.76	5.72

Traits	Marker loci	Chr.	Position	-LogP			R^2(%)		
				E1	E2	E3	E1	E2	E3
	JESPR135	A11(Chr.11)	55.787	ns	5.43	2.34		5.20	2.09
	Gh369	A11(Chr.11)	84.701	3.77	2.09	ns	4.79	3.00	
	NAU1151	A12(Chr.12)	97.965	6.08	ns	ns	5.63		
	NAU3398	A13(Chr.13)	3.311	6.01	2.49	ns	8.19	4.15	
	JESPR204	A13(Chr.13)	59.714	ns	3.68	ns		4.81	
	CIR246	D02(Chr.14)	112.473	4.75	3.14	ns	5.77	4.17	
	BNL3590	D03(Chr.17)	39.284	3.30	2.70	3.47	3.67	3.13	4.26
	NAU2233	D05(Chr.19)	171.278	4.86	2.15	ns	5.96	3.04	
	TMK19	D06(Chr.25)	70.38	4.83	4.02	ns	5.19	4.55	
	NAU3100	D09(Chr.23)	25.262	5.90	2.74	3.47	7.19	3.84	4.93
	NAU2776	D10(Chr.20)	9.452	ns	ns	3.57			4.30
	NAU3917	D10(Chr.20)	31.125	ns	3.66	2.03		4.13	2.45
	BNL1404	D11(Chr.21)	33.571	ns	5.85	2.72		5.64	2.50
	Gh508	D11(Chr.21)	54.48	ns	3.67	3.41		3.38	3.27
	NAU2361	D11(Chr.21)	101.215	6.27	5.16	4.58	9.40	8.45	8.12
SI	NAU493	D07(Chr.16)	113.413	3.70	2.85	5.24	3.85	2.90	5.75

Table 1. SSR marker loci significantly associated with lint yield traits and their explained proportion of phenotypic variation in 3 different environments. LY: lint yield (g/plant); SY: seed cotton yield (g/plant); BN: bolls per plant; BW: boll weight (g); LP: lint percentage (%); LI: lint index (g/100 seeds); SI: seed index (g/100 seeds); E1: Jiangpu in 2009; E2: Dafeng in 2010; E3: Zhengzhou in 2010

To identify favorable alleles, the phenotypic allele effect was estimated through comparison between the average phenotypic value over accessions with the specific allele and that of all accessions:

$$a_i = \sum x_{ij} / n_i - \sum N_k / n_k$$

where a_i is the phenotypic effect of the *ith* allele; x_{ij} is the phenotypic value over the *jth* accession with the *ith* allele; n_i is the number of accessions with the *ith* allele; N_k is the phenotypic value over all accessions; n_k is the number of accessions. If the value of $a_i > 0$, the allele is considered to have a positive effect, if it is < 0, it corresponds to a negative allele. The favorable alleles were then identified according to the breeding objective of each target trait [69, 71]. Phenotypic effects of each QTL allele for the 41 associated loci detected in more than one environment were measured, and 5, 2, 3, 4, 12, 14 and 1 favorable alleles for FY, SY, BN, BW, LP, LI and SI were identified, respectively. Phenotypic effects and representative accessions for each favorable allele are shown in Table 2. Among the favorable alleles, NAU3100-2 had the most positive phenotypic effect for FY and SY, and increased FY and SY by 3.61 g and 7.27 g, respectively; NAU6584-2, NAU3398-2, NAU5166-2 and NAU3917-2 increased BN, BW, LP and

http://dx.doi.org/10.5772/58587

LI by 0.89, 0.42 g, 4.93% and 0.94 g, respectively; while NAU493-1 deceased SI by 0.17 g. Lint yield of cotton is the result of series components and their interactions, such as boll number, boll weight, lint percentage, lint index, and seed index. Developing potentially high-yielding cultivars thus relies to some extent on selecting the appropriate yield components. As some of the QTLs were associated with more than one yield component, favorable alleles must be treated with caution. Positively co-associated genetic loci could simultaneously improve multiple target traits, while negative linkages must be broken.

Traits	Favorable allele	a_i	Accessions	Representative accessions
LY	NAU3269-2	0.27	133	Simian3, Zhongmiansuo9, Huakangmian1
	JESPR204-1	0.70	314	Simian3, Zhongmiansuo9, P164-2
	TMK19-2	1.02	240	Simian3, Zhongmiansuo9, P164-2
	NAU3100-2	3.61	87	Simian3, Zhongmiansuo9, Lumianyan16
	NAU2776-1	0.85	151	Zhongmiansuo9, P164-2, Lumianyan16
SY	NAU3269-2	0.42	133	Zhongmiansuo9, Zhongmiansuo19, Simian3
	NAU3100-2	7.27	87	Zhongmiansuo9, Han4849, Lumianyan16
BN	NAU6584-2	0.89	217	Lumianyan16, Zhongmiansuo44, Zhongmiansuo9
	NAU3269-2	0.08	133	Zhongmiansuo9, Wanmian73-10, Simian3
	TMK19-2	0.45	235	Zhongmiansuo44, Zhongmiansuo9, Wanmian17
BW	BNL1414-2	0.18	93	Zhongmiansuo18, Zhongmiansuo5, I40005
	NAU4047-2	0.03	221	Zhongmiansuo18, Zhongmiansuo5, I40005
	NAU3398-2	0.42	22	Zhongmiansuo5, I40005, Hua101
	JESPR208-2	0.20	86	Zhongmiansuo18, Zhongmiansuo5, I40005
LP	NAU3269-2	0.23	133	Simian3, Ekangmian9, Huakangmian1
	NAU5166-2	4.93	8	Simian3, Huakangmian1, Sumian4
	NAU2508-2	0.36	113	Nannongzao, 86-1, Yu668
	NAU980-3	2.79	9	Ekangmian6, Emian16, Ekangmian10
	JESPR135-1	0.13	343	XiangSC-24, Simian3, Ekangmian9
	JESPR204-1	0.36	309	XiangSC-24, Simian3, Ekangmian9
	BNL3590-1	0.26	327	XiangSC-24, Simian3, Ekangmian9
	TMK19-2	0.58	235	XiangSC-24, Simian3, Huakangmian1
	NAU3100-2	1.55	86	Simian3, Ekangmian9, Nannongzao
	BNL1404-1	0.13	343	XiangSC-24, Simian3, Ekangmian9
	Gh508-1	0.07	347	XiangSC-24, Simian3, Ekangmian9
	NAU2361-3	0.75	73	Ekangmian9, Yu668, Yumian21
LI	NAU3269-2	0.01	133	Huakangmian1, I40005, Ekangmian9

Traits	Favorable allele	a_i	Accessions	Representative accessions
	NAU980-3	0.84	9	I40005, Zhongmiansuo5, Hua101
	JESPR135-1	0.02	343	Huakangmian1, Emian23, I40005
	Gh369-3	0.11	8	Emian16, Ekangmian8, Yumian20
	NAU3398-2	0.80	22	Huakangmian1, I40005, Zhongmiansuo5
	CIR246-3	0.63	16	Hua101, Zhongmiansuo41, Yumian9
	BNL3590-1	0.06	327	Huakangmian1, Emian23, I40005
	NAU2233-1	0.01	212	Huakangmian1, Emian23, I40005
	TMK19-2	0.10	235	Huakangmian1, Emian23, I40005
	NAU3100-2	0.38	86	I40005, Zhongmiansuo5, Hua101
	NAU3917-2	0.94	6	Huakangmian1, Simian4, Sumian9
	BNL1404-1	0.03	343	Huakangmian1, Emian23, I40005
	Gh508-1	0.01	347	Huakangmian1, Emian23, I40005
	NAU2361-3	0.28	73	Emian23, I40005, Zhongmiansuo5
SI	NAU493-1	-0.17	230	Chaoyangmian1, Xuzhou1818, XiangSC-24

Table 2. Favorable QTL alleles, their phenotypic effects (a_i) and representative accessions. LY: lint yield (g/plant); SY: seed cotton yield (g/plant); BN: bolls per plant; BW: boll weight (g); LP: lint percentage (%); LI: lint index (g/100 seeds); SI: seed index (g/100 seeds); Representative accessions are the top-3 entries for the target trait value of accessions with the corresponding favorable allele

Allele frequencies of the 23 favorable alleles in the CK group and the six Chinese historically released cultivar groups are summarized in Table 3. Based on allele frequencies across the different groups, these favorable alleles could be categorized into three classes. The alleles in the first class, such as JESPR135-1, BNL1404-1 and Gh508-1, presented in the founder cultivars and with high frequency in all populations, might have been passed down stably from the original parents and were almost fixed in modern cultivars by selection. Alleles in the second class, such as BNL3269-2, BNL1414-2, NAU3100-2 and JESPR208-2, presented in the founder cultivars and with moderate to low frequency in most populations, should have been underutilized in modern breeding programs. Those in the third class, such as NAU5166-2, NAU980-3, Gh369-3 and CIR246-3, not presented in the founder cultivars and presented at low frequency in modern cultivars, might be from other original parents or could have been generated by mutations and/or recombinations. Favorable alleles, especially of the latter two classes, should have a great potential in future Upland cotton genetic improvement. We suggest that a multi-parent population should be constructed using cultivars that possess most of the favorable alleles, and in the meantime, a ranking system for MAS or genomic selection should be developed based on the results of AM. Favorable alleles that were passed down from the founder parents and have been almost fixed in modern cultivars formed the basis of lint yield of Chinese Upland cotton, and should be treated as fundamental elements in order to reject deleterious alleles at the corresponding loci. Alleles either absent in the founder cultivars or present at moderate to low frequencies in most cultivar groups have been underutilized in modern breeding programs, and should be regarded as essential elements for increasing lint yield potential.

Favorable alleles	CK	I	II	III	IV	V	VI	Total
NAU6584-2	0.3333	0.5000	0.6923	0.7692	0.6747	0.4720	0.7755	0.6096
NAU3269-2	0.6667	0.5769	0.5385	0.6154	0.3976	0.3040	0.1020	0.3736
BNL1414-2	0.5000	0.3077	0.1923	0.4872	0.2410	0.2320	0.1633	0.2612
NAU5166-2	0.0000	0.0000	0.0000	0.0500	0.0000	0.0320	0.0417	0.0225
NAU2508-2	0.4000	0.1200	0.2400	0.2250	0.3012	0.3952	0.4694	0.3333
NAU980-3	0.0000	0.0200	0.0000	0.0256	0.0244	0.0369	0.0000	0.0233
JESPR135-1	1.0000	0.8462	1.0000	1.0000	0.9759	0.9840	1.0000	0.9775
Gh369-3	0.0000	0.0000	0.0000	0.0000	0.0241	0.0480	0.0000	0.0225
NAU4047-2	0.6667	0.5000	0.5769	0.6154	0.5663	0.6400	0.7551	0.6208
NAU3398-2	0.0000	0.0385	0.0000	0.1026	0.0843	0.0720	0.0204	0.0618
JESPR204-1	1.0000	0.8462	0.8077	0.7692	0.8675	0.9200	0.9388	0.8820
CIR246-3	0.0000	0.0000	0.0000	0.0256	0.0241	0.0800	0.0612	0.0449
BNL3590-1	0.5000	0.8077	0.8462	0.8462	0.9036	0.9440	0.8776	0.8904
NAU2233-1	0.6667	0.4231	0.5000	0.3590	0.5542	0.6560	0.8163	0.5955
TMK19-2	0.6667	0.5000	0.5769	0.6667	0.6024	0.7280	0.8163	0.6742
NAU493-1	0.6667	0.5000	0.7308	0.6923	0.6265	0.6800	0.5714	0.6461
NAU3100-2	0.3333	0.2308	0.0769	0.2308	0.2289	0.2400	0.3673	0.2444
JESPR208-2	0.5000	0.3077	0.1154	0.4359	0.2289	0.2240	0.1633	0.2444
NAU2776-1	0.1667	0.4231	0.3462	0.5385	0.4458	0.4480	0.3061	0.4242
NAU3917-2	0.0000	0.0000	0.0000	0.0513	0.0000	0.0240	0.0204	0.0169
BNL1404-1	1.0000	0.8462	1.0000	1.0000	0.9759	0.9840	1.0000	0.9775
Gh508-1	1.0000	0.9231	1.0000	0.9750	1.0000	0.9920	1.0000	0.9888
NAU2361-3	0.2143	0.0769	0.0417	0.1538	0.1125	0.2810	0.3673	0.2066

Table 3. Allele frequency for each favorable QTL allele in historically released Chinese Upland cotton cultivar groups. CK, I, II, III, IV, V and VI indicates the founder parent group (CK), and the Chinese cultivars released in 1930–1960, 1961–1970, 1971–1980, 1981–1990, 1991–2000 and 2000–2005, respectively

3. Favorable QTL alleles for fiber quality traits

With the acceleration of spinning speed, the demand for cotton fiber quality is increasing rapidly [9, 17]. It is important to elucidate the molecular genetics of Upland cotton fiber qualities, and such information would enable the subsequent improvement of cotton cultivars by pyramiding favorable alleles of fiber quality traits. We performed a marker-trait association mapping for fiber quality traits using MLM model implemented in TASSEL [82] with the panel mentioned above [71]. At the α=0.01 (-log$P$=2) level, a total of 59 significant associations were detected between 41 SSR markers and 5 fiber quality traits (Table 4). Among these, almost all of the associations were detected in only one environment, and the proportion of phenotypic variation explained by markers ranged from 1.84% to 7.12%, with an average of 3.53% (Mei et al. unpublished data). If a more stringent threshold with Bonferroni correction [83] was adopted, only 9 associations were found to be significant (Table 4). The result might be caused by low diversity of fiber quality properties existed in the 356-accession panel. Although the yield potential of Chinese cultivars are equal to or a bit higher than those developed in the United States or Australia, the fiber quality traits of Chinese cultivars are not as good as those of American or Australian cultivars [73, 84]. Narrow variation in fiber qualities of Chinese cultivars had severely limited the marker-trait association detection power in association mapping.

Traits	Marker loci	Chr.	Position	-LogP			R^2 (%)		
				E1	E2	E3	E1	E2	E3
FL	NAU845	A07(Chr.07)	54.589	4.16	ns	ns	5.91		
	NAU3398	A13(Chr.13)	3.311	ns	3.15	ns		5.64	
	BNL1707	A13(Chr.13)	104.694	2.39	ns	ns	2.27		
	JESPR152	D01(Chr.15)	110.252	2.59	ns	ns	3.25		
	BNL3359	D06(Chr.25)	140.397	4.3	ns	ns	5.67		
	JESPR297	D07(Chr.16)	43.109	ns	2.18	ns		2.08	
	NAU5418	D11(Chr.21)	75.156	ns	2.08	ns		4.47	
	BNL3537	D12(Chr.26)	39.496	ns	ns	2.06			2.77
	NAU2980	D13(Chr.18)	0	ns	ns	2.02			2.64
FS	NAU6584	A03(Chr.03)	74.975	2.3	ns	ns	3.16		
	NAU2561	A05(Chr.05)	56.73	2.96	ns	ns	3.08		
	NAU3269	A05(Chr.05)	182.215	3.53	ns	ns	3.88		
	NAU3427	A06(Chr.06)	5.598	2.25	ns	ns	2.91		
	NAU3654	A07(Chr.07)	74.363	ns	3.02	ns		4.36	
	NAU5166	A10(Chr.10)	23.423	2.09	ns	ns	1.95		

Traits	Marker loci	Chr.	Position	-LogP			R^2 (%)		
				E1	E2	E3	E1	E2	E3
	BNL1707	A13(Chr.13)	104.694	5.59	ns	ns	6.04		
	BNL2646	D01(Chr.15)	75.614	ns	2.15	ns	2.56	3.44	
	NAU2901	D01(Chr.15)	104.568	2.21	ns	ns	2.09		
	NAU1070	D02(Chr.14)	13.885	3.3	ns	ns	4.3		
	BNL1606	D03(Chr.17)	50.883	ns	2.27	ns		2.92	
	NAU2233	D05(Chr.19)	171.278	2.15	ns	ns	3.42		
	BNL3594	D06(Chr.25)	7.66	ns	2.41	ns		5.4	
	BNL3359	D06(Chr.25)	140.397	3.16	ns	ns	4.23		
	NAU6468	D07(Chr.16)	83.101	2.44	ns	ns	2.36		
FF	JESPR304	A02(Chr.02)	22.517	ns	ns	2.16			3.41
	NAU862	A03(Chr.03)	9.309	2.24	ns	ns	2.21		
	BNL3452	A05(Chr.05)	188.717	2	ns	ns	3.14		
	NAU3427	A06(Chr.06)	5.598	3.82	ns	ns	4.72		
	NAU2935	A10(Chr.10)	51.592	2.55	ns	ns	3.2		
	JESPR135	A11(Chr.11)	55.787	2.34	ns	ns	2.15		
	JESPR204	A13(Chr.13)	59.714	3.81	ns	ns	5.36		
	BNL2646	D01(Chr.15)	75.614	2.54	ns	ns	3.8		
	BNL1604	D07(Chr.16)	36.152	ns	2.85	ns		5.43	
	JESPR297	D07(Chr.16)	43.109	ns	2.03	ns		1.89	
	BNL1694	D07(Chr.16)	52.03	2.11	ns	ns	3.2		
	BNL1404	D11(Chr.21)	33.571	2.72	ns	ns	2.58		
	Gh508	D11(Chr.21)	54.48	3.71	ns	ns	3.68		
FU	NAU3254	A01(Chr.01)	33.644	2.02	ns	ns	2.61		
	NAU2161	A03(Chr.03)	0	ns	ns	2.44			3.83
	NAU3654	A07(Chr.07)	74.363	ns	2.26	ns		3.29	0

Traits	Marker loci	Chr.	Position	-LogP			R^2 (%)		
				E1	E2	E3	E1	E2	E3
	Gh486	A09(Chr.09)	10.554	ns	ns	2.24			4.23
	NAU5428	A11(Chr.11)	155.464	3.91	ns	ns	7.12		
	BNL1231	A11(Chr.11)	169.199	2.77	ns	ns	2.73		
	BNL3261	A12(Chr.12)	40.276	ns	2.08	ns		4.45	
	BNL1606	D03(Chr.17)	50.883	ns	2.48	ns		3.2	
	JESPR297	D07(Chr.16)	43.109	ns	ns	2.57			2.53
	Gh501	D13(Chr.18)	55.386	2.17	ns	ns	2.8		
FSCI	NAU2561	A05(Chr.05)	56.73	2.33	ns	ns	2.31		
	NAU5428	A11(Chr.11)	155.464	2.72	ns	ns	5.34		
	BNL1707	A13(Chr.13)	104.694	3.58	ns	ns	3.68		
	NAU2901	D01(Chr.15)	104.568	2.46	2.27	ns	2.36	2.17	
	JESPR152	D01(Chr.15)	110.252	3.45	ns	ns	4.34		
	NAU1070	D02(Chr.14)	13.885	3.19	ns	ns	4.15		1.99
	BNL1606	D03(Chr.17)	50.883	ns	2.52	ns		3.23	
	BNL3594	D06(Chr.25)	7.66	ns	2.29	ns	3.64	5.2	
	BNL3359	D06(Chr.25)	140.397	3.19	ns	ns	4.25		
	NAU6468	D07(Chr.16)	83.101	2	ns	ns	1.84		
	JESPR208	D09(Chr.23)	118.225	ns	2	ns		2.61	
	NAU2776	D10(Chr.20)	9.452	ns	2.11	ns		2.74	

Table 4. SSR loci significantly (-log$P$≥2.0) associated with fiber quality traits detected in the 356 Chinese Upland cotton cultivars. FL: fiber length; FS: fiber strength; FF: fiber fineness measured by micronaire value; FU: fiber uniformity ratio; FSCI: fiber spinning consistency index; E1: Jiangpu in 2009; E2: Dafeng in 2010; E3: Zhengzhou in 2010

To embrace the genetic diversity of fiber qualities as large as possible, a previous collection comprising 99 Upland cotton cultivars and breeding lines was used for further association mapping. The collection included 63 cultivars and 36 breeding lines with elite fiber quality traits (13 of which were PD lines introduced from the United States), and the fiber properties including fiber length, strength, and fineness were evaluated in 2004 and 2007. A total of 260

SSR markers, including the markers linked to fiber properties reported in previous studies [17-19], were used to screen the 99 accessions, and 97 of which showed polymorphisms [73]. Marker-trait association analysis was performed with the MLM model implemented in TASSEL [82]. At the α=0.01 (-log$P$=2) level, a total of 51 significant associations were detected between 33 SSR markers and 3 lint yield traits, and 7 of the these associations could be detected in both 2 years. The proportion of phenotypic variation explained by markers ranged from 7.76% to 23.99%, with an average of 14.07%. After Bonferroni correction [83], 17 associations were still significant (P≤0.05/97,-log$P$≥3.29). Compared with the results from our previous 356-accession panel, both the number of significant associations and the proportion of phenotypic variation explained by markers were improved in the current panel.

Traits	Marker loci	Chr.	Position	-logP		R^2	
				2004	2007	2004	2007
Fiber length	NAU934	A05(Chr.05)	186.594	2.32	ns	7.83	
	NAU1200	A05(Chr.05)		3.42	ns	17.4	
	NAU1037	A08(Chr.08)	53.526	ns	3.50		17.83
	BNL1317	A09(Chr.09)	88.456	2.62	2.68	12.18	14.12
	NAU2354	A09(Chr.09)	132.251	ns	2.06	10.4	13.32
	JESPR295	A12(Chr.12)	32.732	2.52	2.92	11.56	15.17
	NAU445	A12(Chr.12)	123.764	2.21	ns	10.22	
	JESPR153	A13(Chr.13)	63.046	3.00	ns	13.52	
	NAU2272	D02(Chr.14)	55.105	ns	2.64		16.26
	NAU1102	D05(Chr.19)		2.01	ns	9.32	
	NAU1302	D08(Chr.24)	72.101	ns	3.03		18.24
	BNL1521	D08(Chr.24)	73.477	ns	3.88		16.21
	JESPR78	D08(Chr.24)	75.81	ns	3.88		16.21
	NAU1336	D08(Chr.24)	78.13	ns	3.88		16.21
	NAU1262	D08(Chr.24)	88.599	ns	3.88		16.21
	JESPR127	D08(Chr.24)	97.939	ns	3.88		16.21
	NAU1004	D09(Chr.23)	13.67	2.64	ns	12.23	
	TMO06	D09(Chr.23)	109.242	3.78	3.88	16.86	19.56
	NAU904	D10(Chr.20)	53.078	ns	2.14		13.88
	NAU2443	D13(Chr.18)	62.214	2.30	ns	7.99	

Traits	Marker loci	Chr.	Position	-logP		R^2	
				2004	2007	2004	2007
Fiber strength	NAU934	A05(Chr.05)	186.594	3.82	ns	14.08	
	NAU1200	A05(Chr.05)		2.68	ns	14.5	
	NAU474	A07(Chr.07)	30.627	ns	2.43		17.44
	NAU1043	A07(Chr.07)		ns	2.14		15.86
	BNL1317	A09(Chr.09)	88.456	ns	2.37		12.58
	NAU2508	A10(Chr.10)	126.827	ns	3.29		23.99
	JESPR295	A12(Chr.12)	32.732	2.28	2.72	10.56	14.19
	NAU445	A12(Chr.12)	123.764	2.60	ns	11.96	
	JESPR153	A13(Chr.13)	63.046	5.42	ns	23.3	
	BNL1395	D07(Chr.16)	78.652	ns	2.12		13.62
	BNL1122	D07(Chr.16)	88.995	ns	2.23		14.19
	BNL2634	D07(Chr.16)		2.72	ns	12.47	
	NAU1369	D08(Chr.24)	57.434	2.74	ns	12.13	
	BNL1521	D08(Chr.24)	73.477	ns	2.34		9.26
	JESPR78	D08(Chr.24)	75.81	ns	2.34		9.26
	NAU1197	D08(Chr.24)	77.384	ns	2.01		7.76
	NAU1336	D08(Chr.24)	78.13	ns	2.34		9.26
	NAU1262	D08(Chr.24)	88.599	ns	2.34		9.26
	NAU1322	D08(Chr.24)	89.779	ns	2.04		10.82
	JESPR127	D08(Chr.24)	97.939	ns	2.34		9.26
	NAU780	D08(Chr.24)		ns	3.60		18.14
	NAU816	D08(Chr.24)		3.70	ns	13.6	
	TMO06	D09(Chr.23)	109.242	5.51	3.80	23.66	19.23
	NAU2443	D13(Chr.18)	62.214	6.13	3.16	22.85	13.02
Fiber fineness	NAU934	A05(Chr.05)	186.594	ns	3.074		12.62
	BNL1317	A09(Chr.09)	88.456	4.31	2.31	18.74	9.71
	NAU1162	A11(Chr.11)	99.954	2.05	ns	11.43	
	JESPR295	A12(Chr.12)	32.732	2.87	ns	12.95	

Traits	Marker loci	Chr.	Position	-logP		R^2	
				2004	2007	2004	2007
	BNL3436	D06(Chr.25)	105.073	2.24	ns	9.68	
	TMO06	D09(Chr.23)	109.242	2.85	ns	12.84	
	NAU1004	D09(Chr.23)	13.67	3.03	ns	13.67	

Table 5. SSR loci significantly (-log$P$≥2.0) associated with fiber quality traits detected in the and their explained phenotypic variation in two years

Phenotypic effects of each QTL allele for the 33 significantly associated loci were measured, and 21, 24 and 7 favorable alleles for fiber length, strength and fineness were identified, respectively. Phenotypic effects and representative materials for each favorable allele are shown in Table 6. A wide variation of the favorable alleles processed in the 99 accessions was observed, with an average of 14.84 and a range of 7 to 21 (see reference [73] for details). Most of the representative materials were fiber-elite lines collected from China or introduced from the United States, and some of them, such as Yumian 1 and 7235, were introgression lines and contained more than half of the favorable alleles. For example, 7235 was developed from several hybridizations with multiple parents, such as a *G. anomalum* introgression line, Acala 3080 and PD4381 [85, 86]; Yumian 1 was an introgression line with *G. barbadense, G. arboreum,* and *G. raimondii* as putative donors, which is characterized by high lint yield and high fiber strength [24]. These fiber-elite materials had been used for tagging QTLs underlying fiber quality traits in previous family-based linkage mapping studies [13, 17-19, 24-25; 39]. With the genetic information provided by this and previous studies, MAS should be complemented in the future breeding programs.

Traits	Favorable allele	a_i	Accessions	Representative materials
Fiber length	NAU934-4	1.0498	17	I-62434, 7235, I-62478
	NAU1037-1	4.5458	1	7235
	NAU2354-2	0.3662	10	I-62478, I-62479, PD94045
	BNL1317-3	0.8522	21	I-62434, 7235, I-62431
	NAU445-3	0.7926	31	I-62434, 7235, I-62431
	JESPR295-2	0.8233	31	I-62434, 7235, I-62478
	JESPR153-3	0.8457	16	I-62434, I-62431, Yumian1
	NAU1200-1	0.5373	49	I-62434, I-62478, I-62431
	NAU2272-5	5.8050	1	7235
	NAU1102-3	0.4564	22	I-62431, I-62479, I-62429

Traits	Favorable allele	a_i	Accessions	Representative materials
	NAU1302-1	4.5458	1	7235
	BNL1521-3	5.8050	1	7235
	JESPR78-3	5.8050	1	7235
	NAU1336-3	5.8050	1	7235
	NAU1262-2	5.8050	1	7235
	JESPR127-2	4.5458	1	7235
	TMO06-3	1.3109	19	I-62434, 7235, Yumian1
	NAU904-3	2.3858	1	GA2001163
	NAU2443-2	0.8435	17	I-62434, 7235, I-62431
	NAU780-4	4.5458	1	7235
	NAU1004-2	0.9346	14	I-62434, 7235, TM-1
Fiber strength	NAU934-4	2.6759	17	I-62429, I-62478, PD93019
	NAU474-2	1.0231	31	PD94042, I-62478, PD93019
	BNL1317-3	2.3136	21	I-62429, 7235, I-62433
	NAU2508-1	3.7061	8	7235, PD6992, HS427
	NAU445-3	0.8072	31	I-62429, 7235, I-62433
	JESPR295-2	2.1342	31	I-62429, I-62478, 7235
	JESPR153-3	2.8625	16	I-62429, I-62433, I-62434
	NAU1200-1	0.3169	49	I-62429, PD94042, I-62478
	NAU1043-2	0.9147	29	I-62478, PD93019, Yuwu19
	BNL1395-1	2.2677	12	I-62478, 7235, Yumian1
	BNL1122-1	2.2677	12	I-62478, 7235, Yumian1
	NAU1369-2	1.4296	15	I-62429, I-62433, Yumian1
	BNL1521-3	8.9290	1	7235
	JESPR78-3	8.9290	1	7235
	NAU1197-3	5.6730	2	Xiangmian13, 7235
	NAU1336-3	8.9290	1	7235
	NAU1262-2	8.9290	1	7235
	NAU1322-2	1.7557	17	I-62429, 7235, I-62433

Traits	Favorable allele	a_i	Accessions	Representative materials
	JESPR127-2	8.9290	1	7235
	TMO06-3	3.1629	19	I-62429, 7235, I-62433
	NAU2443-2	3.0749	17	I-62429, 7235, Yumian1
	BNL2634-3	0.8204	26	I-62429, I-62433, Yumian1
	NAU780-1	0.4073	71	I-62429, I-62478, Yumian1
	NAU816-3	1.6559	29	I-62429, PD94042, I-62478
Fiber fineness	NAU934-4	-0.3064	17	Emian11, Emian6, CRI18
	BNL1317-3	-0.3617	21	Jinmian2, Jinmian9, Jimian11
	NAU1162-2	-0.2338	13	Sumian5, CRI16, Yu668
	JESPR295-3	-0.2148	9	Qiannong465, Cangzhou7315-38, Jin185
	BNL3436-3	-0.1132	60	Xiangmian11, Jinmian2, Qiannong465
	TMO06-3	-0.3587	19	Shiduan5, Tai8033-2, Sumian5
	NAU1004-2	-0.1530	14	Qiannong465, Wanmian73-10, Qinli514

Table 6. Favorable QTL alleles for fiber qualities, their phenotypic effects (a_i) and representative materials. Representative accessions are the top-3 entries for the target trait value of accessions with the corresponding favorable allele

4. Favorable QTL alleles for FOV race 7 resistance

Fusarium wilt (FW), caused by *Fusarium oxysporum* f. sp. *vasinfectum* (FOV), is a widespread disease that causes huge losses in cotton (*Gossypium* ssp.) production worldwide [87-90]. Once established in soil, FOV can survive in the field for several years as Chlamydia spores, even in the absence of a host, and is nearly impossible to eliminate. Although both chemical controls and cultural practices have been employed in protecting plants from damage, the most effective and efficient control should be provided through host resistance [87, 89]. In the past several years, eight races (race 1–8) of FOV had been indentified worldwide that use both cotton and non-cotton differential hosts [88]. Three FOV races (race 3, 7 and 8) had been found in China; race 7 possesses the highest virulence and is the most widely distributed race [91]. Recently, DNA-based techniques were employed in conjunction with pathogenicity tests to validate these races and to test new isolates, and highly virulent isolates of FOV were identified in Australia [92] and the United States [93-94]. Host resistance to FOV races has been widely evaluated in cotton germplasm under both field nursery and greenhouse conditions, and many highly resistant cotton cultivars and breeding lines have been developed through conventional breeding [89, 95-96]. However, little is known about the mechanism and genetic basis of FOV resistance. Some early classical genetic studies have suggested that the inheritance of FOV resistance in cotton is determined by a single gene [97-99], while other studies have suggested that FOV resistance is controlled by multiple genes [100-102]. Large-scale resistance evaluations in breeding programs are time-consuming and labor-intensive, and it is not easy to obtain the ideal genotype simply through phenotypic selection. The cultivar development process has been slow in the face of the emergence of new, highly virulent FOV isolates [89-90].

To accumulate useful information for understanding the genetic basis of FOV 7 resistance and identify favorable alleles for facilitating future molecular resistance breeding, we performed a marker-trait association mapping to detect QTLs underlying FOV 7 resistance in Upland cotton [72]. The 356-accession panel mentioned above [71] was used for association analysis and favorable allele mining. Meanwhile, a composite cross population (CP) with three parents was developed for linkage mapping. Three Upland cotton cultivars, Xuzhou 142, Yumian 21 and Shang 9901, were chosen as parents according to many years of FOV 7 resistance evaluation. Xuzhou 142, an obsolete cultivar selected from STV 2B in the 1970s with large boll size and high lint percentage that is severely infested by FOV 7, was selected as the susceptible parent. Yumian 21 was released in 1999 and is currently used as a resistant control in national cotton regional trials due to its extremely high resistance to FOV 7. The cultivar Shang 9901 is an anonymous breeding line with high yield potential and moderately high resistance to FOV 7. Thus serial QTLs for FOV 7 resistance were detected by joint population-based association mapping and family-based linkage mapping. Marker–trait association mapping was performed with the MLM model implemented in TASSEL software [82]. A total of 27 markers were significantly associated with FOV 7 resistance at the at the α=0.01 level (-log$P$=2.0), and were localized to 16 chromosomes (Table 7). Of these loci, 23 were detected under field nursery conditions, 10 were detected in the greenhouse and 6 were detected under both conditions. The proportion of phenotypic variation explained by the markers ranged from 1.48% to 12.99%, with an average of 4.21%. If a more stringent threshold by the Bonferroni correction (P≤0.05/145,-log$P$≥3.46) is adopted [83], only 10 associations were significant (Table 7). Five (*qFW-A3-1, qFW-A12-1, qFW-D3-1, qFW-D5-1* and *qFW-D8-1*) of the 7 QTLs identified by linkage mapping could be detected by association mapping at the α=0.05 level, while only 3 QTLs (*qFW-D3-1, qFW-D5-1* and *qFW-D8-1*) could be detected at the α=0.01 level (see reference [72] for details).

The phenotypic effects of each QTL allele of the 27 associated loci were estimated in both the greenhouse and field nursery evaluations according to the method mentioned above [71], and therefore, favorable alleles for FOV 7 resistance were identified (Table 8). The phenotypic effects of the 27 loci in the greenhouse and field nursery averaged-1.31 and-3.45, with ranges of-3.81to-0.01 and-14.88 to-0.20, respectively. Among the favorable alleles, NAU934-2 had the most negative phenotypic effect in the greenhouse assay and was able to decrease FW DI by 3.8, while NAU6966-3 had the most negative phenotypic effect in the field nursery and was able to decrease FW DI by 14.88. A wide variation of the favorable alleles processed in the 356 accessions was observed, with an average of 14.84 and a range of 7 to 21 (see [72] for details). Pearson correlation analysis between the number of favorable alleles and FW DI was carried out, and highly negative significance was found in both the greenhouse (r=-0.344, P<0.001) and

http://dx.doi.org/10.5772/58587

Marker loci	Chr.	Position(cM)	$-Log_{10}P$		$R^2(\%)$	
			Gh	FN	Gh	FN
NAU2437	A01(Chr.01)	15.248	ns	2.19		5.21
NAU4073	A01(Chr.01)	85.025	2.03	ns	1.48	
JESPR304	A02(Chr.02)	22.517	ns	7.09		9.65
NAU934	A05(Chr.05)	19.421	ns	4.61		5.78
NAU3273	A05(Chr.05)	37.244	ns	2.85		2.81
NAU797	A05(Chr.05)	143.032	2.04	ns	3.22	
BNL3255	A08(Chr.08)	81.913	ns	3.20		4.41
STV031	A10(Chr.10)	12.751	2.09	2.82	3.34	4.34
NAU440	A10(Chr.10)	42.017	2.80	2.57	2.81	2.51
Gh369	A11(Chr.11)	84.701	ns	2.29		3.61
BNL1066	A11(Chr.11)	134.486	ns	2.12		3.94
BNL1707	A13(Chr.13)	104.694	2.29	ns	1.59	
NAU1070	D02(Chr.14)	13.885	2.47	5.89	3.10	7.56
CIR246	D02(Chr.14)	112.473	2.55	3.14	3.65	4.56
BNL3590	D03(Chr.17)	39.284	ns	2.77		3.66
BNL834	D03(Chr.17)	81.098	ns	5.07		5.46
NAU6966	D04(Chr.22)	36.51	ns	2.47		4.16
NAU3095	D05(Chr.19)	10.634	4.20	4.04	5.12	4.99
NAU2816	D05(Chr.19)	160.89	ns	2.62		4.20
BNL3594	D06(Chr.25)	7.66	7.87	4.12	12.99	7.92
NAU3911	D07(Chr.16)	28.658	ns	3.52		3.93
NAU6752	D07(Chr.16)	74.671	ns	3.35		3.44
NAU478	D08(Chr.24)	67.677	2.08	ns	3.86	
NAU3207	D08(Chr.24)	90.625	ns	5.21		5.70
NAU1350	D08(Chr.24)	108.529	ns	4.38		4.69
NAU5418	D11(Chr.21)	75.156	ns	3.71		6.98
NAU3084	D12(Chr.26)	0	ns	2.36		2.27

Table 7. SSR loci significantly ($-logP \geq 2.0$) associated with FOV 7 resistance and their explained phenotypic variation in greenhouse and field nursery evaluations. Gh and FN indicate the results evaluated in greenhouse and field nursery, respectively; ns indicates non-significant at α=0.01 level

the field nursery (r=-0.488, P<0.001) evaluations. The top-3 resistant accessions for each favorable allele were listed as representative materials in Table 8.

Favorable alleles	a_g	a_f	Accessions	Representative materials
NAU2437-4	-3.27	-8.49	26	Yumian21,Xingmian2,Shiyuan321
NAU4073-2	-1.46	-0.68	172	Xinluzao24,Xingmian2,Xinluzao28
JESPR304-1	-0.45	-2.69	316	Yumian21,Jimian14,Xinluzao24
NAU934-2	-3.81	-4.68	39	Xinluzao24,Zhongmiansuo3,Xinluzao28
NAU3273-1	-0.13	-0.79	341	Yumian21,Jimian14,Xinluzao24
NAU797-2	-1.51	-1.03	172	Yumian21,Jimian14,Xinluzao24
BNL3255-1	-0.01	-2.33	284	Yumian21,Jimian14,Xinluzao24
STV031-1	-2.09	-4.91	137	Yumian21,Xingmian2,Zhongmiansuo3
NAU440-1	-0.33	-0.60	347	Yumian21,Jimian14,Xinluzao24
Gh369-2	-1.02	-3.33	10	Xinluzao24,Xinluzao28,Emian13
BNL1066-4	-1.96	-4.14	15	Zhongmiansuo27,Jimian20,Emian13
BNL1707-2	-1.93	-4.79	112	Yumian21,Xinluzao24,Xingmian2
NAU1070-1	-1.73	-5.84	199	Jimian14,Xinluzao24,Xingmian2
CIR246-3	-2.77	-8.65	16	Ejing1,Ekangmian3,Zhongmiansuo49
BNL3590-1	-0.06	-1.04	315	Yumian21,Jimian14,Xinluzao24
BNL834-1	-0.24	-1.70	312	Yumian21,Jimian14,Xingmian2
NAU6966-3	-1.89	-14.88	37	Xinluzao24,Xinluzao28,GK44
NAU3095-1	-2.30	-4.55	192	Yumian21,Xinluzao24,Xingmian2
NAU2816-2	-1.70	-3.43	152	Xinluzao24,Jimian14,Zhongmiansuo3
BNL3594-1	-2.58	-5.23	201	Jimian14,Xingmian2,Zhongmiansuo9
NAU3911-1	-0.33	-1.91	282	Yumian21,Jimian14,Xingmian2
NAU6752-1	-0.14	-0.83	341	Yumian21,Jimian14,Xinluzao24
NAU478-1	-0.21	-0.20	239	Yumian21,Jimian14,Xingmian2
NAU3207-1	-0.17	-2.27	301	Yumian21,Xinluzao24,Xingmian2
NAU1350-1	-0.03	-0.62	348	Yumian21,Xinluzao24,Jimian14
NAU5418-1	-2.90	-2.44	47	Yumian21,Jimian14,Yumian20
NAU3084-1	-0.42	-1.13	326	Yumian21,Jimian14,Xinluzao24

Table 8. Favorable QTL alleles, phenotypic effects (a_i) and their representative materials. a_g and a_f indicate phenotypic effects evaluated in greenhouse and field nursery conditions, respectively; Representative materials are the top-3 accessions with low disease index

Wang and Roberts identified a major resistance gene (*Fov1*) against FOV 1 in *G. barbadense* cv. Pima-S7 and indicated that one or more minor genes in Acala NemX could delay wilt symptoms [54]. Ulloa et al. performed QTL mapping in an F_2 (Pima-S7 x Acala NemX) and a

http://dx.doi.org/10.5772/58587

recombinant inbred line (RIL; *G. hirsutum* TM-1 x *G. barbadense* Pima 3-79) population. The authors detected 6 QTLs (Fov1-C06, Fov1-C08, Fov1-C11$_1$, Fov1-C11$_2$, Fov1-C16 and Fov1-C19) conferring FOV 1 resistance in different genetic backgrounds [58]. Lopez-Lavalle et al. used an intraspecific cross between the Upland cotton MCU-5 and Siokra 1-4 to detected QTLs conferring resistance to Australian FOV races and found that MCU-5 resistance is complex, with 3 QTLs identified in F_3 and 8 ones in F_4. The QTLs were localized to chromosomes A6, D4 and D6 [60]. Very recently, Ulloa et al. investigated 3 intraspecific (*G. hirsutum* x *G. hirsutum* L. and *G. barbadense* x *G. barbadense* L.), 5 interspecific (*G. hirsutum* x *G. barbadense*) and one RIL population in 4 greenhouse and 2 field experiments and identified a set of 11 SSR markers across 6 linkage groups/chromosomes (3, 6, 8, 14, 17 and 25) associated with FOV 4 resistance [59]. Integrating information mentioned above with the QTL mapping results for FOV 7 in our study, it suggests that the inheritance of FOV resistance in cotton should be far more complex than has been elucidated to date. Interestingly, the map positions of some QTLs conferring resistance against different FOV races coincided, suggesting that these genes may play the same or similar roles in the process of different host-pathogen and/or environment interactions. While great differences in the resistance of cotton genotypes against FOV races have been demonstrated in many evaluations worldwide, a genotype with a high level of resistance against all FOV races has not been found. Given that FW is the result of interactions among the host, pathogen and environment, many genes must be involved in this process. The accumulation of resistance alleles, even with relatively minor individual effects, will result in higher levels of resistance. The Upland cotton cultivars from China and Africa have shown more resistance to Australian FOV races [90]. Therefore, the favorable alleles and their typical germplasm resources identified in this study should have great potential for developing highly resistant Upland cotton cultivars in future molecular breeding programs.

5. Discussion and future prospects

Compared to family-based linkage mapping, population-based association mapping offers several advantages such as: (1) the saving of time and money by using existing populations instead of creating cross-controlled populations, (2) analysis of more than two alleles per locus on average, and (3) high expected resolution owing to a short extent of linkage disequilibrium [103]. All these make association mapping an increasingly important tool for complex trait dissection [63, 104].

A suitable association mapping panel should embrace as much phenotypic and genotypic diversity as possible. For example, because the 99-accession panel [73] comprised higher diversity in fiber properties than the 356-accession panel [71] and 81-accession panel [69], both the number of significant associations detected and the proportion of phenotypic variation explained by markers were improved. However, the presence of high diversity from different genetic origins may induce LD between unlinked loci, and consequently result in spurious marker-trait associations [105]. Although several statistical strategies have been developed to account for issues related to population structure and relatedness in order to decrease false positive [106-107], whether these approaches will induce new false negative remain unclear.

Synthetic association populations, such as the multi-parent advanced generation inter-cross (MAGIC) population [108] and the nested association mapping (NAM) population in maize [109], had been used for genome-wide association studies (GWAS); with which both high resolution and better population structure control can be achieved [110-111]. It is certain that such populations had been or are being developed in Upland cotton. Two artificially controlled multiple parent random-mating populations with each comprising more than 800 lines had been developed in our library, which should provide another theoretically ideal panel for association mapping.

The other inherent constraint limiting the successful use of association mapping is rare alleles exiting in natural populations. Given that the number of individuals with a specific genotype is quite small, the effect of rare alleles on mapping can go far beyond the effect of small population sizes [112]. Large population size had been considered as an important factor to improve the QTL detection power in association mapping studies [3, 112]. Many more marker-trait associations for fiber yield were detected in our 356-accession panel [71] than in the 81-accession panel [69] between the same markers and target traits at the same significance level. While family–based linkage mapping can make use of alleles that occur at low frequencies in natural populations by designing crosses to create artificial populations with inflated frequencies of those alleles. So specifically designed mapping populations such as recombinant inbred lines (RIL) and near isogenic lines (NIL) will remain important. Furthermore, joint linkage and association mapping was recommended as an alternative approach to overcome some of the inherent limitations of both linkage and association mapping [105, 112], and this approach has proven to be a powerful tool to detecting architecture of complex traits [72, 113-118].

Recently, two preliminary maps of the whole-genome scaffolds of *G. raimondii* (the putative diploid donor for tetraploid species) were separately released by two different groups [119-120], which will facilitate the tetraploid genome sequencing and assembly. Real genome-wide association mapping will be realized in the near future through resequencing or other high-throughput genotyping technologies [121], which will dramatically accelerate genetic diversity exploitation and favorable allele mining in Upland cotton germplasm resources.

Acknowledgements

We thank all faculties and graduate students in Cotton Research Institute, Nanjing Agricultural University and the other members of the cotton genomics and breeding communities for their contributions, and apologize for not citing many enlightening papers owing to space limitations. This study was supported by grants from 973 (2011CB109300), 863, Jiangsu Province Key Project (BE2012329), and the Priority Academic Program Development of Jiangsu Higher Education Institutions.

Author details

Hongxian Mei[1], Xiefei Zhu[2], Wangzhen Guo[1], Caiping Cai[1] and Tianzhen Zhang[1*]

*Address all correspondence to: cotton@njau.edu.cn

1 National Key Laboratory of Crop Genetics & Germplasm Enhancement, PR China

2 Cotton Research Institute, Nanjing Agricultural University, Nanjing, PR China

References

[1] National Cotton Council, USA. http://www.cotton.org (accessed 10 October 2013).

[2] Zhang HB, Li YN, Wang BH, Chee PW. Recent advances in cotton genomics. Int J Plant Genomics 2008; ID 742304. doi: 10.1155/2008/742304.

[3] Mackay TFC, Stone EA, Ayroles JF. The genetics of quantitative traits: challenges and prospects. Nat Rev Genet 2009; 10: 565–577.

[4] Xu Y, Crouch J. Marker-assisted selection in plant breeding: from publications to practice. Crop Sci 2008; 48: 391–407.

[5] Jannink JL, Lorenz AJ, Iwata H. Genomic selection in plant breeding: from theory to practice. Brief Funct Genomics 2010; 9: 166–177.

[6] Jiang CX, Writght RJ, EL-Zik KM, et al. Polyploid formation created unique avenues for response to selection in *Gossypium* (cotton). Proc Natl Acad Sci USA 1998; 95: 4419–4424.

[7] Ulloa M, Meredith WR. Genetic linkage map and QTL analysis of agronomic and fiber quality traits in an intraspecific population. J Cotton Sci 2000; 4: 161–170.

[8] Ulloa M, Saha S, Jenkin N, et al. Chromosomal assignment of RFLP linkage groups harboring important QTL on an intraspecific cotton (*Gossypium hirsutum* L.) joinmap. J Hered 2005; 96: 132–144.

[9] Kohel RJ, Yu J, Park YH, et al. Molecular mapping and characterization of traits controlling fiber quality in cotton. Euphytica 2001; 121: 163–172.

[10] Saranga Y, Menz M, Jiang CX, et al. Genomic dissection of genotype x environment interactions conferring adaptation of cotton to arid conditions. Genome Res 2001; 11: 1988–1995.

[11] Ren LH, Guo WZ, Zhang TZ. Identification of quantitative trait loci (QTLs) affecting yield and fiber properties in chromosome 16 in cotton using substitution line. Acta Botanica Sinica 2002; 44: 815–820.

[12] Paterson AH, Saranga Y, Menz M, et al. QTL analysis of genotype x environment interaction affecting cotton fiber quality. Theor Appl Genet 2003; 6: 384–396.

[13] Zhang T, Yuan Y, Yu J, et al. Molecular tagging of a major QTL for fiber strength in Upland cotton and its marker-assisted selection. Theor Appl Genet 2003; 106: 262–268.

[14] Wu MQ, Zhang XL, Nie YC, et al. Localization of QTLs for yield and fiber quality traits of tetraploid cotton cultivar. Acta Genetica Sinica 2003; 30: 443–452.

[15] Mei M, Syed NH, Gao W, et al. Genetic mapping and QTL analysis of fiber related traits in cotton (*Gossypium*). Theor Appl Genet 2004; 108: 280–291.

[16] Lacape JM, Nguyen TB, Courtois B, et al. QTL analysis of cotton fiber quality using multiple *Gossypium hirsutum* x *Gossypium barbadense* backcross generations. Crop Sci 2005; 45: 123–140.

[17] Shen X, Guo W, Zhu X, et al. Molecular mapping of QTLs for fiber qualities in three diverse lines in Upland cotton using SSR markers. Mol Breed 2005; 15: 169–181.

[18] Shen X, Zhang T, Guo W, et al. Mapping fiber and yield QTLs with main, epistatic, and QTL x Environment interaction effects in recombinant inbred lines of Upland cotton. Crop Sci 2006; 46: 61–66.

[19] Shen X, Guo W, Lu Q, et al. Genetic mapping of quantitative trait loci for fiber quality and yield trait by RIL approach in Upland cotton. Euphytica 2007; 155: 371–380

[20] Chee P, Draye X, Jiang CX, et al. Molecular dissection of interspecific variation between *Gossypium hirsutum* and *Gossypium barbadense* (cotton) by a backcross-self approach: I. Fiber elongation. Theor Appl Genet 2005; 111: 757–763.

[21] Chee P, Draye X, Jiang CX, et al. Molecular dissection of phenotypic variation between *Gossypium hirsutum* and *Gossypium barbadense* (cotton) by a backcross-self approach: III. Fiber length. Theor Appl Genet 2005; 111: 772–781.

[22] Park YH, Alabady MS, Sickler B, et al. Genetic mapping of new cotton fiber loci using EST-derived microsatellites in an interspecific recombinant inbred line (RIL) cotton population. Mol Genet Genom 2005; 274: 428–441.

[23] Lin ZX, He DH, Zhang XL, et al. Linkage map construction and mapping QTL for cotton fibre quality using SRAP, SSR and RAPD. Plant Breed 2005; 124: 180–187.

[24] Zhang ZS, Xiao Y, Luo M, et al. Construction of a genetic linkage map and QTL analysis of fiber-related traits in upland cotton (*Gossypium hirsutum* L.). Euphytica 2005; 144: 91–99.

[25] Zhang ZS, Hu MC, Zhang J, et al. Construction of a comprehensive PCR-based marker linkage map and QTL mapping for fiber quality traits in upland cotton (*Gossypium hirsutum* L.). Mol Breed 2009; 24: 49–61.

[26] Draye X, Chee P, Jiang CX, et al. Molecular dissection of interspecific variation between *Gossypium hirsutum* and *G. barbadense* (cotton) by a backcross-self approach: II. Fiber fineness. Theor Appl Genet 2005; 111: 764–771.

[27] Saha S, Jenkins JN, Wu J, et al. Effects of chromosome specific introgression in upland cotton on fiber and agronomic traits. Genetics 2006; 172: 1927–1938.

[28] Wang B, Guo W, Zhu X, et al. QTL mapping of fiber quality in an elite hybrid derived-RIL population of upland cotton. Euphytica 2006; 152: 367–378.

[29] Frelichowski JE, Palmer M, Main D, et al. Genetic mapping of microsatellites derived from BAC-end sequences of *Gossypium hirsutum* Acala 'Maxxa' BAC-ends. Mol Genet Genom 2006; 275: 479–491.

[30] He DH, Lin ZX, Zhang XL, et al. QTL mapping for economic traits based on a dense genetic map of cotton with PCR-based markers using the interspecific cross of *Gossypium hirsutum* x *Gossypium barbadense*. Euphytica 2007; 153: 181–197.

[31] Qin H, Guo W, Zhang Y, et al. QTL mapping of yield and fiber traits based on a four-way cross population in *Gossypium hirsutum* L. Theor Appl Genet 2008; 117: 883–894.

[32] Wu JX, Gutierrez OA, Jenkins JN, et al. Quantitative analysis and QTL mapping for agronomic and fiber traits in an RI population of upland cotton. Euphytica 2009; 165: 231–245.

[33] Chen H, Qian N, Guo W, et al. Using three overlapped RILs to dissect genetically clustered QTL for fiber strength on Chro.D8 in Upland cotton. Theor Appl Genet 2009; 119: 605–12.

[34] Luan M, Guo X, Zhang Y, et al. QTL mapping for agronomic and fiber traits using two interspecific chromosome substitution lines of Upland cotton. Plant Breed 2009; 128: 671–679.

[35] Qin YS, Ye WX, Liu RZ, et al. QTL mapping for fiber quality properties in upland cotton (*Gossypium hirsutum* L.). Sci Agric Sin 2009; 42: 4145–4154.

[36] An CF, Jenkins JN, Wu JX, et al. Use of fiber and fuzz mutants to detect QTL for yield components, seed, and fiber traits of upland cotton. Euphytica 2010; 172: 21–34.

[37] Wang FR, Gong YC, Zhang CY, et al. Genetic effects of introgression genomic components from sea island cotton (*Gossypium barbadense* L.) on fiber related traits in upland cotton (*G. hirsutum* L.). Euphytica 2011; 181: 41–53.

[38] Sun FD, Zhang JH, Wang SF, et al. QTL mapping for fiber quality traits across multiple generations and environments in upland cotton. Mol Breed 2012; 30: 569–582.

[39] Zhang K, Zhang J, Ma J, et al. Genetic mapping and quantitative trait locus analysis of fiber quality traits using a three-parent composite population in upland cotton (*Gossypium hirsutum* L.). Mol Breed 2012; 29: 335–348

[40] Ning Z, Chen H, Mei H, et al. Molecular tagging of QTLs for fiber quality and yield in the upland cotton cultivar Acala-Prema. Euphytica 2014; 195: 143–156.

[41] He DH, Lin ZX, Zhang XL, et al. Mapping QTLs of traits contributing to yield and analysis of genetic effects in tetraploid cotton. Euphytica 2005; 144: 141–149.

[42] Wang B, Guo W, Zhu X, et al. QTL mapping of yield and yield components for elite hybrid derived-RILs in upland cotton. J Genet Genomics 2007; 34: 35–45.

[43] Qin YS, Liu RZ, Mei HX, et al. QTL Mapping for yield traits in Upland cotton (*Gossypium hirsutum* L.). Acta Agronomica Sinica 2009; 35: 1812–1821.

[44] Chen H, Qian N, Guo WZ, et al. Using three selected overlapping RILs to fine-map the yield component QTL on Chro.D8 in Upland cotton. Euphytica 2010; 176: 321–329.

[45] Liu R, Wang B, Guo W, et al. Quantitative trait loci mapping for yield and its components by using two immortalized populations of a heterotic hybrid in *Gossypium hirsutum* L. Mol Breed 2012; 29: 297–311.

[46] Shen X, Becelaere GV, Kumar P, et al. QTL mapping for resistance to root-knot nematodes in the M-120 RNR Upland cotton line (*Gossypium hirsutum* L.) of the Auburn 623 RNR source. Theor Appl Genet 2006; 113: 1539–1549.

[47] Wang C, Ulloa M, Roberts PA. Identification and mapping of microsatellite markers linked to a root-knot nematode resistance gene (*rkn1*) in Acala NemX cotton (*Gossypium hirsutum* L.). Theor Appl Genet 2006; 112: 770–777.

[48] Ynturi P, Jenkins JN, McCarty Jr JC, et al. Association of root-knot nematode resistance genes with simple sequence repeat markers on two chromosomes in cotton. Crop Sci 2006; 46: 2670–2674.

[49] Romano GB, Sacks EJ, Stetina SR, et al. Identification and genomic location of a reniform nematode (*Rotylenchulus reniformis*) resistance locus (Renari) introgressed from *Gossypium aridum* into upland cotton (*G. hirsutum*).Theor Appl Genet 2009; 120: 139–150.

[50] Bolek Y, El-Zik Km, Pepper AE, et al. Mapping of Verticillium wilt resistance genes in cotton. Plant Sci 2005; 168: 1581–1590.

[51] Wang HM, Lin ZX, Zhang XL, et al. Mapping and quantitative trait loci analysis of verticillium wilt resistance genes in cotton. J Integr Plant Biol 2008; 50: 174–182.

[52] Jiang F, Zhao J, Zhou L, et al. Molecular mapping of Verticillium wilt resistance QTL clustered on chromosomes D7 and D9 in upland cotton. Sci China C Life Sci 2009; 52: 872–884.

[53] Ning Z, Zhao R, Chen H, et al. Molecular tagging of a major quantitative trait locus for broad-spectrum resistance to Verticillium wilt in upland cotton cultivar Prema. Crop Sci 2013; 53: 1–9.

[54] Wang C, Roberts PA. A Fusarium wilt resistance gene in *Gossypium barbadense* and its effect on root-knot nematode-wilt disease complex. Phytopathology 2006; 96: 727–734.

[55] Chen X, Ge F, Wang D, et al. Mapping of QTLs conferring resistance to Fusarium wilt in cotton. Molecular Plant Breeding 2008; 6: 1127–1133.

[56] Wang P, Su L, Qin L, et al. Identification and molecular mapping of a Fusarium wilt resistant gene in upland cotton. Theor Appl Genet 2009; 119: 733–739.

[57] Wang P, Shi L, Su L, et al. Quantitative trait loci for resistance against Fusarium wilt based on three cotton F_2 populations. Agricultural Sciences in China 2010; 9: 1799–1806.

[58] Ulloa M, Wang C, Hutmacher RB, et al. Mapping Fusarium wilt race 1 resistance genes in cotton by inheritance, QTL and sequencing composition. Mol Genet Genomics 2011; 286: 21–36.

[59] Ulloa M, Hutmacher RB, Roberts PA, et al. Inheritance and QTL mapping of Fusarium wilt race 4 resistance in cotton. Theor Appl Genet 2013; 126: 1405–1418.

[60] Lopez-Lavalle LAB, Gillespie VJ, Tate WA, et al. Molecular mapping of a new source of Fusarium wilt resistance in tetraploid cotton (*Gossypium hirsutum* L.). Mol Breed 2012; 30: 1181–1191.

[61] Rong J, Feltus FA, Waghmare VN, et al. Meta-analysis of polyploid cotton QTL shows unequal contributions of subgenomes to a complex network of genes and gene clusters implicated in lint fiber development. Genetics 2007; 176: 2577–2588.

[62] Lacape JM, Llewellyn D, Jacobs J, et al. (2010) Meta-analysis of cotton fiber quality QTLs across diverse environments in a *Gossypium hirsutum* x *G. barbadense* RIL population. BMC Plant Biol 2010; 10: 132.

[63] Zhu C, Gore M, Buckler ES, et al. Status and prospects of association mapping in plants. Plant Genome 2008; 1: 5–20.

[64] Kantartzi SK, Stewart JMcD. Association analysis of fibre traits in *Gossypium arboreum* accessions. Plant Breed 2008; 127: 173–179.

[65] Abdurakhmonov IY, Kohel RJ, Yu JZ, et al. Molecular diversity and association mapping of fiber quality traits in exotic *G. hirsutum* L. germplasm. Genomics 2008; 92: 478–487.

[66] Abdurakhmonov IY, Saha S, Jenkins JN, et al. Linkage disequilibrium based association mapping of fiber quality traits in *G. hirsutum* L. variety germplasm. Genetica 2009; 136: 401–417.

[67] Zeng L, Meredith Jr WR, Gutierrez OA, et al. Identification of associations between SSR markers and fibre traits in an exotic germplasm derived from multiple cross among *Gossypium* tetraploid species. Theor Appl Genet 2009; 119: 93–103.

[68] Rakshit A, Rakshit S, Singh J, et al. Association of AFLP and SSR markers with agronomic and fibre quality traits in *Gossypium hirsutum* L. J Genetics 2010; 89: 155–162.

[69] Zhang T, Qian N, Zhu X, et al. Variations and transmission of QTL alleles for yield and fiber qualities in Upland cotton cultivars developed in China. PLoS ONE 2013; 8: e57220.

[70] Wang XQ, Yu Y, Li W, et al. Association analysis of yield and fiber quality traits in *Gossypium barbadense* with SSRs and SRAPs. Genet Mol Res 2013; 12: 3353–3362.

[71] Mei H, Zhu X, Zhang T. Favorable QTL alleles for Yield and Its Components Identified by Association Mapping in Chinese Upland Cotton Cultivars. PLOS ONE 2013; 8: e82193.

[72] Mei H, Ai N, Zhang X, et al. QTLs conferring FOV 7 resistance detected by linkage and association mapping in Upland cotton. Euphytica 2014; Doi 10.1007/s10681-014-1063-y.

[73] Cai C, Ye W, Zhang T, et al. Association analysis of fiber quality traits and exploration of elite alleles in Upland cotton cultivars/accessions (*Gossypium hirsutum* L.). J Integr Plant Biol 2014; 56: 51–62.

[74] Breseghello F, Sorrells ME. Association mapping of kernel size and milling quality in wheat (*Triticum aestivum* L.) cultivars. Genetics 2006; 172: 1165–1177.

[75] Jia L, Yan W, Zhu C, et al. Allelic analysis of sheath blight resistance with association mapping in rice. PLoS ONE 2012; 7: e32703.

[76] Huang ZK., editor. The Cultivars and Their Pedigree of Cotton in China. China Agriculture Press, Beijing; 2007.

[77] Du X, Sun J, Zhou Z, et al. Current situation and the future in collection, preservation, evaluation and utilization of cotton germplasm in China. J Plant Genetic Resources 2012; 13: 163–168.

[78] Guo W, Cai C, Wang C, et al. A microsatellite-based, gene-rich linkage map reveals genome structure, function and evolution in Gossypium. Genetics 2007; 176: 527–541.

[79] Pritchard JK, Stephens M, Donnelly P. Inference of population structure using multilocus genotype data. Genetics 2000; 155: 945–959.

[80] Evanno G, Regnaut S, Goudet J. Detecting the number of clusters of individuals using the software STRUCTURE: a simulation study. Mol Ecol 2005; 14: 2611–2620.

[81] Hardy O, Vekemans X. SPAGeDi: a versatile computer program to analyse spatial genetic structure at the individual or population levels. Mol Ecol Notes 2002; 2: 618–620.

[82] Bradbury PJ, Zhang Z, Kroon DE, et al. TASSEL: software for association mapping of complex traits in diverse samples. Bioinformatics 2007; 23: 2633–2635.

[83] Lander ES, Botstein D. Mapping mendelian factors underlying quantitative traits using RFLP linkage maps. Genetics 1989; 121: 185–199.

[84] Wang Y, Yang W, Xu H, et al. The main problems and recommendations in Chinese cotton production. Chin Agr Sci Bull 2009; 25: 86–90.

[85] Qian S, Huang J, Peng Y, et al. Studies on the hybrid of *G. hirsutum* L. and *G. anomalum* Wawr. & Peyr. and application in breeding. Sci Agric Sin 1992; 25: 44–51.

[86] Zhou B, Zhu X, Guo W, et al. Major gene plus poly-gene inheritance of super quality fiber properties in upland cotton introgressed from *Gossypium anomalum* Wawra & Peyritsch. Cotton Sci 2006; 18: 60–62.

[87] Ma C., editor. Researches on Fusarium and Verticillium wilt in cotton. China Agriculture Press, Beijing; 2007.

[88] Davis RM, Colyer PD, Rothrock CS, et al. Fusarium wilt of cotton: population diversity and implications for management. Plant Dis 2006; 90: 692–703.

[89] Ulloa M, Hutmacher RB, Davis RM, et al. Breeding for Fusarium wilt race 4 resistance in cotton under field and greenhouse conditions. J Cotton Sci 2006; 10: 114–127.

[90] Constable GA, Reid PE, Stiller WN. Breeding for resistance to a new strain of Fusarium wilt in Australia. In: Stephens M. (eds.) Proceedings of the World Cotton Research Conference-4, Sept 10-14, Lubbock TX; 2007.

[91] Chen Q, Ji X, Sun W. Identification of cotton-wilt *Fusarium* races in China. Scientia Agricultura Sinica 1985; 6: 1–6.

[92] Wang B, Brubaker CL, Burdon JJ. Fusarium species and Fusarium wilt pathogens associated with native *Gossypium* populations in Australia. Mycol Res 2004; 108: 35–44.

[93] Kim Y, Hutmacher RB, Davis RM. Characterization of California isolates of *Fusarium oxysporum* f. sp. *vasinfectum*. Plant Dis 2005; 89: 366–372.

[94] Holmes EA, Bennett RS, Spurgeon DW, et al. New genotypes of *Fusarium oxysporum* f. sp. *vasinfectum* from the Southeastern United States. Plant Dis 2009; 93: 1298–1304.

[95] Ma C, Jian G, Zheng C. The advances in cotton breeding resistance to Fusarium and Verticillium wilts in China during past fifty years. Scientia Agricultura Sinica 2002; 35: 508–513.

[96] Ulloa M, Percy R, Zhang J, et al. Registration of four Pima cotton germplasm lines having good levels of Fusarium wilt race 4 resistance with moderate yields and good fibers. J Plant Registr 2009; 3: 198–202.

[97] Smith AL, Dick JB. Inheritance of resistance to Fusarium wilt in upland cotton and sea island cotton as complicated by nematodes under field conditions. Phytopathology 1960; 50: 44–48.

[98] Netzer D, Tal Y, Marani A, et al. Resistance of interspecific cotton hybrids (*Gossypium hirsutum* x *Gossypium barbadense* containing *Gossypium harknessii* cytoplasm) to fusarium wilt. Plant Dis 1985; 69: 312–313.

[99] Feng C, Zhang J, Liu J, et al. Inheritance of resistance to Fusarium wilt in several Chinese upland cotton varieties. Acta Agronomica Sinica 1996; 22: 550–554.

[100] Kappelman AJ. Inheritance of resistance to Fusarium wilt in cotton. Crop Sci 1971; 11: 672–674.

[101] Jiao B. Primary research of general combining ability and heritability of resistance to Fusarium wilt and Verticillium wilt in upland cotton. Acta Agronomica Sinica 1985; 11, 267–273.

[102] Wang Z, Ma Z, Qu J. Analysis of gene effect of resistance to Fusarium and Verticillum wilt in upland cotton. Journal of Heibei Agriculture University 1989; 12: 21–25.

[103] Flint-Garcia SA, Thuillet AC, Yu J, et al. Maize association population: a high-resolution platform for quantitative trait locus dissection. Plant J 2005; 44: 1054–1064.

[104] Abdurakhmonov IY, Abdukarimov A. Application of association mapping to understanding the genetic diversity of plant germplasm resources. Int J Plant Genomics 2008; ID 574927. doi:10.1155/2008/574927.

[105] Gupta PK, Rustgi S, Kulwal PL. Linkage disequilibrium and association studies in higher plants: present status and future prospects. Plant Mol Biol 2005; 57: 461–485.

[106] Price A, Patterson N, Plenge R, et al. Principal components analysis corrects for stratification in genome-wide association studies. Nat Genet 2006; 38: 904–909.

[107] Yu J, Pressoir G, Briggs WH, et al. A unified mixed-model method for association mapping that accounts for multiple levels of relatedness. Nat Genet 2006; 38: 203–208.

[108] Cavanagh C, Morell M, Mackay I, et al. From mutations to MAGIC: resource for gene discovery, validation and delivery in crop plants. Cur Opin Plant Bio 2008; 11: 215–221.

[109] Yu J, Holland JB, McMullen MD, et al. Genetic design and statistical power of nested association mapping in maize. Genetics 2008; 178: 539–551.

[110] Buckler ES, Holland JB, Bradbury PJ, et al. The genetic architecture of maize flowering time. Science 2009; 325: 714–718.

[111] Kover PX, Valdar W, Trakalo J, et al. A multiparent advanced generation inter-cross to fine-map quantitative traits in Arabidopsis thaliana. PLoS Genetics 2009; 5: e1000551.

[112] Myles S, Peiffer J, Brown PJ, et al. Association mapping: critical consideration shift from genotype to experimental design. Plant Cell 2009; 21: 2194–2202.

[113] Nemri A, Atwell S, Tarone AM, et al. Genome-wide survey of Arabidopsis natural variation in downy mildew resistance using combined association and linkage mapping. Proc Natl Acad Sci USA 2010; 107: 10302–10307.

[114] Lu Y, Zhang S, Shah T, et al. Joint linkage-linkage disequilibrium mapping is a powerful approach to detecting quantitative trait loci underlying drought tolerance in maize. Proc Natl Acad Sci USA 2010; 107: 19585–19590.

[115] Brachi B, Faure N, Horton M, et al. Linkage and association mapping of *Arabidopsis thaliana* flowering time in nature. PLoS Genet 2010; 6: e1000940.

[116] Pagny G, Paulstephenraj PS, Poque S, et al. Family-based linkage and association mapping reveals novel genes affecting *Plum pox virus* infection in Arabidopsis thaliana. New Phytologist 2012; 196: 873–886.

[117] Korir PC, Zhang J, Wu K, et al. (2013) Association mapping combined with linkage analysis for aluminum tolerance among soybean cultivars released in Yellow and Changjiang River Valleys in China. Theor Appl Genet 2013; doi 10.1007/s00122-013-2082-0.

[118] Cadic E, Coque M, Vear F, et al. Combined linkage and association mapping of flowering time in Sunflower (*Helianthus annuus* L.). Theor Appl Genet 2013; doi 10.1007/s00122-013-2056-2.

[119] Paterson AH, Wendel JF, Gundlach H, et al. Repeated polyploidization of Gossypium genomes and the evolution of spinnable cotton fibres. Nature 2012; 492: 423–427.

[120] Wang K, Wang Z, Li F, et al. The draft genome of a diploid cotton *Gossypium raimondii*. Nat Genet 2012; 44: 1098–1103.

[121] Davey JW, Hohenlohe PA, Etter PD, et al. Genome-wide genetic marker discovery and genotyping using next-generation sequencing. Nat Rev Genet 2011; 12: 499–510.

Chapter 4

Cotton Germplasm in India — New Trends

S.S. Narayanan, Parchuri Vidyasagar and
K. Srinivasu Babu

Additional information is available at the end of the chapter

http://dx.doi.org/10.5772/58622

1. Introduction

Cotton has played a great role in the global and Indian economies since immemorial time. The antiquity of cotton in the Indian subcontinent has been traced to the 4th millennium BC. The fabrics dated approximately 3000 BC, recovered from the Mohenjo-Daro excavations in Sind (Pakistan), were identified to have originated from cotton plants. The close relatedness of those old fabrics to the *Gossypium arboreum* species was reported by Sundaram and his colleagues [1, 2]. The lint-bearing species of the genus *Gossypium* L. are four, out of which the diploid (2n=26) species *Gossypium arboreum* L. and *G. herbaceum* L. are indigenous in Asia and Africa. The history of introduction of the New World cottons (allo-tetraploid species of *G. hirsutum* L. and *G. barbadense* L. with 2n=52) into India dates back to the 18th century AD [3-5]. By the last decade of the 20th century, India had gained a leading position in the global cotton statistics with the largest cropped area of 8.9 million ha in 1996-97, growing the most diverse cultivars in terms of botanical species and composition, producing the widest range of cotton fiber quality suitable for spinning 6's to 120's counts yarn, and supporting the largest agro-based national industry of the country [2, 6].

Cotton is grown globally on an average in about 33-35 million hectares annually representing less than 2.5% of the world's arable land [7], under a great diversity of agro-climatic conditions and widely varied farming practices. Cotton is reported to be grown in more than 100 countries being an important cash crop for the farmers and having great influence on the economy of such countries [4]. More than 120 million family units are engaged directly in cotton production in the world and about 350 million people are estimated to work in the wider cotton industry each year [8]. The most prominent cotton growing countries include Peoples Republic of China, India, USA, Pakistan, Uzbekistan, Tajikistan, Mexico, Brazil, Turkey, Egypt, Sudan, Australia, some African states, Israel, etc., [9].

There are four cultivated species of *Gossypium* Linn., grown for their fibre and also the seed and its by-products. In the world, *G. hirsutum* cotton is predominant with 92-93% area and production, *G. barbadense* is grown for nearly 4-5% and the diploid cottons *G. arboreum* and *G. herbaceum* accounted for less than 2 per cent [4, 10].

The spinnable fibre (lint) is the primary product for growing cotton for textile use. For each kilogram of lint produced, it also results in output of 1.4 to 1.6 kilograms of cottonseed. The estimated recent annual production of cotton fibre in the world is around 25 to 26 million metric tons of lint roughly valued at US$ 40-42 billion [7]. Cotton is the most important natural fibre used in spinning to produce apparel, home furnishings and industrial products and represents about 35-40% of all fibres used in textiles.

As much as 50-55 million tons of cottonseed is produced worldwide annually in recent times valued at US$ 7-8billion [10]. Cotton has become an important oilseed in the world and can be fed as whole seed to dairy cattle (Ruminant animals) or crushed in oil mills to obtain oil, hulls, meal and linters. The oil is used for human consumption after special refining processes to remove the toxic gossypol. The hulls and meals are good sources of vegetable protein for animal and the linters are used as a chemical cellulose source for manufacturing various personal care products and in high quality paper (used for currency printing in USA and EU) [11]. All these add value to cottonseed at each type of product and processing. Cotton has a significant role in meeting essential needs of clothing, besides food and feed and with a projected 9 billion human population and increase in animal production and the global textile fibre requirements projected at 180 million metric tons, the share of cotton should be increased to 40-50 million metric tons by 2050 [8]. Cotton area in India has increased significantly after the transgenic cotton was introduced in 2002-03 and over 90 per cent of the cotton grown is represented by *Gossypium hirsutum* as *G. hirsutum* x *G. hirsutum* hybrids with Bollgard-II (BG-II) type (Cry1Ac+Cry2Ab) and a small percentage as Bollgard-I (BG-I) with Cry1Ac gene. All the cotton hybrids sold in India are proprietary hybrids of different seed companies with varied parents that are not disclosed due to the proprietary nature of the hybrids and hence it is not possible to know the parents / germplasm used.

In this chapter, the information pertaining to germplasm history, contents and location of germplasm resource, funding sources, sharing within India, characterization, evaluation and utilization of germplasm, data bases, novel trends and perspectives and conclusions have been presented.

2. History of cotton germplasm in India

In India, the collection and conservation of plant genetic resources (PGR) of crop species for utilization in crop improvement programmes were initiated with the establishment of the Imperial Agricultural Research Institute in 1905 at Pusa village, Darbhanga District, Bengal (now in Bihar) state. This institute was shifted to New Delhi in 1936 and later in 1947, was renamed the Indian Agricultural Research Institute (IARI). The early conservation efforts of PGR involved frequent multiplication and storage of seeds of crops by the breeders in the

http://dx.doi.org/10.5772/58622

Botany Division of the Institute [12]. To strengthen these efforts, a unit was set up for the assembly of global germplasm in the division in 1941, which was upgraded as the Division of Plant introduction in 1961. The Plant Introduction Division of IARI provided the necessary impetus and leadership at the national level, particularly for the assembly of PGR through introduction from different parts of the world and their subsequent conservation. The establishment of crop(s) based research institutes further extended and strengthened these efforts. The Central Rice Research Institute, Cuttack was established in 1946. Isolated efforts were also being made by the researchers in the State Department of Agriculture, which got a boost with the establishment of the State Agricultural Universities (SAUs). Govind Ballabh Pant University of Agriculture and Technology, the first SAU, came into being in 1960 [13].

Crop improvement research, including PGR management was greatly strengthened and focused with the establishment of multidisciplinary, multicenter "All India Co-ordinated Crop Improvement Projects" starting with that for maize germplasm set up in 1957. The project had coordinated research centres mostly in SAUs and Indian Council of Agricultural Research (ICAR) institutes located in important crop growing areas. Presently, there are 40 multi-crop or single crop-based institutes, project directorates and national research centres, 37 coordinated projects and 31 SAUs. The All India Coordinated Cotton Improvement Project (AICCIP) was established in 1967 with headquarters at Coimbatore, while the Central Institute for Cotton Research (CICR) with headquarters at Nagpur was established in 1976 simultaneously with the CICR Regional Station for South zone at Coimbatore (including AICCIP headquarters), while the CICR Regional Station for the north zone at Sirsa (Haryana State) came into existence by annexing the IARI Regional Station at Sirsa in 1984. The germplasm accessions available at all the cotton breeding stations of the state agricultural university centres all over the country were collected by forming a national germplasm advisory committee at CICR and the collections were also augmented by exchange from other countries, by germplasm surveys and by accessing the elite breeding material available from time to time at various SAU cotton breeding stations. By periodical evaluation, duplicate germplasm accessions were eliminated by growing in the fields of the CICR and its regional stations. The germplasm purification was followed by characterization for 76 characters as per Germplasm Index Card, catalogued, data computerized and seeds conserved in medium term and short term cold storage at CICR and long term storage at the NBPGR New Delhi by depositing selfed (self-fertilized) seeds. Working collections were constituted in all the four cultivated species germplasm and made available to Indian institutions for breeders' use in crop improvement. Thus CICR functioned as "The National Gene Bank of Cotton for India".

These projects, ICAR institutes and SAUs maintained and conserved working collections of germplasm of different crops through frequent seed regeneration and storage under ambient conditions. For example, the Central Rice Research Institute, Cuttack and Indira Gandhi Agricultural University, Raipur conserved rice genetic resources; the "All India Co-ordinated Maize Improvement Project" and the "All India Co-ordinated Wheat Improvement Project", with the headquarters at IARI, maintained maize and wheat germplasm, respectively. The centres of coordinated projects supported these efforts across the country.

At the national level, the ICAR is responsible for research, initial transfer of technology in agriculture and policies related thereto (including PGR management). The ICAR upgraded the Plant Introduction Division, IARI in 1976 to the status of an institute, the National Bureau of Plant Introduction and later, in 1977, renamed it as the National Bureau of Plant Genetic Resources (NBPGR). The NBPGR has the mandate to manage PGR including collection, introduction, exchange, quarantine, evaluation, conservation and use. Thus, NBPGR, under the umbrella of ICAR, functions as the nodal agency for PGR management and closely collaborates with ICAR institutes and SAUs for PGR management, particularly evaluation, characterization and utilization [13].

2.1. Changing species composition

In India, cotton is grown under widely varying agro-climatic conditions represented by regions falling 8°-32°N latitude, 70°-80° E longitude, elevation range of 0-950 meters and annual rainfall range of 250-1500 mm. Cotton has been cultivated since time immemorial in India. Cotton growing, types of cotton grown and cotton textiles produced in Indian subcontinent have earned global fame for over 5000 years. Until the 17th century, India was growing only the diploid (2n=26) cultivated cottons (also referred to as *Desi* cottons) *Gossypium arboreum* L. and *G. herbaceum* L. and the area under these cottons was as much as 95% of the total area of 4.4 million hectares of cotton at the time of partition of India in 1947. Although attempts were made from about 1750s to introduce the allo-tetraploid (2n=52) species of *G. hirsutum* L. (American Upland cotton) and *G. barbadense* L. (Egyptian, Pima and Sea Island cottons), the area under the Upland cottons reached only about 2-3 per cent by 1947-48 in the country. Gradual breeding and extension efforts resulted in increase in area under the Upland cotton replacing the *desi* (diploid cultivated) cottons on a large scale by 1970s and after the introduction of Bt-transgenic cottons of *G. hirsutum* x *G. hirsutum* hybrids in 2002-03, the species composition in India changed drastically. Egyptian cotton *G. barbadense* cultivars suitable for Indian ecologies especially in South India were released in 1968-70s, but the area coverage was small [10].

From cultivation of purebred varieties of various species, it changed from 1970s after the H x H and H x B and even diploid *herbaceum* x *arboreum* (*desi*) cotton hybrids were released for cultivation and both hybrids and pure bred varieties were grown commercially. After the introduction of Bt-transgenic cottons as H x H and to a small extent as H x B hybrids, significant change occurred marginalizing the cultivation of diploid cultivated species cottons. Cottons grown today represents mostly superior medium and long staple cottons all over the country. The short desi (diploid species) cotton production was affected drastically due to large scale replacement with *hirsutum* x *hirsutum* cotton hybrids with Bt-gene(s). Extra-long staple cotton production also dwindled largely due to replacement with *hirsutum* x *hirsutum* Bt-cotton hybrids with superior medium and long staple, apart from virtual decline in area under 'Suvin', the only ELS *G. barbadense* cultivar available and also decline in the ELS *hirsutum* x *barbadense* F_1 hybrids on account of maintenance of seed quality and fibre quality problems especially of the *barbadense* parents. MCU5 cotton of the Upland type with superior long staple also gradually declined due to encroachment of its area by the Bt-cotton hybrids.

http://dx.doi.org/10.5772/58622

The current total area under cotton is estimated as 11.7 million hectares and the output as 6.46 million metric tons of lint (along with estimated 13 million tons of cottonseed) in 2013-2014 [10]. The trend of change in species composition is indicated in Table 1 and Figure 1.

Species	**1947-48**		**1989-90**		**2013-14**	
	Area M ha	**Production MMT**	**Area M ha**	**Production MMT**	**Area M ha**	**Production MMT**
Total of all 4 cultivated species	4.40	0.39 MMT	7.50.	2.17	11.70.	6.46
G. hirsutum (H)	0.133	0.0273	3.15	0.998	10.647	6.266
G. barbadense (B)	-	-	0.025	insignificant	0.001	insignificant
G. arboreum (A)	2.86	0.253	1.275	0.217	1.17	0.129
G. herbaceum (h)	1.408	o.109	0.975	0.130	<0.585	0.0646
Hybrid cotton (Hybrid cotton era from 1970)All hybrids	-	-	2.10	0.825	-	-
hirsutum x hirsutum Hybrid cotton with Bt-gene(s)	-	-	-	-	10.647	6.266
hirsutum x barbadense hybrids with Bt-gene(s)	-	-	-	-	small	small

Table 1. Species composition / contribution in India to cotton area and production

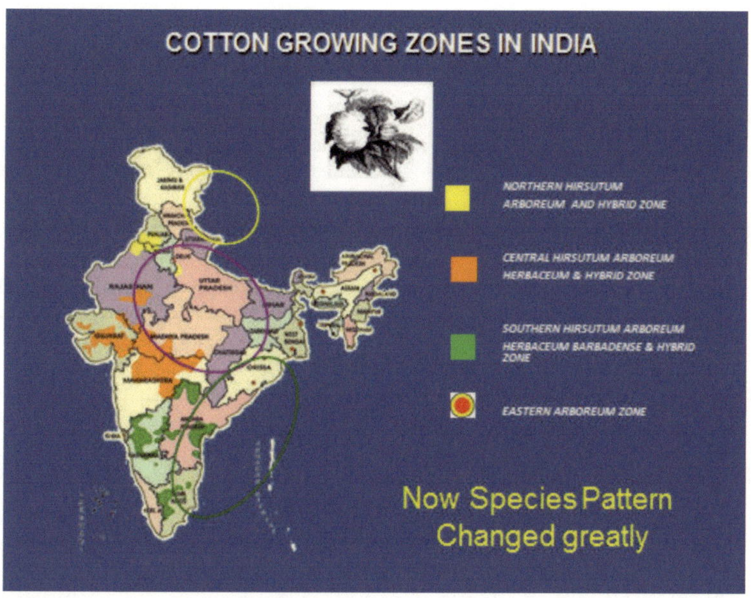

(Adopted from Dr. V. Santhanam, WCRC-5 Mumbai, 2011)

Figure 1. The current species composition of cotton and distribution in India

2.2. Germplasm needs for India's cotton improvement

Germplasm demand depends on various considerations and criteria. Primarily, it depends on the predominant species grown, genetic constitution of the cultivar / hybrid developed for large scale cultivation, the fibre quality requirements of the textile industry and export needs and incidentally various byproduct utility potential. The future attention of the breeders may be more towards the improvement of the *G. hirsutum* cotton because of the changed species composition involving more than 90 per cent area under cultivation of *G. hirsutum* cotton. Some special interest will be shown to the utilization of *G. barbadense* germplasm in cotton improvement because of the need to develop superior cultivars of *G. barbadense* with extra-long staple coupled with better adaptation to Indian conditions and also in the exploitation of the potential of the *G. hirsutum* x *G. barbadense* F_1 commercial hybrids to develop ELS cotton hybrids with high yield potential. Further, the private seed companies holding a major stake in seed business have great role to play in meeting the needs for high quality seeds of superior varieties of the predominant cultivated species preferred by the farmers. The major breeding goals in cotton are based on conventional and changing cropping practices and industry requirements of the 21st century are as follows:

Wide adaptation: agronomic and ecological stability including-Areas of cultivation and their agro-climatic conditions, soil fertility, temperature both day and night temperatures, rainfall characteristics (onset, duration, intensity and occurrence characteristics), adaptation and other factors (like adaptation to various abiotic stresses such as late sowings, droughts, excess rainfall at critical phases of crop growth and major weather aberrations).

Response to advanced production technologies: this will include higher fertilizer use, higher planting densities, mechanization of cultivation practices with insect resistant cotton, chemical herbicide use for weed management and other practices like constraints management, manual and machine picking of cotton, double cropping patterns, continuous improvement in yield per hectare).

Resistance to biotic and abiotic stresses: this includes resistance/tolerance to various kinds of pest and disease reactions and abiotic factors causing serious recurring yield losses and adverse effects on fibre quality.

Cotton requirements for the textile industry: the total quantitative demands of national textile consumption of cotton, extra-factory consumption and export needs (including qualitative needs in terms of share of various staple types like short staple, medium staple, superior medium, long staple and extra-long staple and fibre quality parameters consistent with the desired levels for each of above staple categories besides for various spinning systems).

Improving the utility of cottonseeds: important aspects include elimination of gossypol, increased oil content and improved fatty acid profiles of the oil and protein in seed etc., to improve the utility value of seed and its nutritional qualities for food and feed.

Specialty cotton requirements: these are based on considerations for production of organic cotton and naturally colour-linted cottons with appreciable fibre quality parameters for spinning and weaving, although the market requirement is low at less than 1% of the global production of cotton at present.

Considerations for newer breeding goals: this is specially for India and elsewhere in the world for the demands of the 21st century including suitability of plant architecture for higher plant densities with high yield per hectare for machine harvesting, tolerance to drought and adverse weather situations related to emerging climate change patterns, resistance to sucking pests, mealy bugs and whitefly induced cotton leaf curl virus disease and reducing the duration of cotton for less water use and fitment into double cropping patterns etc. [4,14,15,10,16].

3. Genetic resources of cotton — Content and location

The details pertaining to all cotton genetic resource holdings and their locations, evaluations and conservation are presented below:

3.1. Wild species and related stocks

Cotton plant belongs to the family *Malvaceae* and genus *Gossypium* L., which comprises about 50 species, 45 of which are diploid (2n=2x=26) and the remaining 5 being allotetraploid (2n=4x=52) and whose geographical distribution spans the tropical and sub-tropical regions of the world [17]. The two 'A' genome diploid and two 'AD' genome allotetraploid species are cultivated for their lint fibre. The four species in cultivation have their botanical and geographical races such as (*africanum, acerifolium, wightianum, persicum, and kuljianum under G. herbaceum; races indicum, bengalense, burmanicum, cernuum, sinense, and soudanense under G. arboreum; races latifolium, punctatum, morilli, yucatanense, marie-galante, palmeri and richmondii under G. hirsutum and races barbadense and brasiliense under G. barbadense* as described by Hutchinson, 1951 [3, 17] are available in distinct accessions of germplasm of cotton maintained in gene banks of CICR Nagpur and its regional station Coimbatore and certain other State Agricultural University Centres like UAS Dharwad, GAU Surat, TNAU etc. Intermediary germplasm-genetic stocks and breeding lines developed out of crosses between wild and cultivated species and between cultivated species have been integrated into the maintenance under germplasm for gene banks at CICR and State Agricultural University (SAU) centers and used for crop improvement programmes. The list of *Gossypium* species and those available in India is given in Table 2.

Genome	Species of *Gossypium*	(if available 'Yes')	Genome	Species of *Gossypium*	(if available 'Yes')
Diploid Species 2n = 2x = 26			**Diploid Species 2n = 2x = 26**		
A_1	*herbaceum* L.	Cultivation	K	*costulatum* Todaro	
A_2	*arboreum* L.	Cultivation			
B_1	*anomalum* W&P	Yes	(In C)	*populifolium* Mueller	
B_2	*triphyllum* Hochreutiner	Yes		*cunninghamii* Todaro	
B_3	*capitis viridis* Mauer	Yes		*pulchellum* Fryxell	

Genome	Species of *Gossypium*	(if available 'Yes')	Genome	Species of *Gossypium*	(if available 'Yes')
Diploid Species 2n = 2x = 26			**Diploid Species 2n = 2x = 26**		
?	*trifurcatum* Vollesen			*pilosum* Fryxell	
C_1	*sturtianum* Willis	Yes		*exiguum* Fryxell	
C_1-n	*nandewarense* Dereda	Yes		*nobile* Fryxell	
C_2	*robinsonii* Mueller			*rotundifolium* Fryxell	
D_1	*thurbei* Todaro	Yes		*enthyle* Fryxell	
D_{2}-1	*armourianum* Kearney	Yes		*londonderriense* Fryxell	
D_{2}-2	*harknessii* Brandigee	Yes		*marchantii* Fryxell	
D_3-d	*davidsonii* Kellog	Yes		*anapoides* Stewart	
D_3-k	*klotzschianum* Andersson	Yes			
D_4	*aridum* Skovsted	Yes			
D_5	*raimondii* Ulbrecht	Yes			
D_6	*gossypioides* Standley	Yes	**Allotetraploids 2n = 4x = 52**		
D_7	*lobatum* Gentry	Yes	$(AD)_1$	*hirsutum* Linn.	Cultivation
D_8	*trilobum* Skovsted	Yes	$(AD)_2$	*barbadense* Linn.	cultivation
D_9	*laxum* Phillips		$(AD)_3$	*tomentosum* Nuttal	Yes
D_{10}	*turneri* Fryxell		$(AD)_4$	*mustelinum* Masters	
D_{11}	*schwendimanii* Fryxell		$(AD)_5$	*darwinii* Watt.	yes
E_1	*stocksii* Masters	Yes	Note:		
E_2	*somalense* Hutchinson	Yes	In addition, 82 perennials, 141 land races *(G. arboreum and G. barbadense), 20* distinct *cernuum* race collections with big boll weight , up to 6.4g and 44.4% GOT are available; also 40 synthetic polyploids, 20 male sterile lines from Israel etc., GMS, TGMS and EGMS lines are also maintained at CICR.		
E_3	*areysianum* Deflers				
E_4	*incanum* Hillcoat				
E?	*ellenbickii* Mauer				
E?	*bricchettii* Vollesen				
E?	*benadirense* Mattei				
F1	*longicalyx* Hutchinson & Lee	Yes			
G	*australe* Mueller	Yes			
G	*nelsonii* Fryxell				
G_1	*bickii* Prokhanov	Yes			

Table 2. Species of *Gossypium* and their availability in India (in cultivation or in Species Gardens):-Taxonomic classification of *Gossypium* L. species [18-22].

http://dx.doi.org/10.5772/58622

3.2. Genetic resources of cultivated cottons

The collections-accessions reportedly available mainly in the CICR Nagpur gene bank [or in its regional stations at Coimbatore especially for *G. barbadense* / Sirsa (limited to some diploid cotton accessions] have been described [23, 14, 24, 15]. The total cotton accessions available in India was reported as 7484 in *G. hirsutum*, 263 in *G. barbadense*, 1877 in *G. arboreum* and 530 in *G. herbaceum*, besides wild species and perennials [25]. Additional accessions of *G. hirsutum* and *G. barbadense* acquired after 2011 are to be documented after evaluation and added to the figures; similarly the germplasm additionally available after 2011 for the two diploid species of Asiatic cottons, *G. herbaceum* and *G. arboreum* also have to be incorporated in the total holdings after assessment and characterization. The details of the wild primary, secondary, and tertiary cotton (*Gossypium*) species and the cultivated tetraploid species maintained in several countries has been previously reported [26]. Similar materials of major gene pools including germplasm of the two cultivated tetraploid and the two cultivated diploid species maintained in India are presented in Table 3.

Species	Genome	Collection maintained at CICR Nagpur
Primary gene pool		
G. tomentosum Nuttal ex Seaman	AD_3	1
G. darwinii Watt	AD_5	1
Secondary gene pool		
G. herbaceum L.	A_1	given below
G. arboreum L.	A_2	given below
G. anomalum Wawra	B_1	1
G. triphyllum Hochreutiner	B_2	1
G. capitis viridis Mauer	B_3	1
G. barbosanum Phillips & Clement	B_3?	1
G. longicalyx Hutchinson & Lee	F_1	1
G. thurberi Todaro	D_1	1
G. trilobum (DC) Skovsted	D_8	1
G. davidsonii kellogg	D_2-d	1
G. klotschianum Andersson	D_2-k	1
G. armourianum Kearney	D_{2^-1}	2
G. harknessii Brandigee	D_{2^-2}	1
G. aridum Skovsted	D_4	1
G. lobatum H Gentry	D_7	1

Species	Genome	Collection maintained at CICR Nagpur
G. gossypioides (Ulbrich) Standley	D_5	1
G. raimondii Ulbrich	D_6	1
Tertiary gene pool		
G. sturtianum J.H Wills	C_1	1
G. stocksii Master	E_1	1
G. somalense Hutchinson	E_2	1
G. australe F. Mueller	G	2
G. bickii Prokanov	G_1	1
Cultivated tetraploid species		
G. hirsutum L.	AD_1	
Germplasm		7484
Cultivars		110
Land races/wild stocks		7
Cytogenetic stocks/mutants		32/1
Total		7633
G. barbadense L.	AD_2	
Germplasm		530
Cultivars		3
Land races / wild stocks		1/0
Total		534
Cultivated diploid species		
G. arboreum L.		
Germplasm and all other accessions		1877
G. herbaceum L.		
Germplasm and all other accessions		530

Table 3. Description of the wild primary, secondary, and tertiary cotton (*Gossypium*) species and the germplasm of cultivated cottons of the two cultivated tetraploid and two cultivated diploid cotton species maintained in India

3.3. Germplasm exploration and collection

The exploration of certain regions in India was carried out by the Germplasm Advisory Committee (GPAC) involving the CICR and the NBPGR in seven expeditions. The areas represented formerly predominant areas of Asiatic cotton cultivation in Southern and Central India, NE Hill regions with *cernuum* types of *G. arboreum* and some *G. hirsutum* cotton under the Malwa plateau in Central India representing distinct agro-climate, apart from perennial cottons grown as backyard cottons for house-hold use. Attributes of breeders' interest in the collections included closed boll types in *G. herbaceum* with storm proof nature, big bolls with >6g boll weight, high ginning and high seed number per boll in *G. arboreum* and cold resistance in *G. hirsutum*. The details of the surveys and collections made are given in Table 4.

Year	Organization	Funded by	Regions of expedition	Material collected	Characters observed
1977	CICR/NBPGR	ICAR	Assam and Meghalaya	*Cernuum* types of *G. arboreum*	High ginning, big long bolls, loculi retention after bursting
1978	CICR/GPAC	ICAR	Tinnies tract of Tamil Nadu	Diploid cultivated variants	Introgressed types of early introductions
1979	CICR/ GPAC/UAS/GAU	ICAR	Saurashtra region in Gujarat and Raichur area in Karnataka	*G. herbaceum* types and variants	Closed boll types, round boll, storm proof types
1981	CICR	ICAR	Malwa plateau of Madhya Pradesh	*G. hirsutum*	Local variants, cold resistance
1984	CICR/NBPGR	ICAR	Assam and Manipur	*G. arboreum* race *cernuum*	High seed number per boll, long big bolls, high ginning types
1986	NBPGR	ICAR	Gujarat western tract	*Desi* cotton material	Resistance to moisture stress, high yield potential
1987	NBPGR/CICR	ICAR	Assam regions	*Cernuum* types of *G. herbaceum*	Big boll, higher boll numbers, abiotic resistance

Table 4. Surveys and collections made by the CICR/NBPGR and their description

4. Funding sources for cotton germplasm activities

The Indian Council of Agricultural Research (ICAR), New Delhi is the main funding agency for all the germplasm related activities in cotton and the ICAR is an autonomous body under the Ministry of Agriculture and Department of Agricultural Research and Education (DARE) of the Government of India. The Central Institute for Cotton Research (CICR) Nagpur, the National Bureau of Plant Genetic Resources (NBPGR) New Delhi and also Central Institute for Research on Cotton Technology (CIRCOT), Mumbai are national level Institutes under the ICAR to take care of all cotton research related activities including germplasm related matters. The ICAR may seek collaboration with the FAO in germplasm exploration and collection activities as and when such activities are planned. The responsibility for cotton germplasm is mainly vested with the CICR. The CICR has played a pivotal role in germplasm acquisition, maintenance, evaluation and promoting utilization in breeding and other related researches.

India is probably the third richest country in general and in certain respects probably the richest in the world in its total holdings and diversity of cotton genetic resources including wild species, cultivated species and even certain perennial genotypes of cotton [15]. The National

Gene Bank of Cotton in India is located at the Central Institute for Cotton Research, Nagpur including its regional station at Coimbatore. The total collection represents almost entirely cultivated accessions of *G. hirsutum, G. barbadense, G. arboreum,* and *G. herbaceum*. In addition, the collection also consists of race stock accessions of each cultivated species, 26 wild species, and 32 synthetic introgressed derivatives.

High level of coordination is being achieved in germplasm exchange and utilization with the world level International Institute for Plant Genetic Resources and national level institutions (NBPGR, CICR, CIRCOT and SAUs), The availability of equipment and techniques for mass screening for several parameters in the laboratory, in the fields and glass houses, has made possible to generate precise data in various environments and enabled to have a new-look and re-look at the germplasm for various breeding and gene deployment strategies. It also helped to develop varieties and hybrids for meeting the demands of the farmers, the textiles industry for various end-uses and to overcome inter-fibre competition based on consumer preferences and the cottonseed utilization and biomass utilization industries. Now more information has been accumulated to improve cottonseed yield and quality profile useful for agro-based industrial exploitation. This is to meet human needs for edible oil, protein and cellulose to contribute to enhanced food and nutritional security and also develop various by-products for use as animal feed and further processing in ancillary industries [27, 10].

5. Sharing of germplasm resources

Sharing of germplasm may take place as per Government of India policies and based on inter-country government protocols and exchange programmes on mutual basis of agreements, if any. Within the country, the germplasm is readily available for public sector research institutions carrying out research on cotton and related activities.

6. Characterization, evaluations and utilization

Based on the work done at the CICR in cooperation with the CIRCOT, NBPGR and SAU Centres over the past few decades, the various aspects have been presented below:

6.1. Germplasm Index Card (GIC)

A GIC was designed and distributed for use by cotton breeders all over India. The GIC was designed by the Central Institute for Cotton Research, Nagpur based on the recommendations of the National Germplasm Advisory Committee on Cotton constituted by the CICR under the Indian Council of Agricultural Research (ICAR). This card contains some 76 important characters of cotton plant and produce and is included in the Cotton Genetic Resources Catalogue published by the CICR in 1990 [23] It is based on the International Board for Plant Genetic Resources (IBPGR) model with suitable modifications and various characters, their descriptors and descriptor states for cotton for precise evaluation of genetic resources of cotton.

Common and standard procedures were also provided for recording observations with comparable uniformity over locations. Provision was made for recording data on all quality attributes of fibre (technological characters) as well as cottonseed and biomass, harvest index etc. (Figure 2).

Gossypium hirsutum

Germplasm Index Card

1. CICR Accession No. ....
2. Source Station Code ....
3. Source Designation ....

Race ....

4. Origin/Source ....
5. Pedigree ....
6. Year Received ....
7. Rainfed/Irrigated ....

Year of observation	GROWTH HABIT				STEM			LEAF							FLOWER					BOLL			Card
	Plant type	Plant height (cm)	No. of monopodia	No. of sympodia	Hairiness	Colour	Internode length (cm)	Size	Shape	Lobing	Colour	Surface	Glands	Nectary	Days to 1st flowering	Bracts colour	Petal spot	Petal colour	Pollening	Bearing	Size	Shape No.	Col. (76)
8	9	10	11	12	13	14	15	16	17	18	19	20	21	22	23	24	25	26	27	28	29	30	31

Year of observation	BOLL							SEED										FIBRE CHARACTERS					
	Surface	Glands	1st boll bursting (days)	Opening	Loculi/boll	Seeds/locule	Boll weight (g)	Seed index (g)	Fuzz	Fuzz colour	Oil (%)	Protein (%)	Gossypol (%)	Yield/plant (g)	Duration (days)	Ginning out-turn (%)	Lint index (g)	Lint colour	2.5% span length (mm)	Uniformity ratio	Mature fibres (%)	Fineness (micronaire)	Strength 'O' gauge (g/tex)
32	33	34	35	36	37	38	39	40	41	42	43	44	45	46	47	48	49	50	51	52	53	54	55

Year of observation	REACTION TO PESTS									REACTION TO DISEASES										Card No. Col (76)
	Jassids	Aphids	Thrips	Whitefly	Bollworm			Leaf roller	Others	Bacterial blight	Alternaria	Anthracnose	Wilt		Root-rot	Grey mildew	Myrothecium	Helminthosporium	Others	
					Spotted	Pink	Heliothis						Fusarium	Verticillium						
56	57	58	59	60	61	62	63	64	65	66	67	68	69	70	71	72	73	74	75	76

Index for Evaluation of Characters

GROWTH HABIT		STEM		LEAF						
Plant type	Hairiness	Colour	Internode length	Size	Shape	Lobing	Colour	Surface	Glands	Nectary
1) Compact 2) Lanky 3) Bushy	1) Glabrous 2) Hairy 3) Densely hairy	1) Green 2) Greenish purple (Sun red) 3) Red	1) Short (up to 5 cm) 2) Medium (5.1 - 10 cm) 3) Large (10.1 - 15 cm) 4) Extra-long above 15 cm)	1) Small 2) Normal 3) Large	1) Normal 2) Okra 3) Super-okra	1) Narrow 2) Broad	1) Light green 2) Green 3) Red 4) others	1) Glabrous 2) Hairy 3) Densely hairy	1) Absent 2) Sparse 3) Dense	1) Absent 2) Present

FLOWER				BOLL						
Bracts	Petal Colour	Petal Spot	Pollen colour	Bearing habit	Shape	Size	Surface	Glands	Opening	Boll weight
1) Normal 2) Large 3) Frego	1) White 2) Cream 3) Light yellow 4) Yellow 5) Lavender (pale purple)	1) Absent 2) Small 3) Large	1) Cream 2) Light yellow	1) Sparse 2) Normal 3) Yellow	1) Round 2) Oval 3) Conical 4) Cluster	1) Small 2) Medium 3) Large	1) Smooth 2) Sparsely pitted 3) Densely pitted	1) Absent 2) Sparse 3) Dense	1) Normal 2) Intermediate 3) Closed	Average of 10 healthy bolls

SEED							
Seed index	Fuzz	Fuzz colour	Oil (%) Protein (%) Gossypol (%)	Yield/plant	Ginning out-turn	Lint index	Lint colour
Weight of 100 seeds	1) Naked 2) Sparse 3) Fuzzy	1) White 2) Green 3) Grey 4) Brown (tan)	At 10% moisture basis of seed weight	Minimum 10 plants average	to be obtained from a minimum sample of 100 g	Weight of lint from 100 seeds	1) White 2) Creamy 3) Light brown 4) Brown 5) Others

REACTION TO PESTS AND DISEASES

1) Resistant R
2) Moderately resistant MR
3) Moderately susceptible MS
4) Susceptible S

Figure 2. Germplasm Index Card (GIC) designed by CICR Nagpur for recording data on cotton germplasm

6.2. Cotton genetic resources catalogue

The Germplasm Index Card designed by the CICR was used as the basis for germplasm cataloguing. The Catalogue of Cotton Genetic Resources was compiled based on germplasm data gathered all over the country, particularly at CICR Nagpur, Maharashtra state (Central zone) and its regional centres at Coimbatore in Tamil Nadu (Southern zone) and Sirsa in Haryana state (Northern zone) representing all the three major cotton growing zones of the country. Data for special applications were also recorded by the departments of Pathology, Entomology, Soil Science Agronomy, Physiology, Biochemistry etc. Fibre quality data were generated by the Central Institute for Research on Cotton Technology (CIRCOT), Mumbai and its regional units and that for oil content and seed oil index were obtained at the CICR by using Nuclear Magnetic Resonance (NMR) and other instruments [23].

Close collaboration for data recording and evaluation was ensured between the CICR, the CIRCOT, Mumbai, the National Bureau of Plant Genetic Resources (NBPGR) New Delhi, Indian Agricultural Research Institute (IARI), New Delhi and all the State Agricultural Universities (SAUs) in cotton growing states of the country as partners with the CICR as members of the Germplasm Advisory Committee for Cotton. Average data over 2-3 seasons were taken into consideration for deciding on the potential values of each germplasm accession. The data have been computerized by the CICR. Multi-location data were also generated for field performance, wherever possible and made available to regional breeding centres.

6.3. Selected list of superior germplasm

Based on germplasm evaluation over locations and seasons, the elite accessions for characters of high economic importance in cotton representing all the four cultivated species especially for early maturity, plant architecture, yield influencing attributes like boll number, boll weight and high ginning, seed quality and stress tolerance etc., were sorted out from the total germplasm evaluated. Some of the elite germplasm accessions identified species-wise in the cotton gene pool [15] are indicated in Table 5.

Species	Characters	Elite types identified
G. hirsutum	Early maturity (140-150days)	TXORSC 801-79, Acala 8-1 x Tamcot Sp21, Acala 69/5, D244-10, Riverina poplar. U. aRk, d203-5, d238-13-5,USSR n. Ac.83 (RKS), MCU7, SIMA-1, PKV081, NHS1412, LRA5166, BN, Narasimha, LRK516, PKV442
	Dwarf (below 80cm)	USSR6248, Acala8861 x CA491Early F-8, Acala 1577-7780,TXORSC 80-1-79, TxcaMd21-5-78, SIMA 1, PKV081
	Compact plant type	54727, USSR 6250,PRS72, PRS74,NHS1412, DCI 118
	Bacterial blight resistance	Tx Maroon 2-78, TXORHU1-78, Tamcot CAMDE, Tamcot SP37, Tamcot SP 215, Tamcot SP23, RebaB50, 101-102B, BJA592
	High boll weight "/ >5.5g	T120-76, CP188, Acala 8-1xTamcot SP215, 108F,Hopicala, NC Smooth 1, 133F, Empire WR61, DS56,DS59, Tashkant 1
	High boll number	FTA MDH133, Deltapine 90, MDH 2, LRA 5166, NHS 1412, Narasimha
	High ginning (40%)	Nc177-16-30, Arkot 2-1,Superokra, NC Hairy, IRMA23, U585-12, Half & Half, Kirghis A2, 9030H
	High yield	Reba Pvt9, Delcot 311, Aleppo 40, Deltapine 16, Tashkent 3, Pee Dee 2164, Demeter-iii(1), S1291, 149F, 152F, B4 Empire, DS56, DS 59, SIMA1, LRA5166, MCU5, MCU7, MCU10, F414, NH1412, Suman, Narasimha, Anjali,
G. barbadense	High yield	25-1-3, K3475, CBS34, C 6002-3, ERB4492,ERB 13552, SIV 135, USSR mix 76, CV76, EC I 34390, EC I 32374, SB 289E, SB1085-6
G. arboreum	High seed oil "/ >20%	79/Lohit, Behnoor, AKA12, H4616, Ac733, AKH4, Comilla, 30820, 30840, Gao 16, CB-VIII, Gao 16-CB4, Gao 16-CB7, Coconados 5, Chineese Broad lobe, Chineese Narrow Lobe, Chineese Spotless
	High Yield	G27, Lohit, AKH4, LD 230, LD 133, LD 135, LD 141, LD 143, AKA 28, AKA 8401, H46, H47, Bani 306, Ac types (PAU), Nanded 3883, Desi 52, Coconadas White
	Long staple	LS1, LS2, LS3, 2927, H511,Adonicum, Sel 32-1, K5567, K7, K8, K9, K10
G. herbaceum	General good	5495. Suj M3-3-5, EPSB, Russian 9,Baluchisthan, Kumpta, G. *G. arboreum* COT 11, G. Cot 13, 519-14, Suj 3-3-19, 86-5, 87-2, E2-13-2, 72-34, Suj 22-3-1, LS Early,

Table 5. Some elite germplasm accessions identified for different characters

The estimated numbers of elite types with relatively high performance for various characters in the *Gossypium* gene pool in the CICR were arrived at based on the evaluation in comparison with appropriate local checks (standard cultivars) over seasons with consistent superiority [15] and most of them are included in the breeders working collections for regular use. The details of elite types for various characters are given in Table 6.

Elite character types	***hirsutum***	***barbadense***	***arboreum***	***herbaceum***	**Wild and other stocks**
High stable yield performance	380	16	300	31	-
High boll weight	145	5	150	20	-
High boll number potential	140	3	60	45	2
High seed weight	330	10	40	20	-
High lint index	249	12	30	12	-
High ginning	120	15	150	40	-
Micronaire value (3.5-4.0)	190	30	2	50	4
High span length	220	60	50	40	-
High fibre strength	145	50	180	55	5
Compact to medium plant type	42	5	10	3	-
High sympodial branching	275	12	40	20	2
High seed oil content	75	10	60	25	-
Early maturity	30	3	75	10	-
High biomass potential	400	10	120	45	12
High harvest index	120	1	15	10	-
High seed number per boll	230	2	20	30	-
Long pedicel	35	-	-	-	-
Morphological markers	185	10	30	2	-
Insect pests & disease resistance	280	10	many	many	50
CMS, GMS and Restorer sources	34	-	2	-	3
High coarse absorbent types	15	-	100	10	-
Drought tolerance potential	50	-	300	150	15
Naked seeded types	5	-	1	-	3
Delayed morphogenesis of gossypol	-	-	-	-	3
Chromosomal variants	-	-	-	-	77
Low gossypol gland types	60	-	10	5	-
High fuzzy types	100	-	200	50	4
Working collections	425	10	130	60	perennials

Table 6. Estimated number of elite germplasm accessions with relatively high performance for various characters in *Gossypium* gene pool.

6.4. Range of variability

The extent of variability was assessed for leaf attributes (shape, pattern of lobes and size), calyx shape and size, burst bolls (shape, size, boll opening type and lint colour), seeds (seed size, fuzz content and fuzz colour) and lint (length, density and colour) and the wide range of variability was portrayed in an exhibit form. Some of the wild species especially for delayed morphogenesis, petal spot pattern and colour-linted sample were also included in the exhibit. The range of variability in cotton germplasm accessions of *G. hirsutum* and *Desi* (Diploid) cottons under Nagpur (India) conditions along with some selected wild species and colour lint [23,15] cotton are exhibited in Figure 3.

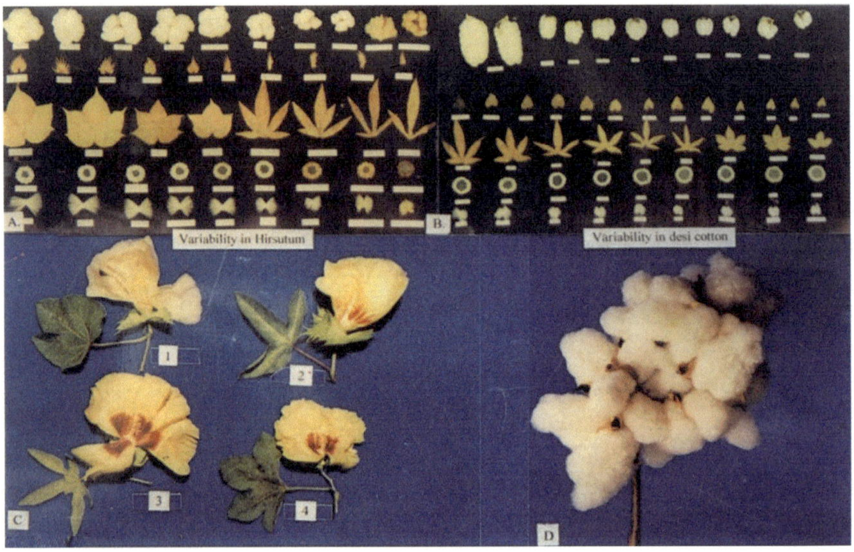

Figure 3. Top: Range of variability in cotton germplasm accessions of A: *G. hirsutum* and B: *Desi* (Diploid) cottons under Nagpur (India) conditions; Bottom: C 1-4 represents selected wild species and D-colour linted cotton.

6.5. Inherent potentiality identified in different wild species

Inherent potentiality identified in different species of *Gossypium* by Indian scientists and others based on [3, 28, 19, 24, 29, 30] for improving the cultivated cottons is briefly summarized in Table 7.

Some useful character transfer into *G. hirsutum* and *G. barbadense* cultivars is described below:

Some useful character transference (introgressions) into cultivars of the two tetraploid species has been achieved and based on [3, 28, 19, 24, 29, 30], some of the achievements include jassid resistance potential from *G. tomentosum*; smoothness for boll weevil resistance from *G. armourianum*; rust resistance from *G. raimondii*; blackarm resistance from *G. arboreum* (into *G. barbadense)*; fibre length from *G. thurberi* and *G. raimondii*; fibre strength from *G. thurberi*; cytoplasmic male sterility from *G. harknessii*; drought resistance from *G. arboreum* and *G.*

http://dx.doi.org/10.5772/58622

Improvement of	Character	*Gossypium species*
Fibre quality	Fibre length	*anomalum, stocksii, raimondii, areysianum, longicalyx,*
	Fibre strength & elongation	*stockssii, areysianum, thurberi, anomalum, sturtianum, raimondii, longicalyx*
	Fibre fineness	*longicalyx, anomalum, raimondii*
	Lint yield	*anomalum, sturtianum, australe, stocksii, areysianum*
	High ginning outturn	*australe*
Insect resistance	Bollworms	*thurberi, anomalum, raimondii, armourianum, somalense*
	Helicoverpa	*somalense*
	Jassid resistance	*anomalum, armourianum, raimondii, tomentosum*
	Whitefly tolerance	*armourianum*
	Mite resistance	*anomalum*
	Aphid resistance	*davidsonii*
Disease resistance	Bacterial blight	*anomalum, armourianum, raimondii*
	Verticillium wilt	*hirsutum (var. mexicanum.nervosum), harknessii*
	Fusarium wilt	*sturtianum, harknessii, thurberi*
	Nematode	*darwinii*
Other attributes	Cytoplasmic male sterility (CMS)	*harknessii, trilobum, aridum*
	Drought tolerance	*darwinii, tomentosum, stocksii, areysianum, anomalum, australe, harknessii, aridum, raimondii*
	Frost resistance	*thurberi*
	Delayed morphogenesis of gossypol glands	*bickii, australe*

Table 7. Inherent potentials in wild species of *Gossypium* identified

herbaceum; fibre length from *G. barbadense* (into *G. hirsutum*); fertility restorer gene from *G. harknessii;* high ginning outturn from *G. arboreum*; hairiness from *G. tomentosum* into *G. barbadense* and caduceus bract from *G. armourianum*.

6.6. Germplasm utilization

In cotton, the approximate number of collections maintained in various centres in the four cultivated species and wild stocks including advanced intermediate breeding lines was estimated at 20,750, but it included duplicates and repeat collections since each Centre maintained as per local breeders' needs [29]. Enormous intra and inter-racial variability occurs in-*Gossypium arboreum* including land races of *bengalense* like *sanguineum*, multani cotton, *roseum* and genotypes characterized by high boiling potential, high yields, low boll weight, medium to high ginning out-turn, fine and long fibre, susceptibility to boll worm and late maturity. The race *cernuum* is extremely coarse-fibred, with very high ginning out-turn (up to 50%), boll weight (4.5-6.0g) and seed number (10-16 seeds/locule). Similarly, *G. herbaceum* grown in Gujarat (Wagad, Broach, Lalio and Goghari Cotton) and Karnataka (Kumpta Cotton) differ from each other in plant habit, maturity, leaf lobation, boll size, lint colour, ginning outturn and seed characters [12].

The Indian *G. hirsutum* types are represented by Punjab American Cotton, Buri types, CTI types, Indo-American types and Madras Cambodia Uganda types. The present day Punjab American Cotton varieties being cultivated in North India are selections from LSS and 216 F (e.g., 320 F, Bikaneri Nerma, H777, F 444, SH 131 etc.). The types Buri 1007 and Buri 0394 are resistant to wilt, jassid and frost. Several CTI varieties (Bandnawar-1, Bandnawar-3 Khandwa-2 etc.) were released through hybridization between Cambodian variety Co.2 with *G. tomentosum* and have high degree of jassid resistance due to hairy leaves. Inter-specific hybridization involving *G. hirsutum* and Asiatic diploid species carried out at Surat in Gujarat gave rise to several Indo-American types (e.g., 170-Co-2, 134-Co 2-M, Gujarat-67, etc.). These varieties are genetically divergent from rest of the *hirsutum* varieties developed in India and are good examples of commercial varieties developed from tetraploid x diploid species for the first time. Pure line selections of Cambodian types at Coimbatore and Tamil Nadu gave rise to variety CO2. This variety was further crossed with two Uganda types, viz. 4-4/4 and A-12, and the selections from these crosses were established as Madras Cambodian Uganda (MCU) types. This resulted in developing long-linted superior quality cottons like MCU-5, MCU-8 and MCU-9.

G.barbadense was introduced in India during the 1930s. However, its cultivation was restricted to limited area in southern states of the country. In 1967, a variety Sujata, a selection from Egyptian variety Karnak, was evolved. The first Indian variety of hybrid origin Suvin was evolved in 1971 from a cross of Sujata and St. Vincent. Therefore, the present day *G. barbadense* cotton in India has these three stocks.

The success in hybrid cotton in India was achieved at Surat where an *intra-hirsutum* cross of Gujarat-67 x American Nectariless (an exotic from USA) was released for commercial cultivation in 1968 as Hybrid 4. The first commercial interspecific hybrid Varalaxmi acceptable to farmers and industry was developed at the University of Agricultural Sciences, Dharwad (Karnataka) in 1972 from a cross between Laxmi (an adapted *G. hirsutum*) and SB 289 E (a Russian *barbadense* variety). Later, a large number of inter-specific hybrids have been developed in India, such as CBS 156, JKHy-1, JKHy-11, Savitri, Godavari, Suguna, H-6, Jayalaxmi, and diploid DDH-2, etc. which are widely grown in different parts of the country [29, 31, 32].

Possession of germplasm in numerical strength in R&D Centres and in a nation is really a great asset. Unless and until the resources are utilized effectively in crop improvement and significant achievements of farming and commercial value is demonstrated, the conservation and maintenance is not really justified. Considering the huge cost involving staff, infrastructure like fields, glass houses and equipment, besides recurring contingencies, a proper strategy should be in place to screen all germplasm and constitute the most elite breeders' working collections for breeders' use. A Memorandum of Understanding (MOU) or Material Transfer Agreement (MTA) basis to enable breeders to obtain germplasm would pay high dividends for the nation in intensifying crop improvement. A suitable global and national policy to share germplasm for breeding requirements may be evolved and adopted for supporting the cotton improvement researches both in the public and private sector R&D Units. Quality of maintenance of germplasm must be kept up at a higher level to maintain purity for the attributes for which each accession is noted for and maintained for original attributes without exercising selection for new attributes [33].

In India, several varieties and hybrid cotton cultivars have been developed through interspecific hybridization and many of them were released for cultivation from time to time in the last sixty years. Some of them also became promising parents for developing superior hybrids. Details of the salient achievements [34] are presented in Table 8.

Cultivars developed	***Gossypium Species involved***	**Research institution involved**
Commercial varieties		
Badnawar 1, Khandwa 1, Khandwa 2	*hirsutum x tomentosum*	JNKVV Indore
SRT1, Deviraj (170 C02), Gujarat 67 (G67)	*hirsutum x arboreum*	GAU Surat
Devitej (134 Co2 M)	*hirsutm* x *herbaceum*	GAU Surat
MCU2, MCU5	*hirsutum* x *barbadense*	TNAU Coimbatore
PKV 081	*hirsutum x anomalum*	Dr. PDKV, Akola
Rajat	*hirsutum* x *(thurberi x anomalum)*	Dr. PDKV, Akola
AKA 8401	*arboreum* x *anomalum*	Dr. PDKV, Akola
Arogya	*hirsutum* x *anomalum*	CICR Nagpur
F1 Commercial Hybrid cottons		
Varalakshmi, DCH 32, DHB 9	*hirsutum* x *barbadense*	UAS Dharwad
DDH2	*herbaceum* x *arboreum*	UAS Dharwad
G. Cot. DH7 & G. Cot. DH 9	*herbaceum x arboreum*	GAU Surat
MDCH 201	*herbaceum* x *arboreum*	MAHYCO Seeds private Ltd Jalna (MS)
NHB 12	*hirsutum* x *barbadense*	Marathwada Aricultural University (MAU) Nanded
TCHB 213	*hirsutum* x *barbadense*	TNAU Coimbatore
HB 224, Shruthi	*hirsutum* x *barbadense*	CICR Regional Station, Coimbatore

Table 8. Some cotton varieties and F_1 hybrids developed through interspecific hybridization and released for cultivation

A large number of *G. hirsutum* x *G. hirsutum* F_1 commercial hybrids and a few *hirsutum* x *barbadense* F_1 commercial hybrids have been released by several private seed companies and marketed as proprietary hybrids during 1980 to 2001. After the introduction of transgenic Bt-cotton in 2002-03, several seed companies developed and marketed as many as 1500 commercial hybrids of *hirsutum x hirsutum* with Bt-background as Cry1Ac (Bollgard-I) and as BG-II (Cry1Ac+Cry 2Ab) and the yield level in the country showed significant increases. Several private H x H hybrids used varieties as superior parents such as-Narasimha, Brahma etc., [31, 24, 15, 10] and the farmers have gotten higher yields and higher income.

The extent of variability in germplasm compared to standard cultivars from agricultural, trade, textile and industrial attributes, approximate number of types with elite performance for various characters of breeding importance in the National Gene Bank have been made accessible to cotton breeders in various centres for guidance and utilization in crop improvement for various agro-climatic zones of India. National Gene Bank of Cotton comprising a significant representation of global pool of genetic variability in India has provided a unique opportunity for cotton breeders and other researcher scientists for accelerating the progress of crop improvement. Studies have been carried out on a significant number of accessions of *G. hirsutum* cotton using the hybrid index scores, metro glyph analysis and Mahalanobis D^2 analysis techniques and the divergent accessions were identified and used in crossing programmes at the CICR, Nagpur, [15]

6.7. Databases of cotton germplasm

The cotton databases are maintained by the CICR, Nagpur. The germplasm holdings maintained undergoes constant change periodically based on additions and deletions. Accordingly, the Cotton Gene Bank of the CICR, Nagpur holds a rich repository and global collection of cotton germplasm numbering 10,597 as reported for 2012-13 including newer accessions consisting geographically and genetically diverse *Gossypium hirsutum* (7542), *G. barbadense* (305), *G. arboreum* (1945) and *G. herbaceum* (566), while another 239 representing about 25 wild species and other wild species, perennials and landraces, races of *G. arboreum, G. hirsutum, G. barbadense* and *G. herbaceum*, inter-specific hybrids and their derivatives are maintained in the wild species garden *in situ* at CICR, Nagpur [42].

7. Cotton genetic resources conservation

After initial evaluation, till now some purified bulk seeds of a significant number of accessions have been deposited at long term storage modules at the NBPGR New Delhi. The working collections and other accessions are periodically rejuvenated under safe conditions and pure seeds maintained in medium term cold storage modules at the CICR. The elite working collections identified from the gene pool are further screened by various departments of the institute for all unsolved and emerging problems and also used for further up-gradation of attribute expressions by breeding and selection. The species and some perennials are maintained in in-situ conditions. The new accessions have been acquired from various sources periodically including survey and collections in cooperation with NBPGR and IPGRI. Detailed account of conservation of germplasm holdings of all crops in India was reported by [35].

8. Novel trends and perspectives

Cotton is being challenged on two fronts: on the production side, cotton is competing with food, feed and biofuel crops for acreage and on the consumption aspects; cotton's textile market share is being challenged by man-made and synthetic fibres, in various ways. Cotton has an image of being renewable, environmentally friendly, traceable and comfortable and has still to compete with man-made fibres and synthetic due to the latter's improving technology and functionality. The global cotton industry has been witnessing very dynamic changes since the turn of the 21st century [17, 36, 41). Cotton is an important global commodity and there are incredible efforts in agriculture and cotton to attend to the social, environmental and economic factors and ensure continual improvement, investment, research and sharing of best practices [36].

8.1. Various new considerations for re-evaluation of germplasm

In the context of changing scenario in various aspects concerning cotton, it has become necessary to evaluate the germplasm for several new parameters and enable their utilization in crop improvement for realizing various targeted goals. Some of the aspects requiring examination of old and new germplasm from these perspectives are suggested in Table 9.

New Considerations	Relevant attributes
Quantum jumps in yield of lint	Plant conformation for higher planting densities, high boll weight, compactness of plant type, shorter sympodial branches with synchronous boll bursting, high ginning outturn, high lint index etc.; high harvest index and cost benefit ratios
Fibre quality for competing / coexistence with man-made / synthetic fibres for improving the share of cotton in textile use	High fibre strength, higher fibre elongation of over 6-7, high level of fibre maturity, amenability for imparting easy care properties
Economics of production especially reducing the cost of production and environmental pollution	High level of resistance to biotic stresses, resistance to reemerging sucking pest complex, mealy bugs and other insect pests like whitefly that acts as a carrier of cotton leaf curl virus disease, ability to withstand weed competition and amenability for herbicide tolerance in cultivar development, improved and consistent yield potential under rain fed conditions under low cost technologies in cultivation, improved competitive ability for yield in relation to competing crops
Sustainability of high production levels	Ability to give stable yields under varied environments, adaptation to low cost technologies of crop management, additional advantages from quality and yield of byproducts derived
Contribution to food security in addition to lint fibre production	Higher seed yield from larger planting density & cultivation of hybrids with high vigour, stable and higher levels of oil content, superior nutritional qualities of oil and protein from seed, freedom from gossypol in harvested seeds, higher biomass with higher harvest index, high seed index, non-fuzzy seeds or with low seed hair density
Suitability for mechanization of harvesting cotton	Ideal plant conformations for irrigated and rain fed cotton cultivars, rapid development of bolls to maturity, appropriate plant height stability with amenability for efficient harvesting, boll weight above 5-6g, and high boll load consistent with higher planting densities

New Considerations	Relevant attributes
Organic cotton production (current demand is low, but may increase over time)	High yield potential and stability of yield under organic farming conditions in rain fed and irrigated areas, development of appropriate fibre quality with organic inputs and management systems,
Naturally colour-linted cotton production under isolation from normal cotton growing areas	Expanding the range and intensity / stability of colours of lint fibres, consistent improvement in the fibre properties desired for better spinning like higher strength, optimum maturity with appropriate Mv. (Micronaire value) and improvement in length of fibres for medium, long and extra-long staple categories, higher ginning outturn
Research & development for improving short and extra-long staple cotton production and removing the imbalance in availability in all classes as per textile industry demands	Higher agronomic adaptability of ELS varieties of *G. barbadense* and *hirsutum* x *barbadense* hybrids for commercial cultivation under certain environment constraints, higher yield potential of short staple cotton varieties, hybrids and transgenic cultivars to increase their preference by the cotton farmers with appreciable cost-benefit ratios, improving the ginning outturn in ELS cotton varieties and hybrids and removing certain deficiencies in Micronaire value (Mv.), maturity, strength etc.
Breeding superior *barbadense* cotton varieties	The *barbadense* cotton suffers from low adaptation to the climatic conditions of peninsular India with potential pockets for cultivation, shows fibre quality deficiencies, and need improvement for boll weight, higher ginning, high fibre maturity and optimum Micronaire value (Mv.), and reduction in crop duration
Pre-breeding *barbadense* germplasm lines with improved properties for use as parents of successful commercial hybrids	Higher boll weight, reduced duration, phenotypic stability of plant conformity, high ginning and short sympodial (fruiting) branches with synchronous boll development pattern.
Pest and disease resistance	Compatible parents for hybrids without susceptibility to New wilt / quick wilt in hybrids judged by physiological and agronomic parameters
Compatibility with competing crops in mixed cropping and multiple cropping situations	Increased early vigour, rapid fruiting ability, resistance to interplant competition in the early stage of mixed crops with cotton, optimum leaf area index and resistance tolerance to moisture stress, high photosynthetic efficiency etc.
Breeding for withstanding drought and other climatic aberrations in the context of climate change	Drought resistance attributes and improved physiologically efficient germplasm with high water use efficiency (WUE), reduced crop maturity duration fitting into rainfall patterns.

Table 9. Certain new considerations for re-evaluation of germplasm and development of superior lines

8.2. Role of private seed companies in germplasm development-a new trend

Prior to the formation of National Seeds Corporation and the State Seed Corporations during the 1960s to 1970s in the Public sector, the entire responsibility of cultivar development, seed multiplication and seed distribution coupled with extension rested with the government agencies and even farmer to farmer seed exchanges. After the Seed Corporations were established, the responsibility for producing breeder seeds rested with the original breeder in the research centres, but the further stages of seed multiplication, quality control and distribution were taken over by State Seed Corporations. With the opening up of breeding and seed development to private sector after 1970s, the private sector started developing hybrid cotton genotypes of a proprietary nature and started the seed business right by establishing their own R&D Units approved by the Department of Science and Technology and ICAR. The parental secrecy was sacrosanct for remaining in seed business and the private seed companies started developing their own parental genotypes and developing superior hybrid combinations and undertook supply of quality seeds to farmers after testing under the "All India Coordinated Cotton Improvement Project" (AICCIP) in multi-locations. In 2002-03, when the transgenic Bollgard-I cotton was introduced and followed later by Bollgard-II cotton in 2006-07, Monsanto, the global seed giant and the owner of the gene patent made suitable arrangements with Mahyco-Monsanto Company to make the gene source available to over 25 cooperating seed companies on sub-licensing basis. At this stage, the publicly bred variety and public sector seed distribution became insignificant. The private seed companies devoted attention to more than 95 per cent transgenic hybrid cotton development, predominantly *hirsutum* x *hirsutum* and a small extent of *hirsutum* x *barbadense* hybrids. The planting seed quality control and commercial seed distribution to cotton growers all over India were also intensified with proprietary hybrids by the seed companies and thereby passed on the reins of seed business to the private seed industry. There are over 650 seed companies in India with about 30-40 of them having a modern to good level R&D and hybrids were released after testing under the aegies of the Genetic and Engineering Approval Committee (GEAC) under the Department of Biotechnology (DBT) and Ministry of Environment and Forests (MoEF) implementing as per EPA regulations.

It was in the last 15-18 years after the post GATT scenario, that the germplasm availability to private seed companies faced constraints, besides non-availability. This came as a promising era to develop their own germplasm by breaking down available hybrids and cross combinations in each Seed Company and reverse pedigree breeding approaches coupled with stringent selection and inter-mating to make new character associations. Many major seed companies thus have made huge germplasm sources maintained as proprietary germplasm. Over 1500 hybrids in transgenic constitution were developed and released by the private seed companies in the last one decade [33, 41].

The character modifications in private seed industry germplasm inter-alia included big (5.5 to 7.2g) and medium boll (4-5g) types, sucking pest resistance, higher boll development with synchrony of reduced plant vegetative duration of 160-170days, long, superior medium and extra-long staple fibre categories, resistance to CLCuV for the northern zone cotton growing areas, moderate drought resistance, high fertilizer efficiency coupled with response for superior management technologies etc., as well as bollworm resistance through BG-I and BG-II Cry gene systems. Even plant type concept has been applied in recent years for higher planting densities and suitability for machine harvesting envisaged for adoption in the next five years or sooner. The Round-up Ready herbicide resistance technology and similar ones are also at its nascent stage in approved seed companies for releasing subject to relaxation of moratoriums by Government and releasing for adoption by farmers.

The private seed companies maintain their own germplasm accessions in cold storage modules and germplasm use as per requirements. Secrecy and privacy is maintained. The seed companies also have their own commercial assessment of germplasm potentials and maintain descriptive records as per business requirements and also as per (Distinctness, Uniformity and Stability) DUS characterization evolved by the PPVFR Authority. It is difficult to acquire information on the wealth of new germplasm developed, utilized and maintained by private seed companies, because of their proprietary nature. However, they are immense in number and variability and serve as the most directly usable material in hybrid development. Competition among private seed companies is acute and hence product development by various seed companies for farmers' use should not only be attractive, but also shine in contrast and popularity compared to those of competitors with high performance potentials. In recent years, big boll hybrids with 6-7.5gram boll weight have been developed by private seed companies as available in hybrids like MRC 7351, Mallika, Sigma, Jackpot, Indravajram, Ajeet 99, RCH 530, and Vikram 5.

Public sector developed varieties were popular and some of them became parents of H x H hybrids and also in H x B hybrids, when the hybrid cotton era dawned for the first time in the world only in India since 1970s. Private seed industry started developing since then and gradually became the dominant developer of proprietary hybrids and primary distributer of quality seeds. With the advent of the transgenic Bt-hybrid cottons from 2002, the private seed industry became the primary source of superior hybrids and total supplier of quality seeds all over the country. In transgenic group, Bunny, Mallika, RCH2, other RCH, Sigma, Dyna, Brahma, MECH-series, Thulasi 4, JKCH99, Ankur 651 and others became popular. In all, 590-600 private seed companies existed and more than 1500 Bt-cotton hybrids were released, but only some 20-25 commanded more than 85% in seed distribution. Prominent Seed Companies including Mahyco, Rasi, Nuziveedu, Vibha Seeds Group, Ankur Seeds, Thulasi Seeds, Bioseeds and certain others are leading in cotton R&D and extent of seed distribution amounting to 30-35 million seed packets (400g transgenic seeds and 50g refugee seeds per packet) per year is estimated at approximately US$ 525 million [41]. With seed rates increasing in recent years, the requirement would increase to 50 million seed packets per year in the next few years.

8.3. Pre-breeding and development of advanced breeding lines from existing germplasm

The public sector institutions like the CICR and SAUs are involved in such basic breeding activities and development of a large number of advanced lines are reported and the effort is continuing. Work is targeted towards big boll, plant type for mechanical harvesting by accommodating denser plant populations, reduction of crop duration, higher level of resistance to sucking pests and new maladies, besides high photosynthetic efficiency for high yields and even resistance to drought stress and restricted water use under emerging climate adversities [37]. Some of the SAUs and the CICR have previously developed superior varieties / germplasm like LRA5166, Narasimha, Brahma, and MCU5 in *G. hirsutum* and Suvin, SB 289E and SB 1085-6 in *G. barbadense,* most of which have served as versatile parents for superior hybrid development. A limited number of *G. hirsutum* germplasm and varieties have proved as proven parents in very many hybrids generated by the seed industry. Development of a large number of improved germplasm lines are in progress in various research centres, but precise information on such results are yet to be made available.

http://dx.doi.org/10.5772/58622

8.4. New techniques and new trends in germplasm assessment

Multi-location evaluation of elite proprietary germplasm is also being adopted by seed companies for precise choice for parents of newer hybrids for different regions. Marker-assisted selection and recurrent selections are adopted by forward looking seed companies for superior parent selection and improvement of fibre quality attributes. Biotechnological tools and scouting for alien gene sources like that of Cry genes for various other envisaged character improvements by the multinational seed companies like Monsanto, Bayer CropScience etc., is also gaining importance in new gene source identification and crop improvement. Traditional applications in germplasm evaluation have undergone significant change and new germplasm developed by private sector and under special programmes in Government R&D centres are targeting the challenging sustainability and competition requirements of the 21st century in the field performance and in industrial applications as issues as discussed in this chapter. In the context of hybrid cottons and in the context of transgenic cotton cultivar *vs.* hybrids, germplasm use requires better understanding of the inherent potentials, their genetic performance under the new circumstances and merit based selection for developing new genotypes. DUS characters developed for cotton by the PPVFR Authority is also being adopted for germplasm characterization [38, 33].

8.5. Gaps in collections (quantitative & qualitative)

There are gaps like (1) augmenting the wild species collections to have as many of the total species as may be available in other country centres, except those, which are not available in live collections elsewhere, (2) augmenting the collections of all important cultivars in all the cultivated species from various cotton growing countries including ELS *G. barbadense* and other material, (3) obtaining on exchange basis, the new collections made through recent surveys by various organizations, and (4) advanced breeding material developed in various SAU R&D Centres after 1990 either in possession or as and when developed also may be obtained and added to the national gene pool at the CICR Nagpur, (5) germplasm enhancement and pre-breeding efforts for future needs may be intensified at the CICR, SAUs and also Private seed companies, [24, 29].

Documented standard control varieties are critical for germplasm evaluations. With the current trend in many crops and cotton particularly toward proprietary germplasm, in the future certain "public" germplasm of known pedigree may be primarily important, not for its outstanding agronomic performance, but for its value as a "control". In addition to helping to distinguish environmental from genetic effects on the phenotype, controls may provide a common denominator for standardizing evaluation reports. Instead of presenting raw data, evaluations can be reported as percentages of controls [33].

Marker-assisted selection (MAS) using molecular markers such as single nucleotide polymorphisms (SNPs), is widely used in different agricultural research centers to design genotyping arrays with thousands of markers spread over the entire genome of the crops, especially in interspecific crosses of *G. hirsutum* x *G. barbadense* for fibre quality attributes and also pest and disease resistance. H x B crosses have resulted in H x B hybrids (F_1) with bigger bolls than of *G. barbadense* parent, ELS (35-38 mm), higher lint index, wider adaptability, yield potential and pest tolerance. Elucidating the genetic control of given traits is important to decide the merit in a specific germplasm. The gene action affecting phenotypes is elucidated by crosses and by recombination in progeny of backcrosses or segregating generations. Dominance becomes apparent in F_1, BC and F_2 generations, as do heritability, and deviations from Mendelian ratios resulting from epistasis, pleiotropic and maternal effects. Molecular-marker characterization can assist with "pyramiding" resistance alleles at different loci to produce more durable resistance to biotic/abiotic stresses. Extensive genome mapping projects of *Gossypium* species *via* the co-segregation of molecular markers and important traits of agronomic value can also help to determine the gene action underlying phenotypes. The need for undertaking planned adoption of MAS systems is emphasized especially for improvement of fibre quality parameters and disease resistance attributes to enable choice selection of germplasm for rapid crop improvement.

More effective accessibility and use of plant genetic resources for crop improvement is essential, since conservation at huge cost without use has little merit. Plant genetic resources of crops especially cotton are conserved for use by people as fibre, food, feed, fuel etc. On the contrary, use without conservation amounts to neglecting the genetic base needed by farmers and breeders alike to increase productivity in the future. To be of use, material held in gene banks must be well documented by adopting all modern techniques as well as field evaluation. Only a very small fraction of the genetic diversity residing in *Gossypium* genus is represented in working collections and improved elite cotton germplasm. Genetic diversity in elite germplasm is reported to be narrow and diversity on the farm is still narrower due to preferential planting of successful cultivars and breeding techniques that tend to promote an over-reliance on a few genotypes. Considering the narrow genetic base of cultivars and commercially elite germplasm, it would be necessary to exploit the diversity residing in wild, commensal, and landrace cottons of six allo-tetraploid and forty-three diploid species of *Gossypium* genus as it may be rewarding. Resources including recombinant inbred line (RIL) populations, back-cross introgression line (BIL) populations, near isogenic introgression line (NIIL) populations, chromosome substitution lines, day-neutral converted race stocks, etc., may also be outsourced from global R & D Centres, conserved and used in Indian gene bank and breeding programmes. The importance of building up new germplasm of breeding value through proper utilization of gene pools has also been emphasized by [39, 40].

8.6. Registration of newly developed germplasm

NBPGR New Delhi has established norms for new germplasm registration by the breeders and it could also be got protected under (Protection of Plant Varieties and Farmers' Rights Act (PPVFRA) especially to protect from poaching and breeders may be encouraged to avail of this and increase their efforts, Guidelines for registration of plant germplasm (revised, 2014) NBPGR, New Delhi. The information could be accessed from NBPGR Website <https://www.nbpgr.ernet.in.>. The information will also be published in the Indian Journal of Plant Genetic Resources functioning at its headquarters by the Member Secretary, Plant Germplasm Registration Committee, National Bureau of Plant Genetic Resource, Pusa Campus, New Delhi-110 012,

http://dx.doi.org/10.5772/58622

9. Conclusion

Cotton is a major global agricultural commodity in the World in over 100 countries including India. Cotton is also a widely preferred natural textile fibre for the industry. India is currently the second largest producer, consumer and exporter of cotton with the second largest textile industry after China. Presently, cotton is produced in a little over 11.5million ha in India and all the four cultivated species (*G. hirsutum, G. barbadense, G. arboreum,* and *G. herbaceum*) are still grown, but *G. hirsutum* cotton predominates in over 90 per cent of the area. From 1970, in addition to varieties, F_1 commercial hybrids of *G. hirsutum* x *G. hirsutum* and in small extent *G. hirsutum* x *G. barbadense* F_1 hybrids were also grown in a sizable area. The diploid interspecies F_1 hybrids of *G. herbaceum* x *G. arboreum* were also developed and made available for cultivation, but their cultivation by farmers remained stagnant due to hybrid seed production constraints. Cytoplasmic male sterility based (*G. harknessii*) source with USA based restorer sources were used for developing few *G. hirsutum* x *G. hirsutum* hybrids with a view to reduce cost of hybrid seed production and this strategy did not meet with the expected level of success in seed production, area coverage and yield gains. USA line "Gregg GMS" based genetic male sterility was also used for developing a few hybrids and the adoption rate was low for various reasons. A local GMS source was identified in *G. arboreum* background for the production of diploid cotton hybrids by the SAU at Hisar (Haryana state), but not much headway was made.

In 2002-2003, the transgenic cotton (genetically modified cotton) was introduced into cultivation in India first with Bollgard-I (Cry1Ac) and subsequently the Bollgard-II (Cry1Ac+Cry2Ab) and the transgenic cottons were all based on proprietary germplasm and hybrids were predominantly of *G. hirsutum* x *G. hirsutum* combinations. As a result, predominantly *G. hirsutum* x *G. hirsutum* based transgenic cotton hybrids are grown in more than 10.0 million ha corresponding to over 90 per cent of the total area under cotton [16].

Since 1960, the Indian collection has grown with the establishment of the Indian Central Cotton Committee, the All India Coordinated Cotton Improvement Project, and the Central Institute for Cotton Research (CICR). In 1976, the Central Institute for Cotton Research was established with a mandate to function as National Centre for Cotton Genetic Resources collection, documentation, and utilization. Hence, the Central Institute for Cotton Research functioning under the Indian Council of Agricultural Research, New Delhi, an autonomous body under the Government of India is looking after the major responsibility for collection, conservation, evaluation, characterization, documentation and utilization of cotton genetic resources in India with the National Gene Bank at Nagpur. The CICR is collaborating with the National Bureau of Plant Genetic Resources (NBPGR) New Delhi for planning germplasm surveys, exchange, collection and conservation under long term storage facility established for all crops at NBPGR. The entire cotton germplasm collection (total cotton gene pool available in India) is primarily maintained in short and medium storage conditions at the Central Institute for Cotton Research (CICR), Nagpur and its Regional station at Coimbatore (additional set of *G. barbadense* collection). Funding for the CICR and the NBPGR is provided by the Indian Council for Agricultural Research that is an autonomous organization of the Indian Ministry of Agriculture-Department of Agricultural Research and Education (DARE), New Delhi.

The total collection exceeding 10, 000 accessions including small additions in the last couple of years represent almost entirely cultivated accessions of *G. hirsutum, G. barbadense, G. arboreum,* and *G. herbaceum*. In addition, the collection also consists of race stock accessions of each cultivated species, 26 wild species, and 32 synthetic introgression derivatives. Long-term storage of cultivated species are managed by NBPGR in New Delhi and maintained at minus 20°C. A working collection of all cultivated accessions, excluding *G. barbadense* accessions, is stored at Nagpur and maintained at 4°C. *G. barbadense* accessions are stored at Coimbatore and maintained. Wild species and race stock working collections are exclusively maintained at Nagpur *in vivo* under natural field conditions as a species garden. Seed of germplasm accessions are renewed by planned seed increases that include forced self-pollination. The accessions are multiplied in phases to keep fresh seeds without losing viability for a period of three years under short term storage and for frequent use by the breeders and other scientists.

Regular collection expeditions were organized by the National Germplasm Centre in collaboration with the NBPGR in various parts of the country. In recent years, plant explorations have covered a large part of India, and several plant exploration trips are planned through in the future. These include exploration of Mizoram, Sundarban (West Bengal), Assam (Kamroop hills and Jayanti hills), Meghalaya (East Garo Hills), and Tripura. The collection has also grown through exchange with the United States of America, France, Uzbekistan, and Czechoslovakia. The FAO-organized germplasm expeditions also provide opportunities to expand the germplasm collection.

Evaluation and characterization of cultivated germplasm accessions are performed based on cotton descriptors and index card developed by the CICR. Evaluation and characterization of cultivated germplasm include morphological, taxonomical, yield, and yield-contributing characters, fiber quality parameters, and reaction to biotic and abiotic stresses. Basic studies are also performed on the structural variation of gossypol and nectar glands, pollen grains, stigma receptivity, cytogenetic studies, and cross-compatibility among various species (wild and cultivated). Accessions of *G. hirsutum* and *G. arboreum* are evaluated in multi-location evaluation trials conducted at three locations within India (Sirsa, North zone-irrigated; Nagpur, Central zone-rain-fed; and Coimbatore, South zone (irrigated). Accessions are evaluated for yield, boll weight, ginning out-turn fiber properties, and reaction to pests and diseases, and promising genotypes are distributed to breeders and researchers at various cotton research stations and government Institutions within India for research purposes only. Germplasm accession data are maintained by the NBPGR and data are freely available only to Indian government organizations. Official germplasm seed requests are made through NBPGR and a special application form is required to procure exotic germplasm. The NBPGR then determines if a Material Transfer Agreement is already available with the requesting country and makes the necessary correspondence. The seed material is subsequently distributed through NBPGR and Central Institute for Cotton Research on the basis of request. New germplasm is also being generated by the CICR and other SAUs and frequently added to the National Gene Bank at CICR. There are gaps, which are sought to be augmented by inter-country exchanges, explorations and from own development through breeding efforts. There is till now no International Institute for Cotton Research under the CGIAR system. In the era of transgenic cultivars/hybrids, the maintenance of original (unconverted) germplasm receives priority attention so as not to lose the valuable germplasm collected and maintained over several decades. Molecular marker tools are recommended for the evaluation of germplasm in India for identification of various hidden potentials and some work has already been initiated by certain private seed companies and the NBPGR / the CICR and certain SAUs in the country.

Acknowledgements

The authors are grateful to anonymous reviewers of the manuscript and the book editor for critically going through the manuscript and offering valuable suggestions and editorial corrections for improving the quality and content of this chapter.

Author details

S.S. Narayanan[1*], Parchuri Vidyasagar[2] and K. Srinivasu Babu[3]

*Address all correspondence to: narayananss@rediffmail.com

1 Central Institute for Cotton Research (CICR), Nagpur, India

2 Vibha Seeds Group Ltd; Hyderabad, India

3 Namdhari Seeds Private Ltd., Bangalore at Hyderabad, India

References

[1] Sundaram V. Antiquity of cotton, In: 50 Years of Research at Cotton Technological Research Laboratory; Indian Council of Agricultural Research, New Delhi, India, 1974 p. 212.

[2] Santhanam V, Sundaram V. Historical perspective of cotton in India, In: Hand book of Cotton in India eds. Sundaram V, Basu A K, Krishna Iyer K R, Narayanan S S, Rajendran T P. pub: Indian Society for Cotton Improvement, Mumbai, 1999, pp.1-17

[3] Sikka, SM. Joshi AB. Cotton breeding-In: Cotton in India, A Monograph-Vol. I. pub: Indian Central Cotton Committee, Bombay, India1960 pp. 137-335.

[4] Fred E Gillham M, Thomas M. Bell, Tijen Arin, Graham A. Matthews, Claude Le Rumeur,, and A. Brian Hear-Cotton Production Prospects for the Next Decade, pub:

The International Bank for Reconstruction and Development / The World Bank 1818 H Street, N.W. Washington, D.C. 20433, U.S.A.1995, p.1-300

[5] Santhanam V. Sundaram V. Agri-history of Cotton in India-An Overview; in: *Asian Agri-History* 1997 Vol.1, No.4, pp. 235-251.

[6] Anupam Barik. Cotton Statistics at a Glance, Pub. Directorate of Cotton Development, Ministry of Agriculture, Government of India, Mumbai and Director, National Centre for Integrated Pest Management, New Delhi; 2010, pp.148

[7] Terry P. Townsend. "A Balanced Perspective on Cotton: Responding to Valid Problems, Challenging Irresponsible Critics" Report of the Executive Director to the 69th Plenary Meeting of The International Cotton Advisory Committee, Lubbock, TX, USA September 20-25, 2010

[8] Agarwal O P. Cotton Economy in India (1780), pub. COTAAP Research Foundation, (Cotton Association of India) MUMBAI, India February 2012, p.1-12

[9] Armelle Gruère. ICAC Reprint from Cotton: Review of the World Situation, Volume 64-No 5 May-June 2011

[10] Narayanan SS. Exploitation of the potentials of *hirsutum* cotton for cottonseed oil and other by-products, Asian Textile Journal, 2014 (*In Press*).

[11] Wikipedia 2013 Euro bank Notes paper and currency economy in the world

[12] Singh M. Raut RN. Genetical research on Cotton and Jute 1983 pp. 154 191; In GENETIC RESEARCH IN INDIA Eds., Jaiswal PL. and Wadhwani AM.). Publications and Information Division, ICAR, New Delhi

[13] Anonymous. 'Research achievements A decade' In: Scientific Monograph No. 11, 1987, Eds. Chandel, KPS &. Singh, BM); pub: National Bureau of Plant Genetic Resources, New Delhi 110 012; India.

[14] Narayanan SS. Singh VV. Kothandaraman R. Cotton Genetic Resources in India; In: Cotton Scenario in India A Souvenir, pub: Central Institute for Cotton Research (ICAR), Nagpur 1990 pp.9 20.

[15] Singh VV. Punit Mohan. Narayanan SS. Cotton Genetic Resources, In: HAND BOOK OF COTTON IN INDIA, Eds: Sundaram V. Basu A K. Krishna Iyer K R. Narayanan S S. Rajendran T P. pub: Indian Society for Cotton Improvement, Mumbai, 1999 p18 40.

[16] Clive James, Global Status of Commercialized Biotech/GM Crops: 2013; Cotton Statistics & News, 2014 No. 51 p1 12

[17] Mare Gilband. Dominique Dessauw. Paulo AV. Barroso. Part 1. Cotton Taxonomy, Breeding & Production Chapter 1. Cotton Taxonomy, Origin and Domestication, In: Cotton Technology for the 21st Century pub: International Cotton Advisory Committee, USA 2010 pp. 5 17.

[18] Fryxell PA. Natural History of the Cotton Tribe, College Station, 1979 Texas A&M University Press.

[19] Narayanan SS. Singh J. Varma PK. Review of genetic wealth in *Gossypium* with special reference to wild species; *Indian society for Cotton Improvement Journal (ISCIJ)*: 1985 p: 51 64.

[20] Fryxell PA. A revised taxonomic interpretation of *Gossypium L. (Malvaceae)*: *Rheedea* 1992: 2(2) p108 165.

[21] Endrizzi JE, Turcote EL, Kohel RJ. Genetics, Cytology and Evolution of *Gossypium Adv. Genet.* 1985 23, 271 335.

[22] Percival AE. Wendel JF. Stewart, JM. Taxonomy and germplasm resources. In: Smith CW and Cothren COTTON: ORIGIN, HISTORY, TECHNOLOGY & PRODUCTION, New York John Wiley & Sons Inc.1990 pp. 33 63

[23] Anonymous. A CATALOGUE OF COTTON GENETIC RESOURCES IN INDIA, Ed. Narayanan, SS. *et al*. 1989 pp.484; pub: Central Institute for Cotton Research, Nagpur (India).

[24] Basu AK, Narayanan SS. Genetics, Cytogenetics and Breeding of Crop Plants (Cotton), Vol.2 Cereal and commercial crops - Cotton, Eds. Bahl PN, Salimath PM and Mandal AK Pub: Oxford & IBH Publishing Co. Pvt. Ltd, New Delhi, 1997 pp: 267 318.

[25] Tripathi KK. Govila OP. Ranjini Warrier. Vibha Ahuja. Biology of *Gossypium spp.* (Cotton): pub: Department of Biotechnology, Ministry of Science & Technology and Ministry of Environment and Forests, Government of India New Delhi 2011 pp:1 50.

[26] Campbell BT, Saha S, Percy R, Frelichowski J, Jenkins JN, Park W, Mayee CD, Gotmare V, Dessauw D, Giband M, Du X, Jia Y, Constable G, Dillon S, Abdurakhmonov IY, Abdukarimov A, Rizaeva SM, Adullaev A, Barroso PAV, Pádua JG, Hoff Mann LV, & Podolnaya L. Status of the Global Cotton Germplasm Resources, *Crop Science,* Vol. 50 July–August, 2010 (*www.crops.org 1179*).

[27] Paopla Fortucci The contribution of cotton to economy and food security in developing countries, Report by ICAC, 2002, p1 10

[28] Narayanan SS. Singh J. Varma PK. Introgressive Gene Transfer in *Gossypium* Goals, Problems, Strategies and Achievement, *Cot. Fib. Tropicales*, 1984 39(4) p123 135

[29] Bhale NL, Narayanan, SS. Need for augmenting Genetic Resources of Cotton Indian Perspective In: "PLANT GENETIC RESOURCES INDIAN PERSPECTIVE" Eds. Paroda RS, Arora RK, Chandel KPS. NBPGR New Delhi 1988 pp.220 231.

[30] Gotmare V. Singh P. Tule BN. Wild and Cultivated Species of Cotton, 2006 *CICR Technical Bulletin* 5, pp.21, Nagpur, India.

[31] Basu AK, Paroda RS. 'Hybrid Cotton in India – A Success Story' Asia Pacific Association of Agricultural Research Institutions, FAO Regional Office for Asia and the Pacific, Bangkok, Thailand, 1995 pp. 38.

[32] Bhale N L. Heterosis Breeding In HAND BOOK OF COTTON IN INDIA eds. Sundaram V. Basu A K. Krishna Iyer K R, Narayanan S S. Rajendran T P. pub: Indian Society for Cotton Improvement, Mumbai, 1999, pp.57 78

[33] Narayanan SS. Innovative research under IP regimes with special reference to cotton *Asian Textile Journal* December, 2013 pp.65 72

[34] Phundan Singh. Narayanan SS. Cotton Improvement Procedures In: HAND BOOK OF COTTON IN INDIA, Eds: Sundaram V. Basu A K. Krishna Iyer K R. Narayanan S S. Rajendran T P. pub: Indian Society for Cotton Improvement, Mumbai, 1999 p.41 56.

[35] Anurudh K. Singh. Dhillon BS. Chapter 52, National Network on Conservation of Plant Genetic Resources SEED IN INDIA, SEED CONSERVATION: TURNING SCIENCE INTO PRACTICE, Eds. Smith RD, Dickie JB, Linington SH. Pritchard HW. and Robert RJ. London: The Royal Botanic Gardens, Kew, 2003 pp. 1023.

[36] Cotton International Annual; New Frontiers envisioning cotton's future, Meister Publication, 2014 pp.145.

[37] Loknathan TR. Phundan Singh. Agarwal RJ. Punit.Mohan. Suman Bala Singh. Vinita Gotmare. Singh VV. Genetic Enhancement of Cotton, 2003, *CICR Technical Bulletin* 26 pp. 16, Nagpur, India.

[38] Rathinavel K. Manickam S. Gururajan N. Deshmukh RK. Shanthy V. Draft National Guidelines for the conduct of DUS Test of Cotton (*Gossypium* Spp.), compiled by AICCIP; 2006 pp1 40, Central Institute for Cotton Research, Regional Station, Coimbatore, India.

[39] Malik SS. Singh SP. Role of plant genetic resources in sustainable agriculture *Indian J. Crop Science*, 2006, 1(1 2) p.21 28.

[40] Percy G. *Gossypium* Germplasm Resources for Cotton Improvement Genomics and Biotechnology, ARS USDA, 2009 pp18.

[41] Parchuri Vidyasagar. "Cotton Improvement in India – Contribution and Perspectives of Private Seed Industry" Dr. V. Sundaram Memorial Lecture Series (2011), 09 June 2011 pp 1 26 pub: Indian Society for Cotton Improvement (ISCI) at Central Institute for Research on Cotton Technology (ICAR) Mumbai (India).

[42] CICR Nagpur "The Cotton Innovate – CICR Newsletter" weekly publication (June 2013) by Central Institute for Cotton Research Post Bag No. 2, Shankar Nagar PO, Nagpur 440010 Phone : 07103 275536 Fax : 07103 275529; email: cicrnagpur@gmail.com; CICR Official website: www.cicr.org.in.

Chapter 5

Usefulness and Utilization of Indian Cotton Germplasm

N. Manikanda Boopathi, S. Sathish,
P. Dachinamoorthy, P. Kavitha and R. Ravikesavan

Additional information is available at the end of the chapter

http://dx.doi.org/10.5772/58619

1. Introduction

Cotton, jute and similar fibre crops are the key money-makers in Indian agriculture sector. India has the largest area of global cotton cultivation that contributes 23% to the global cotton production. Cotton plays a key role in the Indian economy in terms of income generation in the agricultural and industrial sectors. Textiles and related exports account for nearly 33% of the total foreign exchange earnings (~12 billion dollars) of India and it is projected that there will be a significant increase in the coming year [1].

Cotton is cultivated in three different zones (northern, central and southern) of India. Approximately 65% of India's cotton is produced on dry land and 35% on irrigated lands. The northern zone is almost totally irrigated, while the percentage of irrigated area is much lower in the central (23%) and southern zones (40%). Under the non-irrigated conditions, annual rainfall ranges from less than 400 to more than 900 mm coupled with unusual patterns over the years which lead to large-scale fluctuations in cotton production [2].

It is estimated that around 20 million farmers cultivate cotton in India and about 46 million persons are employed directly by the ginning, pressing, trade, knitting, handloom, processing and cotton related textile industry and thus cotton cultivation and textile utilization is the second largest employer after general agriculture. There are more than 2,500 spinning mills and 250 composite mills in India having an installed capacity of approximately 35 million spindles, 1.7 million power looms/handlooms and thousands of garment, hosiery and processing (dyeing and printing) units [3]. The decentralized sector comprising power looms and handlooms, provide employment to over 2.5 million people [4]. Others include thousands of garment manufacturing units, over 3500 ginning and pressing factories and several marketing organizations of raw cotton, yarns, fabrics and garments.

Since India has a large domestic textile industry, the mill consumption of cotton in the country has been continuously on the raise from the beginning of the 1990s. There was a leap in domestic cotton consumption in 2012-13 from 22.9 (in 2009-10) to 27.6 million bales, and in some cases, cotton lint was imported from China [5]. Since the economic liberalization began in 1991, there has been an impressive increase in the export of cotton. In addition to yarns, fabrics and garments, whose exports have been steadily rising in recent years, raw cotton is also permitted to be exported from time to time [6]. Therefore cotton production in India has boundless impact not only on the livelihood of the farmers and economy of the country, but also on international trade. Further, global textile market demands for increased fibre uniformity, strength, extensibility, and novel value added quality. This clearly justify the importance of new and innovative approaches toward evaluating, understanding and utilizing the available cotton germplasm and they are discussed in this chapter.

2. Historical perspectives of cotton germplasm utilization in India

The time when cotton fibre was first used in India for cloth or other textile fabric making could not be dertemined precisely. The first reference to cotton is found in rig Veda hymn [7]. The stages of seed cotton, spinning the lint and weaving the yarn are covered in various religious texts and thus suggest the implicit use of cotton in India by 1000 BC [8]. The cotton textile trade is considered ancient since it was shown that Indian cotton fabrics have been found in the tombs of the Pharaohs [9]. From time immemorial, India was the only country that was known for its cotton fabrics when the rest of the world was being dressed mostly in wool [10]. The fabrics dated approximately 3000 BC recovered from Mohenjo-Daro excavated in Sind were identified to have originated from cotton plants, closely linked to *Gossypium arboreum* [11], thereby confirming that cotton lint was spun and woven into cloth even before 3000 BC. In some of the ancient literatures, perennial cotton trade was reported in the beginning of the Christian era. Colourful and designer handloom fabrics and apparels of India were regularly imported by Egypt, Greece, Rome and China [12]. All Indian cottons in the 13th century were perennials and they were in cultivation until recently. Bushy perennial forms of cotton are still being maintained in remote villages of Rajasthan, Uttar Pradesh and Andhra Pradesh. The East Indian Company (which was the major trader in exporting the Indian cotton to Inter-Asian and European countries [9]) recognized three trade varieties of cotton during the 18th century: 1. *Tinnies* (which is a mixture of *Karunganni* belonging to *G. arboreum* race *wightianum*) 2. *Salems* (which is also a mixture of perennial native cotton *Nadan* (meaning native) belonging to *G. arboreum* race *indicum* and *uppam;* in addition another perennial cotton belonging to the group of *G. hirsutum* L. race *punctatum* introduced by the East India Company in the late 18th Century was also included in this category) and 3. *Karunganni* (which belongs to *G. arboreum*) cotton [12].

Rozi cottons belonging to *G. arboreum* were supposed to be the ancient commercial type. Vizagapattinam of Andhra Pradesh is the place of differentiation of *indicum*. The perennial *Nadan* cotton of the Southernmost part of Tamil Nadu is the progenitor of *Karunganni* variety (belonging to *G. hirsutum*), which has excellent drought tolerance and can provide significant yield under water limited environments. In all the places, selection towards an annual habit type was carried out. Another component is known as *uppam* belonging to *G. herbaceum*. The name *uppam* is synonymous with both *Ukkan* and Udumalpet cottons. Since the early cultivation was centred on Udumalpet in Tamil Nadu, it was named after the place. The other name *Ukkan* has been interpreted to mean that *Vokkalegas* who hailed from Chittaldurg and Dharwad districts of Karnataka and settled in western parts of Coimbatore district in Tamil Nadu, brought the cotton with them during their migration. The women of this community were known to spend their spare time in ginning and spinning cotton. The name *uppam* cotton in Southern tip of Peninsula may have been due to its property of swelling (*uppal* in Tamil) of the kapas by sea breeze (*uppu katru* in Tamil) under whose influence it thrives well in eastern coastal parts of India [12].

Presently, all the four cultivated cotton species (*G. hirsutum, G. barbadense* L., *G. arboreum* and *G. herbaceum* L.) are being commercially cultivated in India. The diploid cotton (*G. arboreum* and *G. herbaceum*) are indigenous to Asia and Africa and are popularly referred to as desi cottons in India. They are mainly cultivated in dry land tracts, though Bengal desi is grown under irrigated situations in the northern states. *G. hirsutum* is known as the American cotton and most popular varieties and hybrids now under cultivation (nearly 90% of plantings) belong to this group. *G. barbadense* is popularly known as the Egyptian cotton and is grown in small area in India. These two new world cottons, i.e., the tetraploid (2n=52) species of *G. hirsutum* and *G. barbadense* were initially introduced into India during the 17th and 18th centuries [13].

Thus it can be clearly conceptualized that the history of cotton and textiles in India is the true representation of the history of the utilization of cotton germplasm and growth of the modern industries in India. It is believed that modern cotton varietal improvement program in India was started as early as 1901. The earlier part of 20th century witnessed cultivation of desi cotton varieties which mature in 200 days and were poor yielding but endowed with resistance to pest, disease and drought. The objectives of breeding program during those days were mainly focused on breeding for short duration and increased yield. Cotton varietal improvement program has employed all the breeding strategies such as introduction, mass selection, pedigree selection, intra-and inter-specific hybridization, backcrossing and induced mutations.

The East India Company made many attempts to improve the native cotton of Tamil Nadu, India. It tried to introduce the American tetraploid cotton. However, all their attempts were unsuccessful. During 1904-05, a chance introduction of an American cotton, cultivated in Cambodia (the present Kampuchea), indicated the possibility of raising it under irrigated conditions. Within three or four years, it spread throughout the Southern Districts of Tamil Nadu and got the name "Tirunelveli American". Later, it spread throughout Tamil Nadu and came to be known as "Cambodia Cotton" in the Southern peninsula and laid the foundation for strong establishment of cotton ginning, spinning and weaving industry in South India [12]. For example, efforts to release American tetraploids were responsible for the release of a cultivar, CO 2 (a pure selection of Cambodia bulk) and several MCU (Madras-Cambodia-

Uganda) series which formed the basis of all cotton improvement programs in Tamil Nadu and other parts of South India [12].

India is the first country to grow hybrid cotton on a commercial scale since the 1970s. During those periods, hybrid seeds were produced by hand emasculation and pollination and the first intra-*hirsutum* hybrid, Hybrid-4, were released from Gujarat Agricultural University, Surat, India in 1971. In subsequent years, it covered 26.8 percent of the total cotton cultivated area in India and contributed 50 percent of the national cotton production [6]. Considering the importance of hybrids in Indian cotton scenario and its market potential in abroad, several hybrids were released such as Varalaxmi, DCH 32 in successive years. In Tamil Nadu, TCHB213 an inter-specific hybrid with high yield potential with superior qualities (such as high elongation percentage that fit to hosiery, resistant to reiniform nematodes and spinning capacity of 100s counts etc.,) was released in 1990.

3. Cotton germplasm at public institutes

Genetic improvement of cotton for higher yield, superior fibre quality, improved agronomic performance and resistance to pest and diseases is the important research agenda in several agricultural Universities and institutes in India. Collection, storage, maintenance and utilization of cotton germplasm activities in the key institutes are described hereunder:

3.1. CICR, Nagpur

With a view to develop a centre of excellence for carrying out long term research on fundamental problems limiting cotton production and also to provide support to research work on cotton, the Indian Council of Agricultural Research has established the Central Institute for Cotton Research (CICR) at Nagpur in April, 1976. The National Centre for Cotton Genetic Resources, which was re-designated as National Cotton Gene Bank, has been established at CICR, Nagpur as *in situ* species garden.

This bank contains totally 10227 accessions including 7484 accessions of *G. hirsutum*, 263 *G. barbadense*, 1877 *G. arboreum*, 530 *G. herbaceum*, 26 wild species, 32 perennials and 15 races of cultivated species and cytogenetic materials. This is one among the globally recognized centres that maintain large collections of cotton germplasm [2]. According to the genomic groupings, germplasm accessions have organized as primary germplasm pools (comprising germplasm accessions with AD genomes), secondary germplasm pools (including germplasm accessions with A, B, F and D genomes) and tertiary germplasm pools (containing germplasm lines with C, G, K and E genomes) [2, 3]. Each pool contains current and obsolete cultivars, breeding stocks, primitive and wild accessions, land races and subspecies. In accordance with the international board of plant genetic resources, the cotton germplasm has been further classified into core collections and working / active collections. The latter are elite stocks of cultivated species and selected cytoplasmic male sterile derived lines that are actively used in breeding and genetic studies. Germplasm banks were also established under AICCIP in important cotton research centres such as Delhi, Surat, Indore, Akola, Nanded, Nandyal and Coimbatore.

Few cytomorphologically stable male sterile plants have been identified from the derivatives of multispecies hybrids involving wild species *G. raimondii, G. thurberi, G. hirsutum* and *G. barbadense*. One hundred and thirty seven *harknessii* cytoplasmic male sterile (CMS) lines, 15 *aridum* CMS lines, 19 genetic male sterile (GMS) lines and 57 restorer lines are being maintained through crossing, sibmating and selfing at CICR. For genetic improvement of CMS and GMS lines, they were treated with physical (gamma rays) and chemical mutagen (ethyl methane sulphonate) and being maintained [16].

Desi cotton species have originated in India, particularly the three geographical races of *G. arboreum* L. namely *bengalense, cernuum* and *indicum* and of *G. herbaceum* L. race *wightianum*. Excavations of Mohenjo-Daro and Harappa have shown that cloth of finest quality of about 300 counts was produced from the *G. arboreum*. Such perennial cotton possesses variability in useful traits like fibre, pest resistance and abiotic stress tolerance. CICR has taken initiative to collect and conserve the landraces of desi cotton and perennials with desirable characters from Maharashtra, Madhya Pradesh, West Bengal, Andhra Pradesh, Mizoram, Meghalaya, Tripura, Gujarat and Tamil Nadu. The important cotton landraces like *Ponduru, Karuganni, Commilla, Uppam* and *Wagad* were collected from different states of India [17].

Seeds of 1517 *G. hirsutum* including 289 exotics and 350 accessions of *G. arboreum* are being maintained at National Bureau of Plant Genetic Resources (NBPGR), New Delhi under long term cold storage, while another set of the same germplasm is being kept in medium term cold storage at CICR, Nagpur. Further, three genetic stocks of *G. arboreum* race *cernuum* immune to grey mildew disease have also been stored at NBPGR, New Delhi.

The germplasm accessions available in the gene bank are regularly being evaluated for major economic characters such as high yield, high boll weight, high ginning out turn and lower maturity period besides their reaction to major pests and diseases. Similarly, the new germplasm lines received every year are also evaluated for a set of agronomic and economic characters. The selected superior accessions will be further evaluated in multi-locations and provided to regional breeding program after validating their usefulness.

3.2. CCS-HAU, Hisar

Evaluation and maintenance of American and Desi cotton germplasm is mandate of CCS Haryana Agricultural University, Hisar. Thirty five genetic male sterile lines have been developed in *G. arboreum* (and six genetic male sterile lines of cotton have been registered with NBPGR, New Delhi) and forty four genetic male sterile lines and forty three cytoplasmic genetic male sterile lines have been developed in *G. hirsutum*. Besides these lines, 55 potential restorers and a large collection of landraces have also been identified and maintained at this University.

3.3. TNAU, Coimbatore

At TNAU, Coimbatore, 1012 accessions of *G. hirsutum,* 149 accessions of *G. barbadense* and wild species of *G. aridum* and *G. hirsutum* race *punctatum* are being maintained and routinely evaluated and used in regional breeding program. Genetic improvement of cotton for improved drought tolerance, pest and disease resistance with better fibre quality traits are being taken up with help of contemporary breeding tools (see below). TNAU's Collaboration with national and international institutes ensured introgression of novel alleles from exotic and other donors.

3.4. UAS, Dharwad

Besides conserving large numbers of *G. hirsutum and G. barbadense* accessions, Regional Research Station – University of Agricultural Sciences, Dharwad maintains several cultures of *G. arboreum* and *G. arboreum* genotypes introgressed with *G. hirsutum* genes. Notable examples in this aspect are cultures DLSA 17 and 19 that are having improved fibre qualities and tolerance to cotton pest and diseases.

3.5. PAU, Ludhiana

An exhaustive germplasm collection, storage and maintenance of several *Gossypium* spp., for fibre yield and superior quality parameters and tolerance to cotton leaf curl virus disease is also in progress at Punjab Agricultural University, Ludhiana and they are regularly being utilized in cotton breeding program.

3.6. Role of AICCIP in germplasm evolution, evaluation and conservation

Launching of All India Co-ordinated Cotton Improvement Program (AICCIP) in 1966 funded by Indian Council of Agricultural Research, New Delhi has been considered as the milestone in cotton genetic improvement efforts in India. The AICCIP in collaboration with State Agricultural Universities made tremendous achievements in cotton production during the last five decades. This program has the following three important mandates: 1) to develop genotypes suitable for different agro-climatic conditions 2) to develop manuals to maximize yield from improved genotypes and 3) to develop effective and economic plant protection measures for location-specific strategies for integrated biotic stress management.

Currently, the AICCIP is in operation with its headquarters at Coimbatore and spread over 21 participating centres involving 16 State Agricultural Universities. They are marked as North (Punjab, Haryana and Rajasthan), Central (Gujarat, Madhya Pradesh, Maharashtra and Orissa) and South Zones (Karnataka, Andhra Pradesh and Tamil Nadu) [3]. The CICR, Nagpur and its Regional Stations at Coimbatore and Sirsa provide basic research support and also take part in some of the strategic research and evaluation activities on Cotton. The Central Institute for Research on Cotton Technology (CIRCOT, ICAR), Mumbai and its regional units are closely associated with AICCIP in assessing the fibre quality parameters of cotton cultures under trial. Major activities of the AICCIP include the evolution of novel varieties and hybrids best suited for different agro-climatic zones, development of sustainable and inexpensive agro-techniques for realizing maximum yields from improved cultivars with economic and effective pest and disease management practices under different environmental conditions.

Numerous agronomical, physiological as well as pest and disease resistance attributes have been studied in detail in the germplasm accessions under AICCIP. Subjective tests like metroglyph analysis, D^2 analysis and combining ability have been done on elite germplasm lines to study the genetic diversity and use the most diverse ones in the breeding programs. There are large variations available in the germplasm for yield attributes, plant traits, flower characteristics, fibre characteristics, oil characteristics, biomass characteristics, leaf characteristics, boll characteristics, seedling characteristics, boll and seed setting efficiency. Several wild species and cultivated species have been utilized to improve the *G. hirsutum* genotypes and bring about both quantitative and qualitative changes in the commercial cultivars [3]. For example, introgression of *G. hirsutum* genes into *G. arboreum* genotype has been successfully attempted at Parphani and Dharwad centres. Similarly, *G. anomalum* genes have been introgressed into *G. arboreum* at Akola. In the same way, *G. aridum* has been successfully utilized in the development of new source of cytoplasmic male sterile lines at Akola and Coimbatore [3].

The germplasm accessions assembled from several parts of the world have also been utilized in India. For instance, Hybrid 4 was developed using the American Nectariless accession. The *G. harknesii* cytoplasm conferring male sterility in *G. hirsutum* genotypes and the restorer genes for *G. harknesii* conferring fertility has been successfully transferred to Indian genotypes and they were utilized for development of cotton hybrids such as PKV Hyb-3. Likewise, *G. aridum* cytoplasm was also utilized to diversify the cytoplasmic male sterility source in several hybrids. Development of varieties such as Deviraj and Devitej (derived from *G. arboreum* and *G. herbaceum*) and MCU5 (derived from *G. hirsutum* and *G. barbadense*) were the result of pioneering research on introgression of favourable alleles from the related species into the elite lines. Similarly, introgression of *G. arboreum* into *G. hirsutum* varieties has resulted in the development of new jassid resistant varieties in *G. hirsutum*. Introduction of *G. barbadense* germplasm in the country as well as their systematic evaluation resulted in the development and release of first *G. barbadense* variety Sujatha by a process of reselection from an Egyptian variety, Karnak in 1969 [3].

In upland cotton, *G. hirsutum*, variety MCU 5 VT resistant to Verticillum wilt was released from CICR, Coimbatore. In *G. arboreum* and *G. herbaceum*, all the varieties released after 1967 are resistant to Fusarium wilt. In *G. hirsutum*, some jassid resistant varieties (B 1007, SRT 1, Khandwa 2, DHY 286, PKV 081) and hybrids (PKV hy2 and NHH 44) have also been released.

Specific varieties and hybrids with wide adaptability have also been released from 1970 onwards. Examples of wide adaptable varieties are Bikaneri Narma, MCU 5, SRT 1 and LRA 5166. Variety Bikaneri Narma was developed in Punjab, which has later cultivated in Haryana, Rajasthan and Northern Madhya Pradesh due to its wide adaptability. By the same token, Variety SRT 1 was released initially for Gujarat; now it is also popular in Maharashtra and Madhya Pradesh. Similarly, varieties MCU 5 and LRA 5166 released for Tamil Nadu, now cultivated in Andhra Pradesh, Maharashtra and Madhya Pradesh by virtue of their wide adaptability. Hybrid H 4 was released for Gujarat state; because of its wide adaptation it spread to other states such as Maharashtra, Madhya Pradesh, Andhra Pradesh and Karnataka. Similarly, hybrid DCH 32 (Jayalaxmi) was released for Karnataka state, but due to its wide adaptability it spread to Tamil Nadu, Andhra Pradesh and Western Maharashtra.

The AICCIP has notified more than 220 cotton varieties and hybrids in 2004 that were released for commercial cultivation with different features such as short and medium duration, leaf curl virus disease resistance, jassid resistance, suitable for rainfed tracts, resistance to Verticillium wilt etc., On the other hand, during 2002, the AICCIP has recommended to de-notify 99 varieties and hybrids that are no longer under cultivation or that are inferior in fibre properties [3].

The problems that impede utilization of germplasm for breeding include photosensitivity, mismatching of blooming period, low fertility index, etc. There is a need for rapid screening of geographically diverse germplasm for useful traits such as low cost technology proposed at CICR, Nagpur for rapid evaluation of germplasm for photo-sensitivity [18]. Equally, genetical studies have been often limited mainly to yield contributing characters and fibre properties and a very little work has been reported on seed oil improvement in cotton. Nevertheless, wide range of genetic variability has been reported (15-33%) for seed oil content in global collection of in Indian germplasm collections [19].

In the recently conducted AICCIP meeting, the breeders are requested to submit two packets of 100 g seeds (in case of varieties) in addition to the number of locations finalized in the panel for long term storage of elite breeding materials. In the panel, detailed discussion was also held for promoting the entries from national trials to the zonal trials. So far, the entries are promoted on the basis of zonal mean to the corresponding zone. It is proposed to promote entries on the basis of 'agro-ecological subzone', henceforth. The draft proposal will be circulated among the breeders and based on the consensus the proposal will be submitted to ICAR, New Delhi for further directives. Detailed discussion was also held on formulating certain index based on seed cotton yield, lint yield, 2.5% span length and bundle strength for promoting the entries from national to zonal trials.

In India, various Transfer of Technology (TOT) programs in cotton have been implemented underlining the importance of problem solving, creating effective scientists and farmers linkage and transferring the latest cotton production technologies to the production line. 'Front Line Demonstration (FLD)' is one of the TOT programs which created remarkable impact on cotton production and facilitated excellent scientist-farmer linkage for the effective transfer of latest cotton protection technologies. In addition to this, the AICCIP is also actively involved in FLDs on improved technologies and organising Kisan Melas (Farmer's day) for effective and speedy dissemination of newer production technologies among farmers. During the year 2012-13, FLDs on cotton production technology and FLDs on cotton integrated pest management (IPM) were conducted by 13 AICCIP centres. The main emphasis was given to the demonstrations for enhancing the production of cotton in low productivity areas / problematic areas with improved package of practices. In addition, the cotton breeder seed production and implementation of "Special Component Plan for Scheduled Caste" and "Tribal Sub Plan for Scheduled Tribes" are also monitored through the AICCIP.

4. *Bt* cotton

The development and commercial cultivation of *Bt* cotton hybrid in 2002 is a revolutionary landmark in Indian agriculture after the green revolution during 1960s. With the introduction of *Bt* cotton in India, which confers resistance to key lepidopteron insect pests of cotton, there has been an incredible increase in the cotton production. India cultivated a record 11.0 million hectares of *Bt* cotton in 2013 with an adoption rate of 95% [14]. There is substantial evidence that the adoption of *Bt* cotton provides economic benefits from increased yields due to limited damage from the bollworm pest complex [American bollworm (*Helicoverpa armigera* Hubner) in particular and other bollworms such as spotted (*Earias vittella* Fab.), spiny (*E. insulana* Boisd.) and the pink (*Pectinophora gossypiella* Saunders), in general] and reducing costs through lower use levels of insecticide [15].

In point of fact, *Bt* cotton developed in India is a combination of transgenic and hybrid technologies. *G. hirsutum* represents 90% of the hybrid cotton in India and almost all the current *Bt* cotton hybrids are *G. hirsutum*. The embedded *Bt* gene acts as an *in situ* biological pesticide factory and hence avoid the need for any chemical spray for the suppression of the lepidopteron pests. In order to have maximum effect of *Bt* gene, the host genotype (one of the parent of the hybrid) chosen from the existing stock of hybrids that have a strong yield potential and popular acceptance (in terms of acreage) of its non-Bt version.

On the other hand, release and widespread usage of *Bt* cotton hybrid has resulted a specific bottleneck. The popular Indian cotton varieties such as LRA 5166, LRK 516, MCU 5, MCU 5 VT, SVPR 2, AKA 081, AKA 7, AKA 8, GCot 11, GCot 13, PA 225, RG 8, Sahana and Surabhi (to cite a few) that were cultivated even in the marginal or low-input supplied regions, have become almost extinct after the introduction of *Bt* cotton hybrids. Undeniably, a *Bt* version of these varieties would have been a benefit for resource-poor regions which cannot be provided by hybrids since they require higher inputs and costlier management practices. Further, fortifying such varieites with drought resistance and fibre quality traits has immense benefits for the Indian farmers, since > 60% of the cotton cultivation is under rainfed conditions (where water availability to the crop growth is always uncertain and water stress can occur anytime during the cropping period that greatly affects the fibre yield and quality). The best national average yield of 17000 Kg seed cotton/ha (with almost the whole crop area being under *Bt* hybrids), seems to be insignificance when many countries harvest about 50000–60000 Kg/ha seed cotton as national average through straight varieties [15]. Thus, there is a great scope for genetic improvement of cotton especially the elite varieties, by utilizing the available rich germplasm.

5. Cotton germplasm in private sectors

There are several national and multinational seed companies in India that focus on breeding, development and commercialization of cotton hybrids, including Bt and other beneficial genes. The cotton plant has been transformed with variety of genes expressing different traits such as insect resistance, herbicide tolerance, drought tolerance, improved fibre quality etc. However, only insect resistance genes have been approved, either individually and/or stacked in various combinations, for commercial cultivation. Each private sector has their own germplasm and breeding materials (since they are under propriety right protection, such breeding materials have not been disclosed to the public). Some private sectors that are actively involved in Bt cotton hybrid development and/or cotton research in India include Mahyco, Rasi Seeds, Nuziveedu Seeds, Ganga Kaveri Seeds, Ajeet Seeds, Tulasi Seeds, Prabhat Seeds, Vikram Seeds, Nath Seeds, Vibha Seeds, Bioseeds, Nandi Seeds, Bayer Crop Science, JK Seeds, Dow Agrosciences, Krishidhan seeds, Zurai Seeds, Navkar Hybrids and DuPont India.

6. Genetic diversity analysis of Indian cotton germplasm

It is increasingly believed that the reason for recent stagnation and/or decline in cotton yield and fibre quality in India was mainly due to declining trend in genetic diversity of released cultivars and breeding stocks, emergence of new menace (such as minor pests become major pests) and a greater than before exposure to environmental hassles such as drought, heat, salinity etc., Research on genetic diversity of cotton cultivars and some of its related species conducted in several global laboratories including India using a range of molecular markers that has clearly shown the narrowness of genetic base of cotton cultivars.

For example, a set of 96 core accessions were screened using the informative polymorphic markers at the CICR, Nagpur. Combination of different type of 46 markers such as simple sequence repeats (SSR), sequence related amplified polymorphism (SRAP) and randomly amplified polymorphic DNA (RAPD) markers were employed to assess the genetic diversity. It was concluded that the available diversity was low and more informative markers are required to understand the genetic diversity among the core accessions [6].

Similarly, the genetic divergence among 19 elite lines of cotton that are more frequently employed in TNAU cotton breeding programs was investigated using morphological (multivariate Mahalanobis D2 statistics) and SSR markers [20]. This study grouped all the 19 *Gossypium* accessions into two main cluster *i.e., G. hirsutum* and *G. barbadense* lines and there were narrow inter-specific genetic diversity. In an another study [21], thirty *G. barbadense* accessions and five *G. hirsutum* cultivars belonging to different institutes of India were genotyped with 88 SSR markers and found to be closely related within the species. Genetic diversity amongst 91 upland cotton accessions (50 maintainer, 'B' and 41 restorer 'R' lines) and three wild species such as *G. aridum, G. thurberi* and *G. anomalum* was analysed using SSR and RAPD markers and also revealed a higher level of genetic relatedness [22].

It should be noted that the low genetic diversity, as mentioned above, was not due to the limitation of marker technology since it was invariably concluded in numerous studies that molecular markers has immense potential in germplasm characterization. For example, all the wild species available in the CICR were efficiently characterized by using simple RAPD and inter simple sequence repeats (ISSR) markers. Further, eleven cotton hybrids along with their parents and 13 cultivars were characterized at the molecular level and specific markers were identified for testing genetic purity. Sequence characterized amplified region (SCAR) markers and specific primers were also designed to identify three cotton hybrids such as Savitha, Shruthi and Surya [6]. Thus, the narrow genetic diversity present in the current cultivars/

hybrids is obviously a great bottleneck for cotton breeding and needs to be widened to meet the demands of both farmers and textile industries.

7. Mapping populations for genetic dissection of agronomic and fibre quality traits

Mapping populations, mainly recombinant inbred lines (RILS), have been developed to genetically dissect the agronomic and fibre quality traits in cotton at several Indian institutes including:

a. TNAU, Coimbatore (RILs derived from 1) *G. hirsutum* var. KC3 and *G. barbadense* var. Suvin 2) *G. hirsutum* var. MCU5 and *G. hirsutum* var. TCH1218 and 3) *G. hirsutum* var. SVPR2 and *G. barbadense* var. Suvin),

b. CICR, Nagpur (RILs derived from 1) *G. arboreum* var. Kwan-3 and *G. herbaceum* var. Jayadhar and 2) *G. hirsutum* var. IRH 1-4-4 and *G. hirsutum* var. AKG 2/50),

c. UAS, Dharwad (RILs derived from 1) *G. hirsutum* var. DS-28 and *G. barbadense* var. SB YF425 and 2) *G. herbaceum* var. jayadhar and *G. arboreum* var. DLSA17) and

d. IARI, New Delhi (RILs derived from *G. hirsutum* var. P56_4 and *G. hirsutum* var. RS 2013).

The above said mapping populations are considered as valuable resources for identification of molecular markers linked to key fibre quality traits such as fibre length and strength besides drought tolerance and cotton leaf curl virus disease resistance traits. The major constraint that hampers the precise and early identification of tightly linked markers is the availability of informative polymorphic markers (due to narrow genetic diversity exist in the above mentioned parents; see above) which are essential for the construction of high-resolution genetic map. To overcome this difficulty, a co-ordinated effort is being formulated with a grateful financial support from Department of Biotechnology, Government of India to constitute a network project on developing saturated genetic linkage maps of cotton using different mapping populations available in India and single nucleotide polymorphism (SNP) chip developed at National Botanical Research Institute, Lucknow (Dr. Samir Sawant, personal communication). Development of such saturated genetic linkage map will eventually be utilized for quantitative trait loci (QTL) identification of cotton fibre yield and quality traits.

Among the different types of mapping population, development and employment of RILs is being pursued in selected cotton institutes including TNAU to utilize donor cotton breeding materials for genetic analysis of the desirable characters (see below). Selected superior recombinant line shall be used in enhancement of genetic stocks through molecular breeding and development of more productive and eco-friendly new varieties/hybrids tailored to fit into the future and existing cropping systems.

At TNAU, Coimbatore evolution of new cotton varieties with drought tolerance, jassid resistance and improved fibre quality traits is the major breeding objective. In particular, there is a need to develop ideotype suitable for rainfed cultivation since large cotton cultivating area is under drought conditions. Seed cotton yield under water stress is determined by a combination of factors: boll number, boll size, seed number per boll, and fibre/seed. Thus the main features of proposed ideotypes for rainfed cultivation includes, earliness (135-165 days), fewer small and thick leaves, compact and short plant architecture, moderately indeterminate habit, sparse hairiness, medium to big boll size, synchronous boll development, high response to nutrients, tolerance to water stress and tolerance to insects and diseases. The RILs derived from 1) MCU 5 and TCH 1218, 2) SVPR 2 and Suvin and 3) KC 3 and Suvin were evaluated with three different water regimes (irrigated control, managed water stress (by withholding irrigation during flowering phase) and rainfed conditions) at several locations of Tamil Nadu (including TNAU, Coimbatore, Cotton Research Station, Veppanthattai, Regional Research Station, Arupukottai and Maize Research Station, Vagarai) for drought tolerance and fibre quality traits. Linkage map was constructed and used for QTL analysis of fibre quality traits under water stress environment (Boopathi et al; under preparation). The important outcome of these evaluation trials (for above said ideotype characters), is identification of promising lines of mapping populations that were shown superior fibre yield and quality traits under water stress conditions. Such lines have been proposed for further evaluation to release as varieties that are suitable for rainfed cultivation.

In another study, we are trying to identify the QTLs linked to jassid tolerance in cotton using a RILs derived from 1) KC 2 and Suvin and 2) MCU 5 and Suvin. *G. hirsutum* cultivar KC 2 and MCU5 had shown tolerance to jassid [23] but with relatively poor fibre quality. On the other hand, the *G. barbadense* cultivar, Suvin, and *G. hirsutum* cultivar MCU 5 was vulnerable to jassid attack; however, they registered better fibre quality traits with good yield. Based on the variability studies of different leaf anatomical features, diversity, correlation and path coefficient analysis conducted at TNAU, Coimbatore, the following conclusion were made to explain jassid tolerance in cotton: i) pubescent nature indicates jassid tolerance ii) lower palisade cells in leaf lamina act as physical barrier for feeding and oviposition iii) thicker laminar coupled with absence of pubescence or lower palisade depicts susceptibility, but with them confers resistance to jassid and iv) higher cortex cell density is indicative of resistance [24, 25]. Hence, RILs that are developed from both of these interspecific and intraspecific crosses are being used for genetic mapping of jassid tolerance in cotton. In a parallel study, two different RILs developed from MCU 5 and TCH 1218 and P 56-4 and RS 2013 at TNAU, Coimbatore and IARI, New Delhi, respectively were evaluated at four different national partner institutes. Preliminary studies have identified several number of major QTLs linked to fibre yield and quality traits and they are being fine mapped using SNPs.

8. Coloured cotton

The vast majority of cotton grown commercially in the world, including India, has white lint, but recently there is a growing interest in coloured linted cotton. During the process of bleaching and dyeing of white lint cotton to impart colours, dyeing and textile units regularly use several toxic chemicals including heavy metal. The water from these units is a main source of pollution in drinking water, soil and environment. Many of these chemicals are carcinogenic

http://dx.doi.org/10.5772/58619

and can cause allergies, skin rashes and other related health problems to human beings. Hence, it is preferred to have garments made from natural coloured cotton which is free from the dangerous textile chemicals. This has provoked many cotton workers into developing eco-friendly coloured cotton and has led to the revival of growing naturally coloured cotton. Further, coloured cotton cultivation should also be encouraged since it possesses resistances to many pests, diseases, drought and salinity [26]. In India, coloured cotton can be cultivated in Andhra Pradesh, Karnataka, Madhya Pradesh, Maharashtra and Orissa. Khadi and Village Industries Commission have experimented producing dress material using coloured cotton. The Maharashtra Hybrid Seeds Company (Mahyco), Mumbai, has initiated coloured cotton-seed production. However, the share of the colour cotton to the total Indian cotton production is very negligible (less than 5000 tonnes).

Up to the middle of the 20th Century, coloured cotton cultivars *Cocanada 1* and *2* were commercially cultivated in Andhra Pradesh and exported to Japan. Similarly, cotton with black, brown, creamy white and khaki linted types were grown in Assam. *Kumta* in Karnataka was the home for *G. herbaceum* with dull white colour. Interestingly, globally acclaimed *Dacca muslin* was made from white and colour linted *G. arboreum* [27]. However, the main disadvantage of coloured cotton is its lower yield, shorter staple length, weaker fibre strength and undesirable micronaire value when compared with white linted ones, limiting its commercial cultivation and utilization [28].

Because of the advancement of spinning and textile processing technologies, there is a need for the production of coloured cotton combining high yield and superior fibre qualities. The F_1s obtained by crossing brown coloured and white linted lines are intermediate between the two parents for colour intensity and technological properties. Significant numbers of colour cotton genotypes are being maintained in India at CICR, Nagpur, UAS-Dharwad and TNAU, Coimbatore. Nearly 40 colour linted cotton germplasm accessions are being maintained at National Cotton Gene Bank, CICR, Nagpur. Scientists at the CICR laboratories and Cotton Research Station at Khandwa in Madhya Pradesh, University of Agricultural Sciences at Dharwad, Karnataka and Panjabrao Krishi Vidyapeeth, Akola, Maharashtra are investigating the agronomic, economic, and technical attributes of these strains for suitable hybrid production. Such studies have resulted in the identification of six cultures with desirable properties such as moderate resistance to pests, large boll size, and good fibre qualities with shades of brown and green. Studies at UAS, Dharwad indicated that colour development in the fibre occurs between 30 and 40 days after boll formation. A collection of 11 coloured cotton *G. hirsutum* genotypes (Higginbotham, Parbhani American, Brymer brown, Hirsutum Tashkent, Lousiana brown, Nankeen brown, Algerian brown, Russian brown, Red 5–7, Arkansas green and Texas green) and four white linted genotypes (MCU 5, 7, 9 and 12) were evaluated by RAPD markers at TNAU, Coimbatore, India. Cluster analysis showed clear-cut separation of the colour and white lint genotypes [29]. It has been recognized in several occasions that exploitation of heterosis might be an effective method for improvement in yield and fibre properties in coloured cotton.

9. Future perspectives

In India, there is a large scope for cotton genetic improvement for value added traits: an example is cotton for floor coverings. Currently, cotton contributes less than 2% of the fibres used in floor coverings, although this industry represents the largest single end-user of fibres in today's market. What is needed to fulfill this niche in the marketplace is to develop cotton fibres that have (1) more flame resistance to meet strict government standards (2) longer with reduced short fibre content to prevent shredding and (3) improved resiliency. It is also imperative to genetically improve the cotton fibre properties for other value added properties such as improved white brightness, increased postharvest properties such as moisture uptake, dye uptake, binding and/or retention and introduction of novel properties such as naturally coloured fibres and antimicrobial fibres for medical and pharmaceutical use.

Physical and chemical mutagenesis provides a powerful alternative to natural, polygenic variation for identifying functional pathways and complex disease genes and more importantly to generate novel cultivars with improved agronomic traits. Though there were some attempts in India, by and large, physical and chemical mutagenesis has not been utilized extensively to create new genetic variation.

The utilization of available germplasm in the national cotton gene bank can be further enhanced by adding the most suitable genetic stocks that can be procured from various international sources. Such activity will be useful in the development of breeding lines by introgressing beneficial alleles from the wild species, races and derivatives. Although elite x elite crosses are typical of traditional plant breeding, interspecific crosses are rarely used in cotton breeding because of numerous barriers. The finding that the *G. hirsutum* allele is favourable at some loci and the *G. barbadense* allele at other loci shows that recombination of favourable alleles from each of these species may form novel genotypes than either of the parental species. Similarly, the genomic exploration of other accessions of these species or other wild tetraploid cottons (*G. tomentosum, G. darwinii,* and *G. mustelinum*), maintained at national cotton gene bank could yield additional valuable alleles.

The most important agronomic traits such as biotic and abiotic stress tolerance, plant development and consumer quality aspects are genetically and physiologically complex. Moreover, because of the polyploid nature of cotton, breeding for such traits is time consuming and difficult. Further, the paucity of information about genes that control important traits and the need for more extensive usage of diverse germplasm hinder the genetic improvement of cotton. The rapidly expanding knowledge on gene function and the availability of whole genome structural features of cotton is expected to offer new perspectives to solve these complex problems and future cotton genetic improvement strategy should integrate such knowledge in the breeding program. Taking up of multi-population analyses (such as NAM, MAGIC, four-way cross, etc.) can unambiguously resolve several issues in QTL models and tests of epistatic interactions of QTL with the genetic background and environment.

Currently, the transgenic approach is feasible to engineer traits that are controlled by one or a few major genes. However, it is not a panacea for all the problems. Quantitative traits like yield

http://dx.doi.org/10.5772/58619

are not easily amenable to improvement through transformation. Further, traits that can be routinely modified via conventional breeding need not be targeted for transformation. Availability of molecular markers to track genes controlling complex traits has further reduced the need for transgenic approach to crop improvement. This, however, does not mean that the transgenic approach is unimportant. Since genes can be sourced from any organism for cotton transformation, novel traits can be engineered with ease. Therefore, from a practical viewpoint, deficiencies that severely limit crop production and for which conventional approaches are inadequate, should be accorded high priority for transgenic improvement. At present, almost all of the Indian cotton transgenic technology and products are in private domain. Hence, there is a general worry that the transgenic crops are being promoted solely with profit motive and not for the good of the public. Thus the opposition to transgenic crops is not only on account of biosafety but also due to IPR, ethical, social, economic and moral issues. For technology to progress and reach the farmers, both public and private investments will be essential.

10. Conclusion

Foregoing section highlighted there are many challenges faced by Indian cotton scientists in creating the next generation of designer cotton plants. Fundamental research is still needed to elucidate biochemical and signalling pathways, as well as acquiring a better understanding of the underlying mechanisms that regulate gene expression in cotton. Further, quick and reproducible protocols for rapid screening of germplasm for biotic and abiotic stress resistance, breeding for drought tolerance, naturally coloured cotton, breeding for cotton varieties that suitable for mechanization and exploiting the genetic potential of wild species require urgent attention.

Acknowledgements

This work is supported by Department of Biotechnology, Ministry of Science and Technology, Government of India. We sincerely apologize for not citing many research papers due to space limitations.

Author details

N. Manikanda Boopathi*, S. Sathish, P. Dachinamoorthy, P. Kavitha and R. Ravikesavan

*Address all correspondence to: nmboopathi@tnau.ac.in

Tamil Nadu Agricultural University, Coimbatore, Tamil Nadu, India

References

[1] Central Institute of Cotton Research. Nagpur, India. http://www.cicr.org.in/pdf/CICR_VISION_2030.pdf (accessed 25 March, 2014)

[2] Khadi BM, Kulkarni VN, Ansingkar AS, Singh VV, Gotmare V. Gene pool concept in diploid cotton. Proceedings of World Cotton Conference: 3, March 9-13, 2003, Cape Town, South Africa; 2003.

[3] Rajendran TP, Jain KC. Achievements in Cotton Research in the All India Coordinated Cotton Improvement Program. CICR regional station, Coimbatore, Tamil Nadu, India. 2004.

[4] ICAR. In: Handbook of Agriculture. Indian Council of Agriculture Research, New Delhi; 2006.

[5] Cotton Corporation of India. http://cotcorp.gov.in/cbs.aspx (accessed 25 March, 2014).

[6] Central Institute of Cotton Research. Nagpur, India. http://www.cicr.org.in/cicr_glance_2011/47_52.pdf (accessed 25 March, 2014).

[7] Khadi BM, Kulkarni VN. Cotton. In: Chopra VL (ed.) Breeding Field Crops. Theory and Practice Oxford & IBH Publishing Co. Pvt. Ltd. Delhi and Calcutta. 2001. pp 531-575.

[8] Sundaram V. In: Antiquity of Cotton: 50 years of research at Cotton Technological Research Laboratory, Indian Council of Agricultural Research, New Delhi, India; 1974. pp 212.

[9] Twomey MJ. Employment in nineteenth century Indian textiles. Explorations in Economic History 1983; 20(1): 37-57.

[10] Dantwala ML. In: A hundred years of Indian cotton. Orient Longmans for the East India Cotton Association, Bombay; 1948. http://books.google.co.in/books?id=x8UzAAAAMAAJ (accessed 25 March, 2014).

[11] Gulati AN, Turner AJ. A note on early history of cotton. Journal of the Textile Institute Transactions 1929; 20: 1-9.

[12] Raveendran TS, Mohan S, Ravikesavan R, Surendran C, Meyyazhagan N, Parthiban VK. In: Cotton, The White Gold. Department of Cotton, CPBG, Tamil Nadu Agricultural University. Coimbatore, India; 2002.

[13] Hutchinson JB. In: The Application of Genetics of Cotton Improvement. Cambridge University Press London, New York; 1959.

[14] James C. In: Global Status of Commercialized Biotech/GM Crops: 2013. ISAAA Brief No. 46. ISAAA, Ithaca, New York; 2013.

[15] Ramasundaram P, Vennila S. A decade of Bt cotton experience in India: pointers for transgenics in pipeline. Current Science 2013; 104(6): 697-698.

[16] http://www.cicr.org.in/CropImprovement.html# (accessed 25 March., 2014).

[17] Saravanan M. Tree cotton and cotton perennials of India – a short note. Cotton Innovate 2013; 3(9): 1.

[18] Mohan P. Low cost technology for rapid screening of cotton germplasm for photosensitivity. Cotton Innovate 2013; 2(10): 1.

[19] Pandey SN. Cottonseed and its utilization. Indian Council of Agricultural research, New Delhi; 1998. pp212.

[20] Thiyagu K, Boopathi NM, Nadarajan N, Gopikrishnan A, Selvakumar P, Santoshkumar M, Ravikesavan R. Sampling and exploitation of genetic variation exist in locally adapted accessions using phenotypic and molecular markers for genetic improvement of cotton. Gene Conserve 2011; 10(40): 129-153.

[21] Boopathi NM, Gopikrishnan A, Jagadeesh Selvam N, Ravikesavan R, Iyanar K, Muthuraman S, Saravanan N. Genetic diversity assessment of G. barbadense accessions to widen cotton (Gossypium spp.,) gene pool for improved fibre quality. Journal of Cotton Research and Development 2008; 22(2):135-138.

[22] Sapkal DR, Sutar SR, Thakre PB, Patil BR, Paterson AH, Waghmare VN. Genetic diversity analysis of maintainer and restorer accessions in upland cotton (Gossypium hirsutum L.). Journal of Plant Biochemistry and Biotechnology 2011; 20 (1): 20-28.

[23] Krishnadoss D, Rajamani A, Ravikesavan R, Muppidathi N, Sankarapandian R, Suresh S, Rajaram V. New jassid resistant cotton variety-KC 2 (Kovilpatti Cambodia – 2). Madras Agriculture Journal 1999; 86: 611-614.

[24] Shimna B, Ravikesavan R. Heterotic expression of leaf anatomical characters for jassid resistance in cotton. Plant Archives 2008; 8 (1): 219-224.

[25] Pushpam R, Raveendran TS. Artificial screening and inheritance studies on resistance to jassid (*Amrasca devastans*) in *Gossypium hirsutum* L. The Indian Journal of Genetics and Plant Breeding 2005; 65(3): 120-125.

[26] Fox S. Naturally coloured cotton. Spin Off. Journal of All India Federation of Cotton Spinning Mills 1987; 15: 48—50.

[27] Murthy MSS. Never say dye: the story of coloured cotton. Resonance 2001; 6(12): 29-35.

[28] Singh VV, Narayanan SS, Kulmethe VM, Anap GR, Nagwekar SN. A brief review on coloured linted cotton documenting selected genotypes of G. hirsutum L. Journal of Indian Society for Cotton Improvement 1993; 18: 91-94.

[29] Punitha D, Raveendran TS. DNA fingerprinting studies in coloured cotton genotypes. Plant Breeding 2004; 123: 101-103.

Chapter 6

Cotton Germplasm of Pakistan

Mehboob ur-Rahman, Zainab Rahmat,
Abid Mahmood, Khalid Abdullah and Yusuf Zafar

Additional information is available at the end of the chapter

http://dx.doi.org/10.5772/58620

1. Introduction

The economy of Pakistan relies heavily on cotton, which contributes ~60% of total foreign exchange earnings (US$ 15 billion in 2012/13). Cotton is grown on about three million hectares annually with average lint production of 670 kg ha^{-1}. Historically the cultivation of cotton can be traced back to 6000 BC with *Gossypium arboreum* L. identified in the ancient remains of Monjadharo (Sindh) [1]. The indigenous cultivated cotton is locally known as Desi cotton, which carries the A-genome [2-3]. Following the industrial revolution in the textile sector, the tetraploid *Gossypium hirsutum* L. gradually replaced *G. arboreum* L., because it generally produces a higher quality lint and has a higher seed cotton yield (SCY) in the Indo-Pak region. These American types originated from New Orleans and Georgia were first introduced in 1818 [4]. This material was primarily a mixture and did not attract the interest of farmers in its initial years of cultivation because of high susceptibility to sucking insects, particularly jassids (*Amarasca devastans* Dist.). Organized selection procedures were adopted to select genotypes suited to the local conditions that laid a concrete foundation for breeding material on the sub-continent.

The four cultivated cotton species can be easily identified based on variations in plant growth habit, leaf shape, boll, flower, seed and fiber features [2-3, 5]. Substantial differences between *G. herbaceum* L. and *G. arboreum* L. have been found based on genetic, cytogenetic, isozyme and genomic data. The two species are easily crossable to produce F_1 hybrids that are fertile and vigorous with high pollen fertility (60%). However, in common with other crops species, genetic incompatibility depresses seed viability and affects plant morphology in segregating generations. Consequently resulting plants resemble one of the parents. One reciprocal chromosomal translocation differentiates the two species [6-8]. Recently eight and 13 unique polymorphic loci of *G. arboreum* L. and *G. herbaceum* L., respectively, have been reported [9].

DNA markers, such as restriction fragment length polymorphism (RFLP), random amplified polymorphic DNA (RAPD), amplified fragment length polymorphism (AFLP) and simple sequence repeat/microsatellite (SSR), have also been utilized to provide genomic polymorphic markers which can distinguish most cotton species [10-12].

Breeders, geneticists, cytogeneticists and biotechnologists have made substantial contribution for the improvement of cotton germplasm conferring resistance and/or tolerance to various stresses including biotic and abiotic, through bridging conventional and genomic tools [13]. Breeding for earliness and photoperiod insensitivity has also been accomplished by introgressing genes from the alien cotton species, which paved the way for not only sustaining cotton production but also provided enough window for cultivating another crop like wheat on the same land, thus laying down a foundation for addressing food security concerns in Pakistan.

2. Germplasm history

When *G. arboreum* L. was first domesticated is unclear but it is believed to have occurred in the Indus valley [14]. The indigenous cotton cultivated in Pakistan is *G. arboreum* L. that evolved from the primitive *G. herbaceum* L. In total, six distinct races of *G. arboreum* L. have been reported; "indicum"—primitive perennial form found in Western India, "burmanicum" —North Eastern India and Myanmar, "soudanense"—evolved in Egypt, Sudan and North Africa, "sinense"—evolved in southern part of China, "bengalense"—developed in Northern part of India and "cernuum"—evolved in the Assam and Chittagang hills of India and Bangladesh.

The annual types belonging to the race "cernuum" evolved independently. The cultivars that are belonging to this race are considered a useful genetic resource for producing big bolls, which are cultivated in the Gharo hills [14-16].The cultivated desi cotton belongs to *G. arboreum* L. "bengalense" in Pakistan and to *G. arboreum* L."cernuum" in Bangladesh.

G. arboreum L. genotypes/cultivars have been characterized at length based on morphological, physiological and agronomical features which suggest that this species can tolerate drought, and resist diseases and insect pests (such as bollworms and aphids). These features allow the *G. arboreum* L. types to adapt to dry and marginal lands [13, 17-19].

2.1. Evolution of *G. arboreum* L. in Pakistan

Historically, farming community of Pakistan has been cultivating *G. arboreum* L. largely on drought prone areas till 1920s which was gradually replaced by the introduction of high yielding Upland cotton varieties. For the last two decades, less than 2% of the total cultivated area of cotton is under *G. arboreum* L. types, which is expected to further decline with the passage of time.

Most cotton varieties/germplasm of *G. arboreum* L. in Pakistan has been bred by selecting variants—resulted due to limited cross pollination or mixing of seeds [20]. Consequently, it resulted in narrow genetic base of the cultivars/genotypes developed by selecting from a single population. The study conducted on 30 *G. arboreum* L. genotypes, largely originated in Pakistan demonstrated a narrow genetic base [20-21]. In this study, two major cultivars Ravi and FDH-228, showed 90.1% genetic similarity in RAPD assay [20]. It has been demonstrated that the narrow genetic base, like many other cultivated crop species, can impede the future breeding progress [13].

2.2. Breeding history of desi cotton cultivars in Pakistan

The initial breeding program for developing high yielding varieties involved selection from the available mixture of various *G. arboreum* L. types. Two cotton varieties Z. Mollisoni and 278-Mollisoni were developed through selections which gradually replaced the old types. The first cotton research station was established at Lyallpur (currently Faisalabad, located in Pakistan), and breeding for developing improved types by making selections from the available cotton varieties/genotypes was initiated by Mr. T. Trought and later continued by Mr. M. Afzal. In 1927, 15-Mollisone cotton line was tested in national trials which was approved for cultivation in 1930 on account of its high ginning outturn (GOT) 35% compared to 34% for "Mollisoni" and 33% for the mixture cultivated in the farmer's field. Another variety 39-Mollisoni exhibited 36-37% GOT versus 35% for 15-Mollisoni. The highest wrap count 8'S was spun by the lint produced of the varieties 39-Mollisoni and 15-Mollisoni (Table 1).

In 1935, efforts for development of elite desi cotton types from the historically cultivated mixture of *G. arboreum* L. biotypes known as "Multani Kapas" for the South West of Punjab—Multan region [22], were initiated through selection. A high yielding variety 119-Sanguineum (119-S), developed in 1936 and approved for cultivation in 1941, demonstrated relatively higher GOT 36.4% compared to 34% of the mixture of various biotypes. Another candidate line 231-R, bred at Hansi Research Center under the administrative umbrella of Cotton Section Lyallpur, was tested in various trials. Testing continued after 1947, and 231-R was ultimately approved for general cultivation in 1959 [23].

The Cotton Research Institute (CRI), Faisalabad carried out breeding for desi cotton at two research stations. Haroonabad was a drought prone area and the major cash crop of this region was desi cotton (60,712 hectares in the early 1950s). Breeding efforts at the Cotton Research Station Haroonabad started in 1952. Four candidate lines were identified based on leaf morphology (broad or narrow) and flower color (white or yellow). One of the varieties, 73/3, showed a higher GOT (42%) with staple length of 13.7 mm compared to a 37-38% GOT and 16-19 mm staple length of the already cultivated mixture. However, the newly developed varieties could match the yield of the already cultivated mixture of desi cotton. Thus breeding efforts, through selection, were abandoned.

The hybridization work at the Cotton Research Station, Faisalabad, started in 1930 to improve fiber quality, especially the staple length, of the existing cultivated desi cotton varieties. Wide crosses were made between 39-Mollisoni and the Chinese variety Million Dollar, resulting in improved strains (called Jubilee strains-D.C.17, D.C.26, D.C.37, D.C.40 and D.C.41). They had improved staple length and a higher GOT but with a lower yield potential over the control variety Mollisoni. Among these, D.C.40 showed improved quality features (staple length=20.3

Serial #	Name of variety	Center of release	Year of release	Pedigree/parentage	GOT %¥	Staple length mm	Fineness µg/inch	Strength tppsi€
1	S.N.R.	ARI, Tandojam	1926 (Sindh)	Selection from Sindh desi types	39.0	17.5	7.8	NK
2	15-M	AARI,Faisalabad	1930	Selection from Local Desi	35.0	17.5	8.0	NK
3	39-M	AARI,Faisalabad	1934	Selection from local Desi mixture	36.0	17.5	8.5	NK
4	119-S	CRS, Multan	1941	Selection from local Desi mixture called Multani Kapas	35.5	17.5	8.4	NK
5	231-R	AARI, Faisalabad	1959	Selection from 39-Mollisoni	40.0	15.9	8.4	NK
6	TD-1	ARI, Tandojam	1963 (Sindh)	Selection from S.N.R.	41.0	15.9	9.4	80.0
7	D-9	AARI, Faisalabad	1970	Bahawalpur Desi – Selection	41.0	14.5	8.2	80.0
8	SKD-10/19	CRI, Sakrand	1975	S.N.R.(single plant selection from S.N.R. G-IV bulked G-4/ NRPT 10 & 19)	40.6	15.5	10.1	80.0
9	Ravi	CRI, AARI, Faisalabad	1982	465 D-selection	40.3	14.9	8.0	80.0
10	Rohi	CRS, Bahawalpur	1986	Haroonabad Local x D- 9	39.0	15.9	8.0	80.0
11	FDH-170	CRI, Faisalabad	1995	D-9 x TD-1	40.3	14.1	8.4	80.0
12	FDH-228	CRI,AARI, Faisalabad	2002	TD-1 x (Commila x FDH-170)	43.5	13.9	7.3	NK

NK: Not known; ¥=Ginning out turn percentage;€=Thousand pounds per square inch

Source: Dr. Akhlaq Hussain, Description of cotton varieties of Pakistan 2004 and Cotton Research and development Memoranda till 60's (Ed. Dr. Mahbub Ali).

Table 1. List of approved *G. arboretum* L. (desi cotton) varieties

mm; highest wrap count=25 and GOT=38.5%) [24]. Efforts to improve staple length of the existing desi varieties continued by crossing one of the Jubilee strains with *G. anomalum* Wawr. and Peyr. that was introduced from Nigeria. Multiple strains were developed using back-crossing followed by selecting plants with improved fertility. These strains were tested in various yield trials in 1944 and demonstrated a substantial improvement in staple length (21.1 to 22.4 mm) particularly for D.C.94 (staple length=22.35 mm, GOT=38.2% and yield per acre=552 kg). These strains have the potential to compete with *G. hirsutum* L. var 4-F for fiber length. However, none of the strains found favor with the farming community. Interspecific crosses were made at Multan between *G. arboreum* L. and *G. thurberi* Tod. followed by two backcrosses with *G. arboreum* L. A few strains with improved staple length were identified; but these did not out yield the existing cultivars. A few strains with shorter staple length (17 mm) showed higher seed cotton yield (125 g/plant) and GOT (42%) over the control 231-R (90 g/plant). Later this germplasm was used for developing improved desi cotton cultivars.

Sindh, another important cotton growing province of Pakistan, is known for having the earliest traces of cotton cultivation-6000 BC at Monjadharo [1]. Efforts were made to develop desi type in the early 20th Century. Seed of an improved cotton variety "Comilla" was imported from the East Pakistan (now Bangladesh). However, due to lack of concerted efforts, no significantly improved germplasm/variety could be developed. A decade later, few plants were selected from *G. arboreum* var neglectum [25] growing in farmer's field, and a variety 27 W.N. was developed in 1922 [26]. This line was released for general cultivation in 1926 with a different name S.N.R., which had a typical morphology (narrow leaves and white flowers) and lint features (GOT=39% and staple length 17.53 mm). This variety covered more than 40468 hectares in Hyderabad Division. Unlike previous varieties, this variety earned high premium in the internal market because of its improved fiber features. In 1963 another variety, TD-I, was approved for general cultivation (Table 1).

Little efforts were made to improve desi cotton in what is now Bangladesh. Only one short staple cotton variety "Comilla" was developed which was known in the market for its roughness.

2.3. Introduction of *Gossypium hirsutum* L.

After the initial introduction of the upland cotton (*Gossypium hirsutum* L.) in Indo-Pak in 1818, the first planned experiments for testing the performance of the upland cotton genotypes were undertaken in 1830 in the Bombay presidency by Dr Lush [23]. It took another almost 50 years for cultivation in farmer's field. Unfortunately, *G. hirsutum* L. varieties could not compete against the indigenous 'desi' cotton (*G. arboreum* L.). These efforts were continued by Benouf and Dobbs under the newly established Agricultural Department in 1906 and later were transferred to Milne in 1908 [22].

Historically, *G. hirsutum* L. was introduced in this region (Subcontinent) ~200 years ago, however, successful cultivation of this species was witnessed only around in 1930s parallel to the revolution witnessed in textile industry in Pakistan [20]. Out of the seven races of G. *hirsutum* L. "latifolium" was extensively used for developing improved cotton cultivars which presently covered ~98% of the total cotton cultivated area in Pakistan. The remaining 2% or even less is under cultivation of diploid cotton species, i.e. *G. arboreum* L. Like Upland cotton, efforts were also made for acclimatizing long staple cotton species (*G. barbadense* L.) but did not capture area in Pakistan because of high photosensitivity resulting in low yields.

Pakistan witnessed a gradual replacement of the *G. arboreum* L. types with the high yielding varieties of *G. hirsutum* L. A number of cotton varieties were also developed through selections but largely by hybridization and a few using mutagens.

3. Maintenance and storage

Short (working collection) and medium term storage facilities have been established at Plant Genetic Resources Institute (PGRI), NARC at Islamabad. Almost 60,000 seed samples (500 gm each) can be stored in the bank [27].

Collection of the crop germplasm is done either by undertaking plant collecting expedition trips or collected from researcher in the country or can be obtained from foreign countries. The health status of germplasm is analyzed upon its arrival and germination and moisture content are monitored. Before getting stored drying, packing and sealing of seed are done. These all activities meet the international standards. The current facilities were acquired through collaboration with Japan International Cooperation Agency (JICA), considering the international standards for seed preservation [27].

On the behalf of Federal Seed Certification & Registration Department, seeds of national approved varieties of cotton are stored at PGRI. At that time storage conditions of Pakistan Central Cotton Research Institute, Multan were not up to mark as PGRI recommendations, allowing medium term storage of genetic stock of cotton. Storage facilities for cotton germplasm at CCRI Multan have recently been established through Pak-US cotton productivity enhancement project (ID=1198). In total, ~30,000 accessions can be stored (Muhammad Idrees Khan, personal communication). This facility would help all cotton breeders for preserving their precious cotton germplasm.

In the botanical garden of CCRI, Multan, 28 cotton species of both cultivated and wild are maintained for utilizing in cotton breeding program of Pakistan. These include *G. barbosanum* (B), *G. anomalum* (B_1), *G. capitisviridis* (B_3), *G. sturtianum* (C_1), *G. nandewarense, G. robinsonii* (C_2), *G. thurberi* (D_1), *G. harknessii* (D_2-$_2$), *G. aridum* (D_4), *G. gossypioides* (D_6), *G. lobatum* (D_7), *G. trilobum* (D_8), *G. laxum* (D_9), *G. stocksii* (E_1), *G. somalense* (E_2), *G. areysianum* (E_3), *G.incanum* (E_4), *G. longicalyx* (F_1), *G. bickii*(G_1), *G. nelsonii* (G_3). All these belong to diploid wild species. Whereas, *G. tomentosum* 2 $(AD)_3$, *G. mustelinum* 2$(AD)_4$, *G. lanceolatum* 2$(AD)_4$ and *G. darwinii* 2$(AD)_5$ are found to belong from tetraploid wild species. Five *G. hirsutum* L. races viz. *latifolium, puncatum, morrilli, palmeri and marie-glante;* one *G. barbadense* L. race *braziliense* (kidney cotton); 13 diploid and 5 tetraploid hybrids; 5 triploid and 2 hexaploid hybrids; 3 pentaploid hybrids and 5 tri and 1 tetra species combinations are also maintained. In total, 62 grafts of out-standing *Gossypium* species and species hybrids were prepared for propagation purpose. These grafts were preserved under green house facility of CCRI Multan.

Though a varietal development procedure in Pakistan ensures enough purity, however, every year variants have been observed in the progenies of a variety developed through single plant selection because of limited natural cross pollination (up to 5%). Sometime, mutation and or mixing of seed during ginning process also contributes very small fraction to exaggerate the problem. In Pakistan, it has been observed that strict rouging is mandatory for maintaining the distinguished features of the variety every year, otherwise after three years the variety would appear like a mixture. In Pakistan, usually the maintenance work has been accomplished so far at the respective breeding center of the variety. Representative plants preferably in thousands are selected from the progeny row block of the best representative families. Ginning out turn percentage and lint quality parameters are measured through high volume instrument (HVI) or conventional tools. Only the plants meeting the set standards (lint percentage=37.50%; staple length=28.00 mm; micronaire value=3.8-4.9 μg inch-1; fiber strength=>92,000 lb psi) are retained for planting progeny rows.

Seed from representative progenies are harvested followed by planting on bigger blocks (~ 0.5 acre). After comparing the yield and lint quality parameters of each of the progeny, families of the best progeny rows are selected for planting on bigger blocks (~10 hectares, depending upon the availability of seed). The seed harvested from the best blocks are multiplied by planting on large scale (1000s of hectares). The seed harvested from this block will make the foundation seed. It is usually accomplished at Govt Farms (preferably at seed corporation farms) or now on private sector farms under the patronage of private seed companies. This seed is exposed to another round of multiplication to raise certified seed which is disposed to farmers for raising the cotton crop. The area under each aforementioned multiplication step can be increased or reduced depending upon the demand of the seed by the farming community. In Pakistan, 65,000 metric tons of cotton seed is needed every year for sowing on 3.2 million hectare. Of this 40-45% was provided through the formal seed sector (certified seed) until 2008. The informal seed sector, that includes farmers, breeders, and shopkeepers, are the major source of uncertified seed. Farmer-to-farmer sale is very popular among the farming community to provide seed to adjoining farms. Also the cotton growers retained a major portion of the seed produced at their own farms for planting in the next cotton growing season. In Pakistan, Plant Breeder Rights have not yet been enforced and the international seed companies, such as Monsanto, Bayer Crop Science and Biocentury, have major concerns pertaining loosing the legal protection of their products (transgenic events, varieties etc.). These are the major factors which hamper the establishment of a dynamic and robust seed industry in Pakistan.

4. Funding sources

Under the umbrella of Ministry of Textile Industry, PCCC established in 1948, is considered as the prime research organization working on cotton encompassing economical, technological and agricultural research. Two main research institutes including Central Cotton Research Institute (CCRI) Multan, Punjab and CCRI Sakrand, Sindh are involved in multidisciplinary research encompassing, varietal development, improvement in all kind of agronomic practices, combating insect pest and diseases, farmer's trainings etc. Under PCCC setup, seven other research stations or sub stations are involved in conducting research in specific area—largely on varietal development in collaboration with Provincial Setup. In total, 44 cotton varieties have been evolved by PCCC (Table 2). These varieties fulfill the requirement of spinners for fineness and strength.

Serial #	Name of variety	Center of release	Year of release	Pedigree/parentage	GOT %¥	Staple length mm	Fineness µg/inch	Strength tppsi€
1	M-4	CRS, ARI, Tandojam	1942	Selection from 289-F	33.0	23.8	4.5	85.0
2	M-100	CRS, ARI, Tandojam	1963	(M-4 x Wilds) x M-4	34.5	27.0	4.0	85.0
3	Qalandri	ARI, Tandojam	1974	(M-4 x *G. anomalum*) x Karnak	34.0	28.6	3.8	92.7
4	Sermast	ARI, Tandojam	1975	(M-4 x Acala) x M-4	34.0	28.6	3.9	92.7
5	K-68/9	CRS, PCCC, Ghotki	1977	(124-F x Babdal) x Wilds	33.0	30.1	4.2	96.0
6	Rehmani	ARI, Tandojam	1985	*G.hirsutum*21 x McNaire TH14920	35.0	27.0	4.4	90.0
7	Shaheen	CRS, Ghotki	1988	GH 7/72 x (DPL-16 x AC-134–F130kr)	35.0	27.4	4.3	94.6
8	Reshmi-90	ARI, Tandojam	1991	Coker 100A x (DPL-16 x AC-134	35.7	31.5	4.1	98.7
9	CRIS-9	CCRI, Sakrand	1993	Rajhans x RA-33-47	34.4	26.3	4.4-4.8	98.0
10	Chandi-95	NIA, Tandojam	1996	(DPL-16 x AC-134-(F_1 30kr, 300Gy gamma rays)	35.0	29.0	4.2	97.0
11	CRIS-5A (Marvi)	CCRI, Sakrand	2001	{(M-4 x *G. anomalum*) x Karnak} x 9L-34 ICCC	34.5	26.5	3.9	96.0
12	CRIS-134	CCRI, Sakrand	2001	(DPL-16 x AC-134)-F_1 Irradiated-30 kr Gamma rays (60 Co) x DPL-70	34.8	22.5	4.0-4.5	98.0
13	CRIS-467	CCRI, Sakrand	2001	LRA-5166 x CRIS-9	37.5	27.5	4.6	98.5
14	Shahbaz-95	ARI, Tandojam	2001	{(M-4 x *G. anomalum*) x Karnak} x Acala 1517	33.5	27.5	4.2	94.6
15	Sohni	NIA, Tandojam	2002	NIAB-78 (300 gy)	37.5	27.5	4.5	98.0
16	CRIS-121	CCRI, Sakrand	2006	NIAB-78 x B-909	34.8	26.1	4.6-4.9	98.0
17	Hari Dost	ARI, Tandojam	2006	Sarmast x Deltapine	38.0	27.4	4.3	97.0
18	Sadori	NIA, Tandojam	2006	F_1[(Shaheen x DPL-14) Gamma rays 250 GY]	37.2	27.8	4.4	97.0
19	Sindh-1	ARI, Tandojam	2010	NIAB-78 x Stoneville	37.0	28.0	4.5	97.0
20	Malmal	ARI, Tandojam	2010	CIM-70 x Reshmi	38.0	30.0	4.0	97.0
21	NiaUfaq	NIA, Tandojam	2010	DEM-84(R-RAUS 250 GY CO 60 source)	38	28.5	4.3	97.0

¥=Ginning out turn percentage; **€**=Thousand pounds per square inch

Source: Dr. Akhlaq Hussain, Description of cotton varieties of Pakistan 2004, Cotton Research and development Memoranda till 60's (Ed. Dr. Mahbub Ali), approval documents of cotton varieties released after 2004 and personal communication with breeders of the cotton varieties.

Table 2. List of approved *G. hirsutum* L. (upland cotton) varieties (non-GM) for Sindh

The establishment of Punjab Agricultural Research Board (PARB) as an autonomous body under PARB Act, 1997 for fostering an integrated approach for research planning and efficient allotment of research resource so that the agriculture innovation system of the province can generate appropriate solutions of the issues faced to various stakeholders in the food and fiber chain [28]. The vision of the PARB is to support scientific innovations for the prosperity of Agricultural Stakeholders in Punjab. Ministry of Food, Agriculture and Livestock (MINFAL, desolved after 18th amendment) was also remained actively involved in improving agricultural studies in Pakistan by providing funds.

Presently, a project on cotton productivity enhancement has been initiated by the generous support of the U.S. Department of Agriculture, Agricultural Research Service; under agreement No.58-6402-0-178F (operating through ICARDA Pakistan). Major theme of the project revolves around the characterization of the various viral strains, screening of US cotton germplasm in Pakistan, transferring of new sources of resistance into adapted varieties of Pakistan, etc. [29].

A project "Sustainable Control of the Cotton Bollworm, *Helicoverpa armigera*, in Small-scale Cotton Production systems" was sponsored by the Common Fund for Commodities to be executed by China, India, Pakistan and UK. The overall objective of the project was to develop, apply, and disseminate cropping systems and pest management practices for cost-effective and sustainable control of the cotton bollworm *Helicoverpa armigera*. The project aimed to build on existing knowledge and experiences for the further development of efficient methods, resulting in substantially reduced uses of hazardous pesticides and increased profitability for cotton producers.

5. Sharing

In Pakistan, germplasm (conventional) can be shared for utilizing in local cotton breeding programs without imposing any kind of restriction. However, for utilizing in breeding program outside the country, one must get permission from the developer provided the venture is commercially driven. However, two organizations like NIBGE and CEMB are involved in the introduction of alien genes through utilizing genetic engineering approaches. In this regard, for example, CEMB has restricted the utilization of its material through signing MTAs with the private seed companies. Similarly, these two organization also got their novel genes patented (national and or internationally) which itself restrict the use of the genetic material.

Since 1992, Pakistan is signatory to UN convention on biological diversity (CBD), ITPGRA, and International Technical Conference on Plant genetic Resources, Lipzig, Germany. Thus country grant permission for accessing PGR on jointly agreed provisions subjected to pre informed approval of contracting bodies. Also, the contracting bodies are supposed to share the results of research and developments and the benefits that are achieved by exploring such resources. In order to utilize the germplasm, the access to PGR is a mandatory step. In Pakistan, Biodiversity working group of Ministry of Environment has prepared draft Biodiversity law 2005 and was circulated to all stakeholders for safe sharing of germplasm.

6. Characterization, evaluation and utilization

Germplasm characterization and evaluation are the key elements for determining the characteristics of the germplasm. The newly introduced material, if not in sufficient quantity, first its seed quantity is multiplied. In the next normal cotton growing season, the material is planted and data of various characters including plant height, flowering time, number of bolls and their weight, fiber characteristics and yield potential are collected. However, screening to cotton leaf curl disease remains the major focus of all the breeders in the country.

There are two categories for germplasm evaluation. The first category comprises systematic collection of descriptors that is chiefly conducted by the guardian of the working collection of the National Collection of *Gossypium* Germplasm, largely by PCCC. These second evaluations usually involve germplasm collection in varying sizes subsets and often are neither systematic nor exhaustive in their approach. Such investigation is being leaned towards goal. University and federal investigators often undertake evaluations for studying the various aspects of cotton plant biochemistry and physiology especially after exposing to various abiotic stresses. Following research institutes are involved in taking notes of various cotton plant characters:

1. Morphological and agronomic trait evaluations: Agronomy section AARI Faisalabad, CRI AARI Faisalabad (including its stations), NIBGE Faisalabad, NIAB Faisalabad, NIA Tandojam and institutes of PCCC.
2. Cytogenetic: CCRI Multan, CRS Multan and NIAB Faisalabad.
3. Biochemical (gossypol): NIAB Faisalabad
4. Quantification of Bt toxin: CEMB Lahore, NIBGE Faisalabad, ABRI Faisalabad, NIGAB Islamabad.
5. Seed Quality: FSC&RD Islamabad
6. Disease resistance: PCCC, NIBGE Faisalabad, AARI Faisalabad
7. Stress evaluation: NIBGE Faisalabad, UAF Faisalabad, CCRI Multan and AARI Faisalabad.
8. Fiber properties: CCRI Multan, NIBGE Faisalabad, CRS Multan and CRI AARI Faisalabad.

The accessions are hybridized with the adaptive cotton variety. After, fixing all the traits of interest, breeder of the line develops a descriptor. This line is then submitted for registration to FSC&RD and also for testing in the National Coordinated Varietal Trials (NCVTs). Federal Seed Certification and Registration Department conducts these CVRTs for two successive years. The data of various characters of the advanced line is compared with the data given in the descriptor. Salient features of the cotton varieties released till present are documented by the FSC&RD in a book "Cotton Varieties of Pakistan" which provides information about the descriptions of the varieties that is primarily based on stability, uniformity and distinctness, and also on the studies conducted for two successive years under field and laboratory conditions [30].

Recent challenge for evaluation of the newly released cotton varieties is narrow genetic base that is limiting future breeding progress against various stresses. Mainly selection and crossing of well adapted cotton parent genotypes for developing new varieties are the main causes of yield stagnation in the country. It can be partly overcome by involving genetically diverse parent genotypes in the genealogy of a new variety. For example, genes conferring resistance to abiotic stresses especially drought, and biotic stresses especially resistance to the CLCuD can be introgressed from *G. arboretum* L. and or *G. herbaceum* L. into the cultivated *G. hirsutum* L. cotton species. For undertaking this process on massive scale, tissue culturing tools may help in overcoming the phyletic barriers. Preliminary steps have already been taken for introgressing useful genes into the cultivated cotton varieties at CRS Multan and CCRI Multan. Similarly, QTLs/genes conferring high quality traits have been transferred into the cultivated cotton species using DNA markers at NIBGE Faisalabad. All these experiments would help in widening the genetic base of the cultivated cotton varieties in the field. Another strategy for creation of genetic variability is the deployment of various mutagens (radiations and chemicals). In this regard, leading genotypes of *G. hirsutum* L. and *G. arboreum* L. have been treated with EMS for developing TILLING populations that would help in understanding the genes involved in conferring various traits of interest. The preliminary genomic information from model species such as Arabidopsis and cacao genome can be instrumental in exploring the conserved but complex pathways in least possible time.

DNA fingerprints by deploying SSRs of all the leading cotton cultivars including germplasm and also the extent of genetic divergence among the genotypes should be made available to the cotton breeders. This information can be used in planning crosses. Secondly, involving of more than two parent genotypes preferably conical crosses should be made which may help in increasing the genetic window among the newly developed cotton varieties [31].

6.1. Utilization of germplasm for the development of Upland cotton varieties in Pakistan

The variety 268-F, bred at research sub-station Jhang, was early maturing and was approved for cultivation in 1948 because of the superior physical properties of its fiber (could spin up to 41 counts) over the existing strains/varieties (4-F, L.S.S., 289-F/43 etc.). However, ultimately 268-F was banned because of its poor germination rate [32].

The cotton variety L.S.S. was extensively used in hybridization in Pakistan. A cotton variety 362-F, developed by selection from the population of L.S.S. was approved for general cultivation in 1958 because of its earliness trait exhibited in the Lyallpur region. However, this variety showed adaptability only in the 'Thal' region (a sandy, rain fed area). The variety was of the bushy type but was not adopted in other cotton growing districts (Table 3).

Serial #	Name of variety	Center of release	Year of release	Pedigree/parentage	GOT %¥	Staple length mm	Fineness µg/inch	Strength tppsi€
1	3-F	CRI, Faisalabad	1913	Selection from varieties introduced from USA by East India Company	33.0	20.6	4.9	85.0
2	4-F	CRI, Faisalabad	1914	Selection from stray plants of American Cotton	32.0	20.6	5.0	85.0
3	289-F	CRI, Faisalabad	1921	4-F-Selection, Natural hybrid- an off type plant found in the 4 F field	32.0	25.0	4.5	95.0
4	289 -F/K25	BCGA, Khanewal	1930	289-F bulk selection	33.5	23.8	4.5	95.0
5	L.S.S.	CRI, Faisalabad	1934	Selection from 4-F-a single plant variant (natural hybrid) in the 4-F field	32.2	23	5.0	85.0
6	289-F/43	CRS, AARI, Faisalabad	1934	Selection from 4-F-natural hybrid, an off-type plant in the 4-F field	31.0	23.8	4.5	95.0
7	124-F	CRI, AARI, Faisalabad	1945	Selection from 289-F/43	33.0	24.6	4.8	96.0
8	216 -F	CRI, AARI, Faisalabad	1946	Selection from 4-F	33.0	23.8	4.5	90.0
9	199-F	CRI, AARI, Multan.	1946	Selection from 4-F-98 (material from Sakrand)	35.0	24.6	4.5	90.0
10	238-F	CRI, AARI, Faisalabad	1948	Selection from 289-F/43	31.5	23.8	4.5	88.0
11	Lasani-11	CRS,AARI, Faisalabad	1959	Selection from 181-F	34.5	28.6	4.0	90.0
12	AC-134	CRI, AARI, Faisalabad	1959	148-F x 199-F	34.5	26.5	4.5	93.5
13	362-F	CRI, AARI, Faisalabad	1959	Selection from 289-F	33.0	23.8	4.5	93.0
14	BS-1(13/26)	CRS, AARI, Khanpur	1962	Selection from M-4	33.8	26.0	4.2	94.2

Serial #	Name of variety	Center of release	Year of release	Pedigree/parentage	GOT %¥	Staple length mm	Fineness µg/inch	Strength tppsi€
15	MS-40	CRS, AARI, Multan	1970	(124-F x 181-F), a single variant plant (natural hybrid) selected from AC-252 field	34.0	31.3	4.0	89.4
16	MS-39	CRS, AARI, Multan	1970	Natural hybrid in L-11 field	33.5	31.8	3.6	87.5
17	149-F	CRS, AARI, Multan	1971	124-F x Babdal	34.5	28.0	4.0	97.0
18	B-557	CRI, AARI, Faisalabad	1975	268-F x (45-F x L.S.S)	35.9	28.1	4.5	93.0
19	MNH-93	CRS, AARI, Multan	1980	(124-F x Babdal) x (MS-39 x Mex 12)	37.5	28.6	4.5	94.2
20	NIAB-78	NIAB, Faisalabad	1983	DPL-16 x AC-134)-F_1 Irradiated-30 kr Gamma rays (60 Co)	37.0	27.0	4.6	92.0
21	MS-84	CRS, AARI, Multan	1983	(124-F x 181-F) x DPL-16	34.0	33.3	3.9	91.3
22	SLH-41	CRS, PCCC, Sahiwal	1984	(289-F x Mysor American) x (124-F x Babdal) x Mex 68)	36.7	27.8	4.4	95.8
23	Rehmani	CRS, AARI, Tandojam	1985	*G. hirsutum* 21 x McNaire TH-14920	35.0	27.0	4.4	90.0
24	MNH-129	CRS,AARI, Multan	1986	{(124-F x Babdal) x (MS-39 x Mex 12)} x DPL-16	38.5	28.7	4.4	95.0
25	CIM-70	CCRI, PCCC, Multan	1986	Coker 8314 x (124-F x Babdal) x Coker 100 WA)	31.1	28.6	4.2	92.5
26	S-12	CRS, AARI, Multan	1988	{(124-F x Babdal) x (MS-39 x Mex 12)} x 7203-14-4-Arizona	41.3	28.0	4.6	93.0
27	FH-87	CRI, AARI, Faisalabad	1988	AC-134 x Paymaster	36.8	27.8	4.2	96.0
28	RH-1	CRS, AARI, R.Y. Khan	1990	LH-62 x W-1104	31.8	29.8	3.9	103.7
29	NIAB-86	NIAB, Faisalabad	1990	(DPL-16 x AC-134-F1 30kr) x Stoneville-213	34.5	29.0	4.3	95.0

Serial #	Name of variety	Center of release	Year of release	Pedigree/parentage	GOT %¥	Staple length mm	Fineness µg/inch	Strength tppsi€
30	Gohar-87	CRS, PCCC, Bahawalpur	1990	(124-F x Babdal) x B-557	36.0	28.0	4.5	98.6
31	CIM-109	CCRI, Multan	1990	(DPL-16 x AC-134 – F1 30kr) x A89/FM	35.0	27.3	4.4	91
32	Reshmi -90	CRS, ARI, Tandojam	1991	Coker 100A x (DPL-16 x AC-134 – F1 30kr)	35.7	31.5	4.1	98.7
33	NIAB -26N	NIAB, Faisalabad	1992	(DPL-16 x AC-134-F_1 irradiated 30kr) x DPL-NSL	37.5	28.0	4.4	95
34	MNH -147	CRS, AARI, Multan	1992	[{(124-F x Babdal) x (L -11 x Lankart 57)} x {(124-F x Babdal)} x Mex Pollen) x MS-64)] x {B-557 x (124-F x Babdal) x DPL-16)}	41.3	28.5	4.2	95.5
35	FH -682	CRI, AARI, Faisalabad	1992	(B-557 x Ala (68)1) x Lankart-57	37.0	28.5	4.3	95.7
36	CIM-240	CCRI, PCCC Multan	1992	Coker 8314 x (124-F x Babdal) x Coker 100 WA) x W 1104	36.5	27.8	4.7	94.0
37	BH-36	CRS, PCCC, Bahawalpur	1992	M-4 x T x Bonham-76C	38.7	27.8	4.3	100.5
38	Gomal -93	CRS, PCCC, D.I. Khan	1993	387-F x AC-134	34.5	26.5	4.5	93.0
39	SLS-1	CRS, PCCC, Sahiwal	1995	SLH-19 x SLH-19 x (DPL-16 xAC-134 – F1 30kr)	35.0	27.4	4.5	95.3
40	S-14	CRS, AARI, Multan	1995	{(124-F x Babdal) x (AC-252 x DPL-16) x DPL-16) x Lankart 4789 A} x {(124-F x Babdal) x (AC-252 x DPL-16) x Coker. (F_1 x F_1)}	43.0	29.5	4.2	93.0
41	RH-112	CRS, AARI, R.Y. Khan	1996	(124 -F x Babdal) x Delfoss) x (AC-134 x C.T.)	34.3	27.6	4.6	95.0
42	MNH-329	CRS, AARI, Multan	1996	{(124-F x Babdal) x (MS-39 x Mex 12)} x {B-557 x (124-F x Babdal) x DPL-16)}	41.0	28.5	4.2	96.0

http://dx.doi.org/10.5772/58620

Serial #	Name of variety	Center of release	Year of release	Pedigree/parentage	GOT %¥	Staple length mm	Fineness µg/inch	Strength tppsi€
43	NIAB-Karishma	NIAB, Faisalabad	1996	{(DPL-16 x AC-134-F_1 30kr) x Stoneville 213)} x W 83-29 Mex	37.4	28.6	5.0	93.3
44	FH-634	CRI, AARI, Faisalabad	1996	CEDEX x B-557	36.3	28.5	4.1	95.1
45	CIM-1100	CCRI, PCCC, Multan.	1996	(W-1104 x {(124-F x Babdal) x (MS-39 x Mex 12)} x 7203-14-4-Arizona) x CP 15/2	38.0	29	4.0	94
46	CIM-448	CCRI, PCCC, Multan	1996	{(124-F x Babdal) x (MS-39 x Mex 12)} x 7203-14-4-Arizona (sister line CIM-1100)	38.0	28.5	4.5	93.8
47	FVH-53	CRS, AARI, Vehari	1998	KIVI 1021 x {(124-F x Babdal) x (MS-39 x Mex 12)} x 7203-14-4-Arizona	38.4	28.6	5.2	98.5
48	CIM-446	CCRI, PCCC, Multan	1998	CP-15/2 x {(124-F x Babdal) x (MS-39 x Mex 12)} x 7203-14-4-Arizona	36.1	27	4.7	97.4
49	CIM-443	CCRI, PCCC, Multan	1998	(DPL-16 x AC -134 – F_1 30kr) x A-89/FM x LRA-5166	36.5	27.6	4.9	96.1
50	MNH -554	CRS, AARI, Multan	2000	{(124-F x Babdal) x (L-11 x Lankart-57) x 4-C} x (C-603 x Mex 3) x LRA -5166	41.3	28.0	4.2	94.0
51	MNH -552	CRS, AARI, Multan	2000	(124-F x Babdal) x LRA -5166	40.0	27.5	4.9.0	95.0
52	FH-901	CRI, AARI, Faisalabad	2000	{Coker 8314 x (124 -F x Babdal) x Coker 100 WA) x W 1106} x {(W 1104 x {(124-F x Babdal) x (MS-39 x Mex }	38.0	27.5	5.2	92.0
53	FH-900	CRI, AARI, Faisalabad	2000	(FH-672 x AET-5) x (B- 557 x LRA- 5166)	38.0	28.5	4.3	95.1
54	CIM-482	CCRI, Multan	2000	{(DPL -16 x AC -134 – F_1 30kr) x ALS 15(CIM -39 x ALS -15} x CP-15/2	39.2	29.0	4.5	98.0

Serial #	Name of variety	Center of release	Year of release	Pedigree/parentage	GOT %¥	Staple length mm	Fineness µg/inch	Strength tppsi€
55	BH-118	CRS, Bahawalpur	2000	(T x 339 x ST-7A) x (ST-7A x AET- 5)	38.5	28.0	4.6	98.0
56	CIM-473	CCRI, Multan	2002	[{(Coker 8314 x (124 -F x Babdal)} x {Coker 100 WA) x (CIM- 46 x (AC -134 x (DPL- 16 x AC- 134-F_1 30kr)}] x LRA -5166	39.7	29.5	4.3	95.0
57	NIAB-999	NIAB, Faisalabad	2003	(DPL -16 x AC -134-F_1 30kr) x LRA- 5166	36.5	28.7	4.6	98.0
58	FH-1000	CRS, AARI, Faisalabad	2003	[{(124 -F x Babdal) x (MS- 39 x Mex 12)} x 7203-14-4-Arizona] x [{(124 -F x Babdal) x (MS- 39 x Mex 12)} x 7203-14-4-Arizona]	38.8	29.5	4.6	96.9
59	CIM-499	CCRI, Multan	2003	CIM-433 x 755-6/93	40.0	29.6	4.4	97.3
60	CIM-506	CCRI, Multan	2004	CIM-360 x CP-15/2	38.6	28.7	4.5	98.9
61	CIM-707	CCRI, Multan	2004	CIM-243 x 738-6/93	39.0	32.2	4.2	97.5
62	NIAB-111	NIAB, Faisalabad	2004	F_1seed 300 Gy gamma radiation 0R (NIAB-313/12 x CIM-100) F_1 300 Gy	37.5	30.5	4.4	218.8
63	BH-160	CRS, Bahawalpur	2004	Cedix FDW 946 x 673/93	39.0	29.5	4.2	95.1
64	CIM-496	CCRI, Multan	2005	CIM-425 x 755-6/93 (1993)	41.1	29.7	4.6	93.5
65	CIM-534	CCRI, Multan	2006	Hybridization of local line 5-4/94 with locally developed variety CIM-1100	40.32	27.9	4.5	97.2
66	MNH-786	CRS, Multan	2006	(S-14 x CIM-448) x (MNH-564 x MNH-516)	38.7	27.2	5.1	95.0
67	NIBGE-2	NIBGE, Faisalabad	2006	S-12 x LRA- 5166	36.2	28.6	5.0	100.0
68	NIAB-846	NIAB, Faisalabad	2008	NIAB-78 x REBA-288 Pollen irradiated (10Gy) with gamma rays	38.5	29.8	4.7	96.0
69	CIM-554	CCRI, Multan	2009	2579-4/97 x W-1103	41.5	28.5	4.7	96.8

http://dx.doi.org/10.5772/58620

Serial #	Name of variety	Center of release	Year of release	Pedigree/parentage	GOT %¥	Staple length mm	Fineness µg/inch	Strength tppsi€
70	NIAB-777	NIAB,Faisalabad	2009	NIAB-78 x Reba-288	38.8	28.9	4.4	93.0
71	CRSM-38	CRS, Multan	2009	583-85/99 x FH900 583-85/99 = LRA5166 x BJA592	39.5	29.0	4.5	95.0
72	NIBGE-115	NIBGE, Faisalabad	2012	S-12 x LRA-5166	38.15	29.51	4.93	93.1
73	BH-167	CRS, Bahawalpur	2012	VH-53 x BH-142 (Hybridization)	41.2	29.1	4.8	92.7
74	FH-942	CRI, AARI, Faisalabad	2012	FH-900(S) x CIM-121(hybridization)	38.01	29.63	4.28	95.1
75	NIAB-852	NIAB, Faisalabad	2012	NIAB-78 x REBA-288 Pollen irradiated (10Gy) with gamma rays	37.8	31.6	4.5	91.2
76	CIM-573	CCRI, Multan	2012	H-2118 x H-2119 (cross in 2000-01)	39.34	31.61	4.64	90.2
77	SLH-317	CRS, Sahiwal	2012	{LRA-5166 x (SLH-205 x LRA-5166)}	38.0	29.8	4.4	96.7
78	NN-3	NIBGE, Faisalabad	2013	S-12 x LRA-5166	38.14	30.17	4.63	93.6
79	NIAB-Kiran	NIAB, Faisalabad	2013	NIAB-98 x NIAB-11I	38.96	30.41	4.61	93.8
80	NIAB-112	NIAB, Faisalabad	2013	NIAB-111 x NIAB-999	38.3	28.6	4	90.0
81	CIM-608	CCRI, Multan	2013	2(*G. hirsutum*/*G.anomalum*)x G^3-*hirutum*	40.3.	29.88	4.78	95.4
82	GS-14	Gohar Seed Corporation, Multan	2013	CIM-448 x exotic variety Acala SJ-2 (USA)	40.82	28.04	5.88	96.0

¥=Ginning out turn percentage; **€**=Thousand pounds per square inch

Source: Dr. Akhlaq Hussain, Description of cotton varieties of Pakistan 2004, Cotton Research and development Memoranda till 60's (Ed. Dr. Mahbub Ali), approval documents of cotton varieties released after 2004 and personal communication with breeders of the cotton varieties.

Table 3. List of approved *G. hirsutum* L.(upland cotton) varieties (non-GM) for Punjab

In the mid-1960s, efforts were made to grow cotton varieties previously recommended for cultivation in various countries especially in the USA. Deltapine, a smooth leaf variety, was introduced in Multan and Sheikhupura. In total, 16-17 insecticides sprays were applied on these newly introduced varieties, and 922 kg/hectare seed cotton yield was harvested, demonstrating a limited scope of the introduced cotton varieties in this region. In the same normal cotton growing season, a number of exotic cotton varieties like Tide Water, Stoneville-213, Stoneville 7-A, Acala P-5, Carolina Queen, Dixie King, Express H3-P1, Defos 44, Deltapine Smooth Leaf and Coker Wild along with AC-134 and L-11 (local controls) were planted at the CRS Multan. The yield of some of these varieties was comparable with the control AC-134. Breeding efforts for overcoming the menace of insect pests infestation were made through selection, but went fruitless because of a limited genetic diversity available in the exotic germplasm. Hybridization of the exotic germplasm with the locally adapted cultivars/germplasm was remained the only strategy for improving the local cotton varieties by introducing high yielding genes of the exotic material into local cultivated cotton varieties [33]. Big boll trait was transferred from Lankert-57, and compactness and earliness from Babdale. The major limitation of big boll variety was susceptibility to insects. The newly developed strains derived from these crosses out yielded the standard AC-134. The other advantages over the indigenous cultivar AC-134 were drought tolerance and earliness in maturity. The upland cotton varieties developed till 1990s were dominantly of open type. Boll size was relatively smaller than the present day varieties. Emphasis was given to improve boll size especially after the introduction of Bt cotton varieties in Pakistan. Earlier, all successful varieties till the evolution of S-12, bred for large number of bolls rather than boll size for compensating the boll damage done by bollworms infestation. NIAB-78, proved to be the most successful variety, bears large number of bolls with small to medium sizeed boll. Later, the best extension services provided by public sector organizations and especially the private sectors, dominantly pesticide companies, educated farmers for eradicating pest population through chemical means.

In Pakistan, one of the main objectives is to develop a variety that matures early than that of the varieties released before 1980s. Such early maturing varieties help farmers to sow wheat- a major staple food crop in Pakistan. However, very early maturing varieties are not suitable because high temperature early in the cotton growing season may affect boll opening which ultimately may cause significant reduction in seed cotton yield [26]. Best suitable time for cotton maturity in Pakistan is between November 15-30—enough time to harvest high yield and good quality lint without compromising the cultivation of wheat crop. For addressing this issue, breeders have been successful in releasing cotton varieties like NIAB-78, S-12, CIM-496, IR-NIBGE-3701 and MNH-886, etc. which allows farmers to plant wheat in time. Further efforts for releasing varieties which mature in mid of Nov. through exploiting the available germplasm, resulted in the development of an advance line IR-NIBGE-5, flowers five and seven days earlier than IR-NIBGE-3 and IR-NIBGE-3701, respectively. However, such kind of genetic material requires unusually much more water and nutrients. Thus, a comprehensive breeding approach by bridging molecular and conventional tools is needed for releasing highly adaptive cotton varieties.

6.1.1. *Leading G. hirsutm L. cultivars of Post-CLCuD Era*

Leaf curl disease on cotton was first time reported in 1912 from Nigeria, and then it spread in many other cotton growing countries such as Pakistan, India and China. This disease is of viral origin and transmitted by a vector whitefly (*Bemisia tabaci* Gennadius), which may cause 30-70% or even more depression in seed cotton yield. It was first time appeared on few plants in 1967 in Pakistan. Typical symptoms of the disease are small and large veins thickening and upward or downward curling of the leaf. Under high infection, a small leaf like structure—called enation underneath of the leaf has been observed (Figure 1).

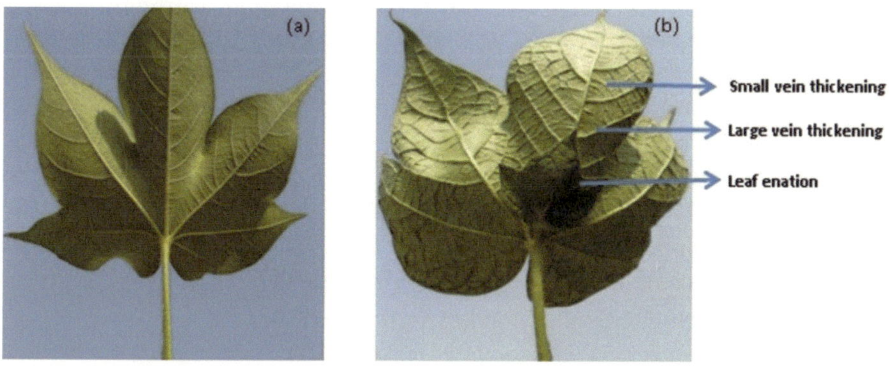

Figure 1. Comparison of healthy (a) versus infected cotton leaves showing symptoms of cotton leaf curl virus disease

Efforts were made for combating the disease by finding resistance sources from the available cotton germplasm. In this regard, more than 1000 cotton lines available in the gene pool of CCRI Multan were screened under natural conditions (Muhammad Afzal, CCRI Multan, personnel communication). Three genotypes LRA-5166, CP-15/2 and Cedix were identified. However, LRA-5166 and CP-15/2 were used extensively for deriving resistance into the cultivated susceptible cotton cultivars through various hybridization breeding procedures. In this regard, CIM-1100 was the first resistant cotton varieties released from CCRI Multan in 1997 followed by a series of resistant cotton varieties by CCRI Mutlan and few from other cotton breeding research institutes (Table 3). Deploying of the two sources of resistance in breeding program has created a major genetic bottleneck in evolution.

Resistance to the Multan strain of virus was controlled by two genes [33]. This resistance was overcome in within five years because of the evolution of new strain of virus called Burewala strain. Till today, none of the variety was found completely asymptomatic. However, high tolerance or field resistance was observed in few cotton genotypes, viz. NIBGE-2472, NIBGE-3661, NIBGE-115 [34], FH-142, and NN-3[35]. Cotton germplasm (3000 accessions of *G. hirsutum* L. and introgressed lines) received through the United States Department for Agriculture (USDA) has also been screened. Initial studies have shown that Mac-07 and approximately 95 lines are resistant to the disease. These newly identified sources can be used extensively in improving the cotton germplasm/varieties resistant to the CLCuD.

Introgression breeding procedures have been deployed to introgress important traits from *G. arboreum* L. like, resistance to CLCuD, tolerance to drought etc. into the cultivated *G. hirsutum* L. cotton varieties. In these experiments, chromosome of *G. arboreum* L. was doubled by applying colchicine followed by hybridization with the allotetraploid *G. hirsutum* L. under natural conditions. Exogenous treatment of hormones 50 mg/L gibberellic acid and 100 mg/L naphthalene acetic acid were applied for overcoming the problem of boll shedding. It has been demonstrated that the percentage of pollen viability in F_1s was 1.90% in 2(*G. arboreum*) x *G. hirsutum* versus 2.38% in *G. hirsutum* x 2(*G. arboreum*). Further confirmations were made through cytological studies; found that all F_{1s} were sterile. All the F_1 plants exhibited resistance to the CLCuD after exposing through grafting of the infected buds, indicating the chances of success for transferring resistance into the cultivated tetraploids [36]. Currently the progenies/advance generations are being screened against the disease at CCRI Multan (Project PI Mr. Zahid Mehmood, Pr Scientist) and CRS Multan (Project PI Dr. Saghir Ahmed, Botanist). Similarly, emphasis was also made for improving quality parameters of the local cultivated species var FH-1000 by crossing it with the *G. barbadense* L. The introgressions of the DNA fragments from *G. barbadense* L. were monitored through SSR markers [37]. The resultant hybrids or progenies had two types of leaves, narrow versus broad lobed types. It was reported that bolls of the narrow lobed types did not mature due to bad opening. However, the broad lobed types were found comparatively high yielder but poor in lint quality. Efforts on various fronts are going on for evolving useful germplasm or varieties.

7. Databases

In early seventies, activities related to the collection as well as conservation of germplasm have been started in Pakistan. In this regard, cotton germplasm have been collected from various countries largely of upland cotton. Recently, more than 3000 accessions have been imported from US under the Pak-US cotton productivity enhancement project. Before this, cotton material (accessions of *G. hirsutum*) was imported from different countries including USA, Uzbekistan, and France, etc. Most of the accessions are available with CCRI Multan, and maintained descriptions of each accession both hard as well as soft copy which can be obtained upon the request. However, no website is available showing the description of the cotton germplasm in Pakistan.

Efforts for conservation of genetic material are also under way at PGRI, Islamabad. Passport data of around 75% of the accessions of different crops has been entered in the form of dBase files. Users can get information in the form of computer print outs on request. However, local scientists on a limited scale can get direct on-line access to the files. Consultation of data books that are maintained by the institute can be done at any time by local scientists. Linkage of documentation section with all PGRI laboratories is made sure by availability of a local network that is not in working condition yet. However, currently there are no options available for networking with other gene banks for the data exchange on crop basis as well as regional basis. The process of data base and information system establishment is on the move. PGRI has plans for its connection to other gene banks in future.

http://dx.doi.org/10.5772/58620

8. Novel trends and perspectives

Exotic Bt cotton strains were first cultivated in Sindh in 2000. This introduced material showed high susceptibility to sucking insect pests and CLCuD. Breeding to introgress the *Bt* gene (*Cry1Ac*) by backcross hybridization was initiated in 2000 by various public and private sector organizations of Pakistan but resulting lines could not be tested in the field due to the suspension of biosafety rules in Pakistan. The National Institute for Biotechnology & Genetic engineering (NIBGE) initiated development of Bt cotton and field testing under the "voluntary code of conduct" issued by the Ministry of Environment. A huge quantity of data for the safe release of Bt cotton in the field was generated using rabbit as an experimental animal, and also the impact of Bt cotton residues on weed and soil microbial populations. It was demonstrated that the cultivation of Bt cotton is safe to wild as well as domesticated animals, and its impact, if any, will be low or negligible. This approach for characterizing risk is consistent with the accepted risk assessment procedures and shared similarities with the previous assessments over a wide range of situations (Zaman & Co-workers, unpublished).

The area under Bt cotton cultivation has been increased dramatically. Around 40,000 kg of seed of the Bt cotton strains IR-FH-901 (later approved as IR-NIBGE-901), IR-NIBGE-2 (later approved as IR-NIBGE-1524 in 2010), IR-CIM-448 (later approved as IR-NIBGE-3701) and IR-CIM-443, was provided to farmers and was grown on over 3,238 ha (hectares) in 2005-2006 [38]. IR-NIBGE-1524 was approved for general cultivation in 2010 and 2011 for Punjab and Sindh (Table 4). This variety was drought tolerant, with an open canopy and bears small bolls. It was planted on a large area (more than 5%) in 2007 and retained ~2% of the area, particularly in the drought prone, each year until 2012 in Punjab. In Sindh, it was planted on ~10% of the area in 2012 (Director General Agriculture Sindh). The NIBGE Bt cotton strains were used extensively in breeding programs as a source for developing Bt cotton varieties by various research organizations, and established the foundation of Bt cotton cultivation in Pakistan.

In post-Bt era, preference for cultivating compact to semi-compact varieties has been given for sowing in normal season. Earlier, semi-compact to compact type cotton varieties like CIM-448, CIM-497, NIAB-111 and BH-160 were released for general cultivation but could not capture significant area. There were two major reasons. Firstly, it is difficult to control insect pests especially bollworms in compact shaped plant versus open type plant. Secondly, compact shaped plant does not compensate for low population density compared to the open shaped plant. Before Bt cotton cultivation, major area >10% covered by open type varieties, viz. B-557, NIAB-78, MNH-93, S-12, CIM-240, NIAB-Karishma, CIM-473 and CIM-496 etc. Bt cotton varieties offered inbuilt resistance to *Heliothus*, spotted and marginally to pink bollworm. Thus one of the disadvantages of cultivating compact shaped varieties has been addressed. First Bt cotton variety, IR-NIBGE-3701—semi-compact shaped variety, tested for yield in National Coordinated Bt Trials (NCBT) in 2009, out yielded all candidate lines and standard cotton variety CIM-496. IR-NIBGE-3701 formed the basis for cultivation of compact shaped variety among the farming community. Later on, CIM-886 dominantly a compact shaped variety covered a significant area in 2012.

Serial #	Name of variety	Center of release	Year of release	Pedigree/parentage	GOT %¥	Staple length mm	Fineness µg/inch	Strength tppsi€
1	IR-NIBGE-3701$	NIBGE, Faisalabad	2010	Selection from IR-CIM-448	43.23	27.52	5.43	90.2
2	IR-NIBGE-1524$	NIBGE, Faisalabad	2010	Transgenic line as a donor parent for Bt gene.NIBGE-2 as an adapted parent	38.55	30.15	4.73	92.5
3	Neelum-121	Neelum Seeds Corporation	2010	A-92 x exotic variety	41.87	28.70	4.81	29.5
4	FH-113	CRI, AARI, Faisalabad	2010	FH-925 x Bollgard	38.13	28.61	5.00	24.85
5	AA-802	Ali Akbar Seeds, Multan	2010	[{(FH-1000 x HK-303) x LRA-5166} x Linea-100]	43.26	29.49	4.77	92.8
6	AA-703	Ali Akbar Seeds, Multan	2010	CIM-482 x Exotic Line	38.8	29.8	4.45	99.98
7	MG-06	ThattaGurmani Research Center, KotAdu, Muzafarghar	2010	CIM-443 x IR-448	38.0	29.32	4.7	28.7
8	Sitara-008	Agri Farm Research Center, Multan	2010	NIAB-III x IR-448	40.0	27.3	4.6	95.9
9	IR-NIBGE-901£	NIBGE, Faisalabad	2011	Transgenic line as a donor parent for Bt gene. FH-901as an adapted parent, used in backcrossing	38.86	27.06	5.38	90.8
9	MNH-886	CRS, Multan	2012	FH-207 x MNH-770 x Bollguard-1	41.01	28.21	4.95	99.5
10	Bt. CIM-598	CCRI, Multan	2012	CIM-446 x IR-CIM-448	41.82	29.03	4.38	94.8
11	Tarzen-1	4-Brothers Seed Corporation, Multan	2012	{(CIM-496 x hk 303) x Linea-100}	42.6	29.15	4.96	95.0
12	Neelum-141	Neelum Seeds Corporation	2012	IR-448 x C-2-2	41.05	29.0	4.9	101.5

Serial #	Name of variety	Center of release	Year of release	Pedigree/parentage	GOT %¥	Staple length mm	Fineness µg/inch	Strength tppsi€
13	FH-114	CRI, Faisalabad	2012	Non-*Bt* early maturing cotton lines FH-925 with Australian *Bt* variety Bollgard-1(*Cry1Ac*)	39.64	28.12	4.85	95.5
14	IR-NIBGE-3	NIBGE, Faisalabad	2012	Developed through selection from IR-NIBGE-2381);Bt version of FH-1000	38.68	28.3	4.96	97.6
15	Sitara-009	Agri Farm Research Center, Multan	2012	{(CIM-496 x Sitara-008) x MNH-786}	39.8	25.7	4.87	97.6
16	A-One	Weal Ag Corporation, Multan	2012	{FVH-53 x Exotic *Bt*}	38.01	29.91	4.56	96.6

$=Approved for Punjab and Sindh provinces while rest of the varieties are only approved for Punjab; £=Approved for Sindh province only; ¥=Ginning out turn percentage; €=Thousand pounds per square inch

Source: Minutes of 42nd meeting of Punjab Seed Council at Lahore dated Feb 16, 2012, approval documents of cotton varieties and personal communication with breeders of the cotton varieties.

Table 4. List of approved Bt-cotton varieties

Now the emphasis is on releasing varieties with a high boll count and a low shedding rate. It has dramatically been changed after the introduction of Bt cotton as it offers inbuilt resistance to the cotton plant; otherwise this trend has not been observed in varieties released before the Bt-era. Also, spring cultivation is gaining popularity in the Punjab province. Around 5-10% of the area is sown early (Feb-March) because of the Bt varieties are not prone to early infestation by bollworms.

9. Conclusions

In Pakistan the provision of high quality seed has been a major issue that emerged after the first epidemic of CLCuD. The informal seed sector (growers/breeders/private seed companies) profited by selling unapproved seed of advanced resistant lines resulting in the release of unstable cotton lines in early 1990s and onward. This situation was further exaggerated after the introduction of Bt cotton varieties. Thus a number of varieties, not properly bred, have been released in a very short time period, which accelerated the varietal replacement rate. All these issues hampered the process of production of certified seed.

The low germination of most cotton varieties, particularly in the post-Bt cotton era, is another area of concern for growers, regulators and policy makers. The germination rate can be improved by avoiding the use of early opened bolls and seed cotton exposed to excessive rain. Similarly, proper control of the moisture content of seed and proper storage conditions can also ensure the good health of cotton seed.

For Bt-cotton, the mixing of various types, mixing of non-Bt seed with the Bt variety, and the expression level of Bt genes in different varieties are the major issues which need to be addressed. The marketing of earlier released cotton varieties/strains under different names in the market is another area of concern which has affected the reputation of the cotton seed industry. In this regard, FSC&RD must ensure the distinctness of each of the newly developed varieties and or advanced strains with authenticated pedigree that may be verified by the use of DNA fingerprinting.

The deterioration of a cotton variety leads to reduced seed cotton yield. One of the major causes of this is a high natural cross pollination rate, largely by honeybees, in the Bt cotton era due to a reduction in the number of insecticide applications. Most of the breeding centers are located near urban areas where farmers also grow fodder and vegetable crops which provide alternative hosts for pollinators. Under such circumstances, selfing of plants is recommended on the representative plants of the variety/genotype which would help in maintaining the typical features of the variety.

Cultivation of hybrid cotton showing heterosis for seed cotton yield has remains a major challenge in Pakistan. Conventional methods of hybrid seed production (manual emasculation of floral buds), low seed setting, high cost of production resulting in high cost of seed and purity of seed are the major issues for cultivating hybrid cotton on significant area. Though limited efforts by the private sector (Mr Siddique Akbar Bukhari spent ~30 years; Guard and Four Brothers Seed Corporation Pakistan.) and public sector organizations (CCRI Multan, CRI Faisalabad, NARC Islamabad etc.) have been made, but are unable to provide seed which can cover even one percent of the total cotton growing area of Pakistan. In this regard, the development of male sterile and restorer lines, deployment of new genomic tools (such as RNAi technology), and also chemical emasculation, are the most plausible approaches for overcoming the issue surrounding the widespread adoption of hybrid seed.

Cultivated cotton has a narrow genetic base which limits future breeding progress. The selection and crossing of well adapted cotton varieties for developing new varieties are the main causes of the narrow genetic base. This problem can be partly overcome by involving genetically diverse parent genotypes in the genealogy of a new variety. For example, genes conferring resistance to abiotic stresses, particularly drought, and biotic stresses, particularly resistance to CLCuD, can be introgressed into *G. hirsutum* L. from *G. arboreum* L. and or *G. herbaceum*L. Tissue culture tools may help in overcoming the phyletic barriers. Preliminary steps have already been taken for introgressing useful genes into the cultivated cotton varieties

http://dx.doi.org/10.5772/58620

at CRS Multan and CCRI Multan. Similarly, QTLs/genes conferring high quality traits have been transferred into *G. hirsutum* L. using DNA markers at NIBGE, Faisalabad. Another strategy for the creation of genetic variability is the deployment of various mutagens (radiation and chemical). In this regard, leading genotypes of *G. hirsutum* L. and G. *arboreum* L. have been treated with EMS to develop TILLING populations—would help in understanding the genes involved in conferring various traits of interest.

The introduction of new genes from distantly related species using gene cloning and transformation approaches has emerged as a revolutionary genomic tool worldwide. In common with many other major cotton growing countries, the public sector in Pakistan has made substantial investment in developing GM-cotton conferring resistance to biotic and abiotic stresses. Bt cotton containing *Cry1Ac* gene is cultivated on 82% of the area of Pakistan. The first step towards the introduction of two genes (*Cry1Ac* and *Cry2Ab*) has been taken at CEMB Lahore and NIBGE Faisalabad. The material is being tested in multiple trials. For commercialization of advanced cotton lines containing these two genes, proposals for approval from the National Biosafety Committee have been submitted. Secondly, the expressing transgenes in different genetic backgrounds should be quantified to identifying genotype (s) best suited for commercial cultivation. This practice will reduce the possibility of resistance against the target pest developing—will help in formulating IPM strategies. Thirdly, Bt toxins are lethal to insects belonging to different orders. Hence, proper characterization of Bt gene cultivars is imperative before their release into the environment. To evaluate the possible impact of transgene containing cotton, or their byproducts, it is important to establish dedicated biosafety labs, which are lacking at the moment in the country, Ethyl methanesulfonate to ensure the safe release of GM crops and their products.

Abbreviations

AARI	Ayub Agricultural Research Institute
AFLP	Amplified Fragment Length Polymorphism
ARI	Agricultural Research Institute
CBD	Convention on Biological Diversity
CCRI	Central Cotton Research Institute
CEMB	Centre of Excellence in Molecular Biology
CLCuD	Cotton Leaf Curl Disease
CRI	Cotton Research Institute
CRS	Cotton Research Station
DAS	Days After Sowing
EMS	
GM	Genetically Modified

GOT	Ginning Outturn
HVI	High Volume Instrument
IR	Insect Resistance
ITPGRA	The international Treaty on Plant Genetic resources for food and Agriculture
NARC	National Agriculture Research Centre
NARS	National Agricultural Research System
NIAB	Nuclear Institute for Agriculture & Biology
NIBGE	Nuclear Institute for Biotechnology and Genetic engineering
PAEC	Pakistan Atomic Energy Commission
PARB	Punjab Agricultural Research Board
PARC	Pakistan Agricultural Research Council
PCCC	Pakistan Central Cotton Committee
PGR	Plant Genetic Resources
RAPD	Random Amplified Polymorphic DNA
RFLP	Restriction Fragment Length Polymorphism
SSR	Simple Sequence Repeat/Microsatellite
TILLING	Targeting Induced Local Lesions in Genome

Acknowledgements

I am extremely grateful to Prof Rob W Briddon for editing this chapter in least possible time. We cordially acknowledge a number of cotton breeders of PCCC especially Muhammad Idrees Khan, Muhammad Afzal and Ms. Rehana Rajput for providing us useful information for writing this chapter. We are also grateful to Dr Sajjad Haider for providing us information about the NIAB-based cotton varieties. We are also grateful to the cotton breeders of Provincial Govt of Punjab (Dr Saghir Ahmed, CRS Mutlan) and Sindh (DG Agri Dr Atta Muhammad Somroo) for sharing useful data and experiences which have been included in this manuscript. Similarly, information regarding seed quality related issues was provided by Ch Abdul Ghaffar, Punjab Seed Corporation Khanewal. Information pertaining to the development of hybrid cotton in Pakistan was kindly provided by Dr. Shaukat Ali, NARC Islamabad. This work is also partly supported by the U.S. Department of Agriculture, Agricultural Research Service; under agreement No.58-6402-0-178F through two subprojects entitled "Germplasm Evaluation (ICARDA-ID-1198-5 and Gene Mapping (ICARDA-ID-1198-6)". Any opinions, findings, conclusions or recommendations expressed in this manuscript are those of the author(s) and do not necessarily reflect the views of the U.S. Department of Agriculture". We dedicate this chapter to Dr. Mahbub Ali (Scientist Emeritus, Govt. of the Punjab), born on August 13, 1923 and did his Ph.D at Texas A & M University, USA. He has been involved in breeding cotton varieties and unraveling the genetics of various traits of cotton using conventional approaches over the last six decades.

Author details

Mehboob ur-Rahman[1], Zainab Rahmat[1], Abid Mahmood[2], Khalid Abdullah[3] and Yusuf Zafar[4]

1 Plant Genomics & Molecular Breeding (PGMB) Lab, National Institute for Biotechnology & Genetic Engineering (NIBGE), Jhang Road Faisalabad, Pakistan

2 Ayub Agricultural Research Institute (AARI), Faisalabad, Pakistan

3 Textile Industry Division, and Pakistan Central Cotton Committee (PCCC), Islamabad, Pakistan

4 Permanent Mission of Pakistan to the IAEA, Vienna, Austria

References

[1] Moulherat C, Tengberg M, Haquet JF, Mille B. First evidence of cotton at Neolithic Mehrgarh, Pakistan: analysis of mineralized fibres from a copper bead. Journal of Archaeological Science 2002; 29(12) 93–1401.

[2] Fryxell PA. The natural history of the cotton tribes. Texas A and M University Press College Station. USA; 1979. XVII p 245.

[3] Fryxell PA. A revised taxonomic interpretation of *Gossypium L. (Malvacea)*. Rheedea. 1992; 2(2) 108–165.

[4] Hutchinson JB. The application of genetics to cotton improvement. Empire Cotton Growing Corporation. University Press, Cambridge, 1959.

[5] Hutchinson JB, Silow RA, Stephens SG. The evolution of *Gossypium* and the differentiation of the cultivated cottons. Oxford University Press, London 1947.

[6] Gerstel DU. Chromosome translocations in interspecific hybrids of the genus *Gossypium*. Evolution 1953; 7 234–244.

[7] Gerstel DU, Sarvella PA. Additional observations on chromosomal translocations in cotton hybrids. Evolution 1956; 10 408–414.

[8] Phillips LL. The cytogenetics of speciation in Asiatic cotton. Genetics 1961; 46 77–83.

[9] Wendel JF, Olson PD, Stewart JMcD. Genetic diversity, introgression and independent domestication of old world cultivated cottons. The American Journal of Botany 1989; 76 1795–1806.

[10] Khan SA, Hussain D, Askari E, Stewart JMcD, Malik KA, Zafar Y. Molecular phylogeny of *Gossypium* species by DNA fingerprinting.Theoretical and Applied Genetics 2000; 101 931–938.

[11] Rana MK, Bhat KV. A comparison of AFLP and RAPD markers for genetic diversity and cultivar identification in cotton. Journal of Plant Biochemistry and Biotechnology 2004; 13 19–24.

[12] Tabbasam N, Zafar Y, Rahman M. Pros and cons of using genomic SSRs and EST-SSRs for resolving phylogeny of the genus *Gossypium*. Plant Systematics and Evolution 2013; DOI 10.1007/s00606-013-0891-x.

[13] Rahman M, Shaheen T, Tabbasam N, Iqbal MA, Ashraf M, Zafar Y, Paterson AH. Genetic resources in cotton and their improvement. Agronomy for Sustainable Development 2012; 32 419–432.

[14] Hutchinson JB. New evidence on the origin of the old world cotton. Heridity1954; 8 225–241.

[15] Silow RA. The genetics of species development in Old World cottons. Journal of Genetics 1944; 46 62–77.

[16] Brubaker CL, Bourland FM, Wendel JF. The origin and domestication of cotton. In: CW. Smith and JT. Cothren. (Ed.) Cotton origin, history, technology and production. John Wiley, New York; 1999. p 3–31.

[17] Stewart JM. Potential for crop improvement with exotic germplasm and genetic engineering. Challenging the future: Conference-1 proceedings, 1994, Brisbane Australia, GA Constable and NW Forrester (ed.) CSIRO, Melbourne, Australia, 1994.

[18] Mehetre SS, Aher AR, Gawande V, Patil VR, Mokate AS. Induced polyploidy in *Gossypium*: a tool to overcome interspecific incompatibility of cultivated tetraploid and diploid cottons. Current Science 2003; 84(12) 1510–1512.

[19] Chandra M, Sreenivasan S. Studies on improved *Gossypium arboreum* cotton: Part I—Fibre quality parameters. Indian Journal of Fibre & Textile Research 2011; 36 24-34.

[20] Rahman M, Tabassum N, Ullah I, Asif M, Zafar Y. Studying the extent of genetic diversity among *Gossypium arboreum* L. genotypes/cultivars using DNA fingerprinting. Genetic *Resources* and *Crop* Evolution 2008; 55 331–339.

[21] Shaheen T, Zafar Y, Rahman M. Detection of single nucleotide polymorphisms in the conserved ESTs regions of *Gossypium arboreum*. Electronic Journal of Biotechnology 2010; 13(5) doi: 10.2225/vol13-issue5-fulltext-3.

[22] Afzal M. Growth and development of cotton plant and its improvement in the Punjab. Govt. printing Press, Lahore 1947.

[23] Ali M. Cotton varieties in Pakistan. Cotton Research and development Memoranda till 60's. Pakistan Academy of Sciences; 2007.

[24] Ahmad N, Akram M. An estimate of water consumption by sugarcane, cotton and wheat crops under high water-able condition and its effect on their yield. Engineering News, West Pakistan Eng. Congress, Lahore 1966; 6(3 & 4) Sep.-Dec, 1986, p 32-53.

[25] Ansari MAA. Maintenance of purity in improved cottons. Pakistan Cotton Bulletin 1952; I.

[26] Memon AM, Bloach MA. Cotton Breeding achievements in Hyderabad Region. West Pakistan, (Government Information Deptt., West Pakistan) 1959; 2(8).

[27] Punjab Agricultural Research Board. PARB. http://parb.punjab.gov.pk/ (Accessed 9 April 2014)

[28] ICARDA.http://www.icarda.org/blog/%5Bnode%3ABlog%20type%5Dpakistan-us-cotton-productivity-enhancement-program. (Accessed 16 April 2014)

[29] Anwar R. International Technical Conference on Plant Genetic Resources, Leipzig, Germany, 17-23 June 1996. Pakistan: country report to the FAO international technical conference on plant genetic resources. Leipzig 1996.

[30] Hussain A, Ibrahim M, Naz AM. Cotton varieties of Pakistan. Ministry of Food, Agriculture & Livestock, Govt. of Pakistan, Islamabad May 2004; 1-166.

[31] Rahman M, Hussain D, Zafar Y. Estimation of genetic divergence among elite cotton (*Gossypium hirsutum* L.) cultivars/genotypes by DNA fingerprinting technology. Crop Sciences 2002; 42 2137–2144.

[32] Khan and Din MS. Cotton varieties. Kapas Bureau of Agri. Inf, West Pakistan, Lahore 1964; 109.

[33] Waddle WM. Accelerated cotton improvement reports West Pakistan. Report No.4. Cotton. Recommendations for cotton improvement programme in West Pakistan. Planning Cell Agriculture Department, Government of West Pakistan, Lahore, October 30, 1966.

[34] Rahman M, Zafar Y. Registration of NIBGE-115 Cotton. Journal of Plant Registrations 2007; 1 51-52.

[35] Rahman M, Zafar Y. Registration of NN-3 Cotton. Journal of Plant Registrations 2012; 6 (3) 342-347.

[36] Ahmad S, Mahmood K, Hanif M, Nazeer W, Malik W, Qayyum A, Hanif K, Mahmood A, Islam N. Introgression of cotton leaf curl virus-resistant genes from Asiatic

cotton (*Gossypium arboretum* L.) into upland cotton (*G. hirsutum* L.). Genetics and Molecular Research 2011; 10 (4) 2404-2414.

[37] Mumtaz H. Identification of structural and functional genomic markers for fiber quality traits in cotton using interspecific population (*G. hirsutum* x *G. barbadense*). MPhil thesis. Quaid-i-Azam University Islamabad Pakistan; 2007.

[38] Haq MA. Development of Mutant Varieties of Crop Plants at NIAB and the Impact on Agricultural Production in Pakistan. In:QY. Shu (ed.) Induced Plant Mutations in the Genomics Era. Food and Agriculture Organization of the United Nations. Rome; 2009. p 61-64.

Chapter 7

The U.S. National Cotton Germplasm Collection – Its Contents, Preservation, Characterization, and Evaluation

Richard G. Percy, James E. Frelichowski,
Mark D. Arnold, Todd B. Campbell, Jane K. Dever,
David D. Fang, Lori L. Hinze, Dorrie Main,
Jodi Scheffler, Monica A. Sheehan, Mauricio Ulloa,
Jing Yu and John Yu

Additional information is available at the end of the chapter

http://dx.doi.org/10.5772/58386

1. Introduction

The early history of the cotton industry in the U.S. was, for the most part, a story of importation and adaptation of cottons from Mexico, Guatemala, and the tropics of the Western Hemisphere. By the 19th century there were two distinctive types of upland cotton, with distinctive origins, being grown in the U.S. One type, known as green-seeded cotton, was from southern Mexico. The other dominant type of upland, white-seeded cotton, had its origins in the central plateau of Mexico [1,2]. Although these cottons were grown extensively, no coordinated efforts were made to maintain the original stocks or their progeny. Modern, systematic collection and preservation of cotton in the U.S. only began in response to the outbreak of the boll weevil in the 1880's [3]. Three collection trips between 1902 and 1906 were responsible for the introduction of two cottons, Acala and Kekchi, which would contribute significantly to the development of modern U.S. cultivars [4]. From these initial collecting trips and ensuing trips, federal, university and state experiment stations began to assemble the germplasm collections. Also from these efforts there sprang collaborative efforts that were formalized into U.S. regional projects involving scientists and members from all aspects of the U.S. cotton industry. The first Regional Research Project was S-1 in 1950 (succeeded by many) and it established a priority of acquiring and studying diverse germplasm for cotton improvement [5-7]. Increased organization and centralization of germplasm activities was necessary to manage and increase cotton germplasm resources. Plant Introduction centers were established with the Agricultural Marketing Act of 1946 and a National Seed Storage Laboratory (now the National Center for Genetic Resources and Preservation or NCGRP) was established in 1958 for long term backup storage of germplasm. Federal funds and staff also were committed to create working collections throughout the U.S. to specialize in crops. In 1960, the cotton sub-collections were deposited at NGCRP with their passport data, and in the early 1980's they were consolidated in College Station, TX, USA. Increased staff, greenhouses, seed processing and storage facilities were added. The curators continued to add germplasm from publicly donated cultivars and germplasm lines, explorations and exchanges with other collections and to record descriptors on new and existing germplasm. The International Board for Plant Genetic Resources (now Bioversity International) established a set of cotton descriptors in 1980 to serve as a guide for data collection for the U.S. and other collections [8]. Databases for the National Plant Germplasm System (NPGS) and the collection are managed online by the Germplasm Resources and Information Network (GRIN).

2. Content, preservation, and distribution

The U.S. National Cotton Germplasm Collection (NCGC) currently has approximately 10,000 accessions covering 45 species of *Gossypium* as described by Fryxell [28]. Representation of species within the collection varies significantly, and to some extent reflects historical opportunities for collecting or exchange with other collections (Table 1.) However, there has been a conscious effort to focus on fiber producing species that readily hybridize with the cultivated cottons. Accessions of the collection are officially recognized by Plant Introduction (PI) numbers in the NPGS, which maintains a permanent long-term backup inventory, or base collection, in the NCGRP in Fort Collins. However the working, or active, collection in College Station, TX further subdivides the collection to reflect historical organization and taxonomic classification. This additional step facilitates easy organization and retrieval of seed from the temperature controlled vault. The working collection is under the care of a full-time curator and supporting staff with the ARS-SPARC in College Station, Texas and it is the source of *Gossypium* germplasm distributed to the public.

The collection is subdivided to seven different sub-collections that consist of: 1) variety sub-collection, primarily *G. hirsutum* (prefixed by SA-), 2) landrace sub-collection, primarily *G. hirsutum* (prefixed by TX-), 3) *G. barbadense* sub-collection, (prefixed by GB-), 4) Asiatic (A-genome species) sub-collection, (prefixed by either A_1-or A_2-for *G. herbaceum* or *G. arboreum* respectively), 5) wild species sub-collection (prefixed by a taxon specific genome letter-number combination [9]), 6) genetic marker sub-collection, and 7) a base sub-collection (i.e. NCGRP) of all materials in sub-collections1-6 and new plant introductions [3,10]. Sub-collections 1-5 constitute the "working collection", which is routinely seed propagated and distributed by the USDA-ARS at College Station, Texas. Seed of the working collection is maintained at 4°C and 23% relative humidity [11]. Sub-collection 7 is housed at the NCGRP in Fort Collins, CO under conditions more favorable for long-term storage (-20°C, ~5% seed moisture content [12]). The SA sub-collection is short for Stoneville Accession and represents the obsolete cultivar collection originally started at the Delta Branch Experiment Station in Stoneville, MS. The TX (or TEX) sub-collection was started on the campus of Texas A&M University, College Station, TX, to catalogue *G. hirsutum* landraces and various genetic stocks and is the format continued to the present day, exclusively for *G. hirsutum* photoperiodic landraces or tropically collected material. The GB sub-collection originated from *G. barbadense* accessions curated at Phoenix, AZ, and after consolidation with the main collection, it has continued to expand as new acquisitions have been made.

	ARS								Texas A&M Agrilife[5]			
	Working Collection[1]					CGRU[2]	SC[3]	CSRL[4]				
Gossypium genome/species	Accessions	Distribution 1987-2013	Seed Increase 2011-2013	Characterization, Digital Imaging 2011-2013	SSR, Seed Oil/Protein Evaluation	CLCV Evaluation	Landrace Evaluation	Salt/Drought Evaluation	Characterization, Digital Imaging	Abiotic Evaluation	Biotic Evaluation	Phenotypic Evaluation
(AD) *hirsutum* total	6302	42659	2878	3731	1541	631	1380	440+	700+	290	473	400+
(*hirs.* landraces)	(2522)	-	(1220)	(1174)	-	(510)	(1380)	(440+)	-	-	-	-
barbadense	1584	5502	340	328	430	23	42	20	5	-	25	-
tomentosum	16	98	3	5	2	-	-	-	-	-	3	-
mustelinum	19	125	4	4	7	-	-	-	6	-	6	-
darwinii	138	80	8	4	4	-	-	-	9	-	-	-
(A) *herbaceum*	194	1487	129	129	49	194	-	20	26	-	2	-
arboreum	1729	4287	1729	1729	145	1729	-	20	24	10	4	-
(B) *anomalum*	7	95	3	3	5	-	-	-	2	-	-	-
capitis viridis	1	36	1	1	-	-	-	-	-	-	-	-
triphyllum	2	14	0	1	-	-	-	-	1	-	-	-
(C) *nandewarense*	6	11	1	1	1	-	-	-	-	-	-	-
robinsonii	3	31	0	1	-	-	-	-	1	-	-	-
sturtianum	7	103	1	2	3	-	-	-	-	-	-	-
(D) *aridum*	14	135	4	2	4	-	-	-	-	-	-	-
armourianum	10	115	1	2	2	-	-	-	-	-	-	-
davidsonii	31	140	4	2	9	-	-	-	2	-	1	-
gossypioides	8	135	4	4	7	-	-	-	-	-	-	-
harknessii	19	72	0	1	-	-	-	-	1	-	1	-
klotzschianum	59	52	1	1	1	-	-	-	2	-	-	-
laxum	2	3	1	1	1	-	-	-	-	-	-	-
lobatum	4	61	1	1	1	-	-	-	-	-	-	-

	ARS								Texas A&M Agrilife[5]			
	Working Collection[1]					CGRU[2]	SC[3]	CSRL[4]				
Gossypium genome/species	Accessions	Distribution 1987-2013	Seed Increase 2011-2013	Characterization, Digital Imaging 2011-2013	SSR, Seed Oil/Protein Evaluation	CLCV Evaluation	Landrace Evaluation	Salt/Drought Evaluation	Characterization, Digital Imaging	Abiotic Evaluation	Biotic Evaluation	Phenotypic Evaluation
raimondii	56	315	3	2	4	-	-	-	3	-	-	-
schwendimanii	2	1	1	-	-	-	-	-	-	-	-	-
thurberi	41	268	20	11	9	-	-	-	5	-	1	-
trilobum	11	118	4	3	6	-	-	-	-	-	-	-
(E) *areysianum*	2	13	1	1	1	-	-	-	1	-	-	-
incanum	4	22	1	1	-	-	-	-	-	-	-	-
somalense	3	65	1	1	1	-	-	-	1	-	-	-
stocksii	4	65	2	2	1	-	-	-	3	-	-	-
(F) *longicalyx*	4	213	4	4	4	-	-	-	3	-	-	-
(G) *australe*	11	103	2	2	3	-	-	-	3	-	-	-
bickii	5	82	1	1	4	-	-	-	3	-	-	-
nelsonii	2	11	2	1	1	-	-	-	-	-	-	-
(K) *costulatum*												
exiguum	1	-	1	-	1	-	-	-	-	-	-	-
marchantii	2	-	2	2	1	-	-	-	-	-	-	-
nobile	2	-	2	2	1	-	-	-	-	-	-	-
populifolium	4	2	1	1	1	-	-	-	-	-	-	-
pulchellum	1	3	1	1	1	-	-	-	-	-	-	-
rotundifolium	1	-	1	-	-	-	-	-	-	-	-	-

[1] Southern Plains Agricultural Research Center, USDA-ARS, College Station, TX

[2] Crop Genetics Research Unit, USDA-ARS, Stoneville, MS

[3] Coastal Plain Soil, Water and Plant Research Center, USDA-ARS, Florence, SC

[4] Cropping Systems Research Laboratory, USDA-ARS, Lubbock, TX

[5] Texas A&M Agrilife, Lubbock, TX, data compiled from 2005-2013

Table 1. *Gossypium* germplasm accession holdings, distribution, seed increase, characterization, digital imaging, and evaluation activities of the U.S. National Cotton Germplasm Collection (NCGC) at College Station, USDA-ARS collaborators, and Texas A&M.

To meet the goal of renewing seed of the collection every ten years or less and to ensure the availability of viable seed for distribution, storage, and backup at the NCGRP, accessions of the collection are grown in the Cotton Winter Nursery (CWN) in Tecoman, Mexico, in a local nursery in College Station, or in greenhouses. The majority of the working collection, including photoperiodic and many perennial accessions, are grown, force self-pollinated, and seed increased at the tropical CWN nursery. A large portion of the TX and GB sub-collections are of tropical origin, uncultivated, and are short-day flowering types that require a tropical nursery or a winter greenhouse to induce flowering and reproduction. Wild diploid species (sub-collection 5 of the collection) and recalcitrant accessions with critically low seed numbers must be seed increased in College Station. These high maintenance accessions typically exhibit characteristics such as a perennial growth habit, exerted stigmas, or prerequisite environmental stimuli to induce flowering, to name a few. These accessions are typically grown year round in greenhouses to target seed yields of at least 3000 seeds. Accessions are replenished on a 10 year cycle, as determined by viability studies of cottonseed under storage conditions of the working collection, or as indicated from germination testing on the base collection by the NCGRP.

	2007	2008	2009	2010	2011	2012
U.S.	768/59	1,537/90	2,300/101	1,702/78	3,200/83	4,900/128
Int'l.	919/26	546/18	450/12	65/10	1,254/10	1,100/12
Total	1,687/85	2,083/108	2,750/113	1,767/88	4,454/93	6,000/140

Table 2. Number of accessions/orders distributed from the National Cotton Germplasm Collection (NCGC) in College Station, TX, to requestors from the U.S. and internationally (int'l) in the past six years.

Germplasm users in all countries have equal access to the U.S NCGC, and distributions are limited only by the availability of the germplasm at the time of the request and by proper adherence to customs and phytosanitary laws of the U.S. and the requesting country. The policy of free access has grown out of the belief that germplasm is a world heritage to be freely shared. Seed distribution is provided from the working collection at College Station and shows an upward trend in number of requests and amount of accessions distributed yearly (Table 2). Information regarding materials available can be found online at GRIN-GLOBAL (http://distribution.grin-global.org/gringlobal/search.aspx).

Seed samples are supplied in amounts of 25 self-pollinated seed per sample, if sufficient seed is available for distribution (accessions with a minimum of 500 seed). Cooperators requiring more than 25 seeds must arrange for their own seed increase and in some cases are asked to return excess seed generated (if they are acquiring rare or difficult to manage accessions and can increase seed under controlled conditions with careful self-pollination in greenhouses). Some seed requests go unfilled due to critically low seed amounts, repeated germination difficulties with the seed, or because users request materials that are unavailable (e.g. germplasm under patent protection or accessions not present in the collection). Some accessions prove difficult to germinate from original or even increased seed, and require treatments such as seed scarification or hot water baths to achieve germination. Regular re-inventory of the critical and/or difficult to manage accessions indicate if they need to be re-established from backup seed at the NCGRP, or through a repeated exploration or germplasm exchange with the host country.

3. Collecting and exchange

Although domestic upland (*G. hirsutum)* cotton dominates world production (around 95%), it is generally accepted that its genetic diversity is very low [13-16]. Various bottlenecks and restrictions to genetic variability have occurred during the breeding history of upland cotton that have led to the low diversity currently seen in commercial cotton [17,18]. However, our germplasm collections have historically served as reservoirs of diversity for the breeding community; providing useful variation for disease and insect resistance, fiber quality improvement, and resistance to environmental stress. Collecting and exchange efforts are necessary to maintain and increase the genetic diversity of our collections [18,19]. In addition to early collecting trips that provided the foundation for the germplasm collection, numerous sponsored plant exploration trips and germplasm exchange efforts have occurred since the mid-twentieth century [10,20,21] and continue to occur. In 1982 the sovereign rights of countries over their germplasm was recognized [22,23] and many countries have become signatories to the International Treaty on Plant Genetic Resources for Food and Agriculture, implemented on 29 June 2004. This treaty states as a goal "the conservation and sustainable use of plant genetic resources for food and agriculture and the fair and equitable sharing of the benefits arising out of their use, in harmony with the Convention on Biological Diversity, for sustainable agriculture and food security". The acquisition of germplasm through collection has become the subject of extensive negotiation with host countries, and often includes the topics of benefit sharing and agreements on proprietary rights of host countries to products originating from germplasm. The latter topic has become a major stumbling block to collecting for the U.S. NCGC. In the past, the collection has only acquired germplasm that could be distributed free and clear of proprietary obligations, and the collection remains committed to this policy. Careful bilateral negotiation with individual nations, assuring mutual benefit, has led to limited germplasm acquisitions by the U.S. national collection in the latter half of the twentieth century. Since 1985 twelve acquisition trips have been made by U.S. scientists to collect germplasm. Ten of the trips were used for *in situ* explorations, while two of the trips were conducted to exchange germplasm with India, China, Russia, and Uzbekistan respectively [24]. Continued collection and germplasm exchange is essential to address gaps in individual collections worldwide and to conserve *ex situ* germplasm threatened by development [25].

The two most recent collecting efforts that resulted in germplasm acquisition by the U.S. collection were to Mexico in 2004-2006 and to Puerto Rico in 2013. Mexico encompasses the species range of several diploid cotton species, and Mexico-Guatemala is the recognized center of origin of *G. hirsutum,* the most widely cultivated species in the world. Mesoamerica is the center of morphological diversity for *G. hirsutum* [26]. Collecting efforts in Mexico during the last century are not well documented, and published information is limited. A series of collection/exploration trips were made in southern Mexico and Central America in the mid-twentieth century by T.R. Richmond and C. W. Manning in 1946, S. G. Stephens in 1947, and J. O. Ware and C. W. Manning in 1948 [21]. From the germplasm collected in these trips, a series of eight 'landraces' was established that generally corresponded to areas of native production or geographic occurrence. N. Lemeshev (USSR) and Q. Obispo (Mexico) in 1977-1978 made several collection-expeditions covering 16 Mexican states, from the peninsula of Baja California to the state of Yucatan. They collected several landraces and seed of seven *Gossypium* species (*G. armourianum* Kearney, *G. harknessii* Brandegee, *G. trilobum* (DC.) Skovsted, *G. aridum* (Rose &Standley) Skovsted, *G. lobatum* Gentry, *G. laxum* Phillips, and *G. gossypioides* (Ulbrich) Standley) [26]. P.A. Fryxell from 1968 to 1975 made several collection-expeditions in the country, providing a larger number of specimens to herbaria (MEXU and XAL) with clear and precise descriptions of habitat and location of collected accessions [27]. He made the most recent taxonomic classification of *Gossypium* species [28,29]. A. E. Percival and J. M. Stewart of the USDA-ARS, and A. Hernandez and F. de Leon of the Instituto Nacional de Investigaciónes Forestales Agricolas y Pecuarias (INIFAP) made several collection-expeditions throughout the states of the Yucatan Peninsula and in parts of the states of Tamulipas, Veracruz, Tabasco, Oaxaca and Chiapas in 1984 [10]. Also, A. E. Percival (USDA-ARS), J. M. Stewart (Univ. of Arkansas), E.A. Garcia, and L. Peréz (SAGAR-INIFAP Mexico) made additional collection expeditions in the state of Baja California Sur and parts of Sonora and Sinaloa states in 1990.

The most recent collecting efforts in Mexico for the collection were made by M. Ulloa (USDA), J.M. Stewart (Univ. of Arkansas), and several researchers from Mexico's INIFAP. These collecting efforts covered the Pacific west coast of Mexico, from the state of Sonora (North) to the state of Chiapas (South) and included several trips from 2002-2004 [19,26]. As a result of these efforts, a significant number of additional *Gossypium* accessions from various parts of Mexico are now available for evaluation, including several accessions of each diploid species of the D genome [19,26]. The cooperative collecting efforts of 2002-2006 also led to a significant number of additional *Gossypium* accessions of the subgenus *Houzingenia* from various parts of Mexico being placed in a nursery or botanical garden in Iguala Guerrero Mexico, including several accessions of each of the arborescent species for ex *situ* conservation [19,26]. This botanical garden was supported from 2006 through 2009 by additional funding from Cotton Incorporated (Cary, NC, USA) provided by J. M. Stewart to INIFAP. Today, Mexico maintains this *Gossypium* nursery in Iguala Guerrero (C. Perez-M. *personal communication*).

Since the first collecting trips were made in Mexico, the *in situ* survival of Mexican cotton germplasm has been threatened with increasing human population, modernization of agriculture and urbanization. New roads and population growth continue to increase. At this point, one species (*G. aridum*) of the subsection *Erioxylum* appears not to be threatened, probably because of the great diversity (botanical and geographic) encompassed by this species [26]. However, some of the most recent collected and non-described taxons (e.g., US-72) or ecotypes of the *G. aridum* species [19,26] may be in the process of becoming extinct in the wild. In addition, the D_8 *G. trilobum* species is almost extinct or already extinct. The natural habitat of this species has been replaced by intense and extensive agricultural production of guava (*Psidium* spp.). We speculate that the crop of guava and *G. trilobum* must have very similar environmental requirements, particularly as influenced by altitude (around 4,000 feet). Whereas in the past *G. trilobum* was considered to be a common, widely distributed species, based on surveys (J.M. Stewart and M. Ulloa, 2004 expedition), we are of the opinion that urbanization and agricultural development have very severely eroded its habitat, and that the species is becoming extinct in the wild (Drs. Stewart and Ulloa *personal communication*). Within the eight races described in *G. hirsutum*, much of the original diversity existing *in situ* appears to have been lost. According to information obtained from local sources, eradication of naturally occurring landrace, feral, and dooryard cottons was attempted in areas of southern Mexico in the 1980's in efforts to remove perceived insect reservoirs. Apparently all attempts at commercial cotton production since then have been abandoned. No commercial fields of cotton were encountered during expeditions between 2002 and 2004 in the central and southern part of Mexico [19,26]. Currently, with the exception of the northern cotton production regions of Mexico, the diversity of the *G. hirsutum* is limited to feral plants that occur opportunistically in waste areas and as occasional home garden plants maintained by rural peoples or village residents [26].

Due to its relative proximity to the U. S. and its status as a U.S. territory, Puerto Rico (PR) was a target of opportunity for collecting efforts in 2013. Puerto Rico was revisited in the most recent germplasm collecting effort by James Frelichowski, the curator of the U.S. collection, Louis Prom, of the USDA-ARS, College Station, TX and by collaborators from the USDA-ARS Tropical Agriculture Research Station (TARS) in Mayaguez, PR. Previous reports on wild cotton in the Caribbean [30,31] and the recent taxonomic identification of a new species in the Dominican Republic [32] justified continued exploration for *Gossypium* in Puerto Rico. The current collection inventory indicates 49 accessions originally collected from Puerto Rico and surrounding islands, but GPS locations and details on habitats are lacking. Judging from the limited passport data, the trend was for wild cotton to occur in areas with drier climates in or near coastal regions. Only four Puerto Rican accessions in the collection were observed to have maturity and productivity ratings similar to cultivar checks in the CWN. The Puerto Rican accessions were more characteristic of landrace cottons, and suggest that cotton in Puerto Rico is likely native or is cotton of tropical origin that has become naturalized.

In the most recent collecting efforts in Puerto Rico, attempts to address gaps in the knowledge of the island's diversity and diversity structure were addressed through tagging of all collection sites and resulting accessions with GPS coordinates and with geographic mapping of native cottons. Seventy-nine cotton plants or populations were photographed and tagged with GPS coordinates to give a detailed map based survey of PR. Numerous other cotton plants or populations were sighted and recorded on a GPS map, but not collected due to time restrictions or safety or access concerns. Southern Puerto Rico was much more populated with cotton than the north, but morphological diversity was seen throughout the island and justified the wide search of the island for wild cotton. Differences in fiber length, quality, seed fuzz, and leaf pubescence were evident during collection, and sometimes individual traits were observed to vary among neighboring plants. This confirms the need to collect from individual

http://dx.doi.org/10.5772/58386

plants and to document their locations carefully. A local botanist, Duane Kolterman and the curator of the Puerto Rico Herbarium, Jeanine Velez Gavilan, indicated that two species inhabit PR, *G. hirsutum* and *G. barbadense* with probable species introgression in discovered specimens. Only one clear cut *G. barbadense* was seen and it was a dooryard cotton, which we were not able to access. Most of the observed cotton plants were similar to collection accessions classified as race 'marie galante'[31], which is typical of the Caribbean and often produces good fiber. However these plants were not as strongly arborescent as the classic 'marie galante' accession. In addition these plants had characters, such as tapering boll shapes, which were typical of *G. barbadense*, and therefore warrant further inspection. In the southwest portion of Puerto Rico, in the Cabo Roja region, the cotton plants were more variable. In the salt flats at the southwest tip of Puerto Rico, the dominant cotton plant had shorter, coarser and darker fibers than that typically observed on the remainder of the island, and were more characteristic of accessions classified as race 'yucatanense'[31]. The southwest portion of PR faces the Dominican Republic where a sixth tetraploid species is proposed, and a priority site for further exploration and collection. Dooryard cottons were in low frequency on the island and may be declining as cotton products and substitutes become more available for purchase. One resident extolled the virtues of natural cotton because of lack of chemicals used on them, and she demonstrated how they were propagated via cuttings, which may be indicative of a hard seed coat frequent in wild cottons. The digital data collected allows us to assemble a vivid description of wild cotton in Puerto Rico in what appears to be an ever changing landscape and justifies exploration to ensure their *ex situ* preservation.

4. Phenotyping and characterization

Phenotypic characterization of the national collection has historically served dual purposes. Until the very recent past (when molecular tools became available), phenotypic descriptors were the primary means of describing the diversity contained in the germplasm collection and rationally classifying that variability. The second role of phenotypic descriptors was to assist breeders and others in identifying germplasm of interest in genetic improvement efforts. However, to be useful, phenotypic descriptors needed to be well defined and universally applied. Throughout the history of the collection, this has been a goal that has been striven for but not completely attained. The convention in the past has been to follow, as much as possible, the guidelines set by Bioversity International (formerly IBPGR) in 1980 [33], revised in 1985 and again in 1995 [34] in creating descriptors. Prior to the universal adoption of computers, the internet, and electronic databases, descriptor data files of the collection's holdings were periodically published, with the last publication occurring in 1987 [10]. Presently, data files of descriptors for accessions of the collection can be found in GRIN-GLOBAL at http://distribution.grin-global.org/gringlobal/search.aspx or in the CottonGen database at www.cottongen.org. Descriptors and descriptor sets for phenotyping the collection have not remained static over time, but have evolved as their use has evolved. In 2009, the Cotton Crop Germplasm Committee [14] summarized the need to expand the collection's databases with morphological, agronomic, molecular, and priority trait evaluations to improve user utility of the collection.

Of particular interest to the breeding and crop improvement community was the addition of traits of agronomic value, to supplement traits of a primarily botanical or taxonomic nature adopted from Bioversity International.

Within the collection, a goal has been set to routinely characterize or re-characterize approximately 1,000 accessions (or a tenth of the collection) annually in the CWN, or in local fields or greenhouses at College Station, TX. Although the photoperiodism of a large portion of the collection requires that it be renewed in the tropically located CWN, collecting descriptors at that site has been challenging, due to travel costs and time limitations. With the great diversity of accessions being grown in the CWN, and their variable maturation rates, collecting complete descriptor sets for accessions has been a lengthy, multi-year process. To aid in the description of the collection, digital imaging has been adopted. An immediate concern has been to develop a pictorial reference of the descriptor scores in order to establish clear standards and reduce subjectivity that occurs when scoring descriptors on such a spectrum of diversity in the collection. Mackay and Alercia [35] have described the use of digital imaging to document variation in germplasm, and this approach has been used in several collections [36,37]. Digital imaging can be tailored with software to detect minute differences among accessions and to determine duplicates [38]. Digital photography to document *Gossypium* diversity has been used by collaborators [38,39] and recently by the NCGC staff during descriptor collection. Currently within the collection, digital imaging has been concentrated upon plant structures that are most informative in differentiating and classifying the diversity of the genus. Samples of typical leaves, flowers, and bolls are gathered per accession, tagged, and quickly assembled under high resolution digital cameras. Only mature, fully expanded leaves (below the fifth main stem node) are photographed. Cotton flowers are photographed on the day of anthesis to reveal flower color, petal spots, pollen color, and stigma length. Fully expanded, mature but non-cleft bolls are photographed to reveal shape and locule number. To obtain photographs, several cameras are fixed with tripods, some for an overall view of size of plant tissues and others for a close up of minute leaf hairs, nectaries, and glands. All images are produced with a measured grid background for a consistent size reference. Portable shade is constructed at the CWN or in the local field to stabilize lighting conditions and reduce wind disturbance. Images are identified by photographed tags, and then named according to accession inventory number, year/environment of planting, and a code for the plant tissue or structure photographed.

To date (2011-2013), standardized descriptors and digital images have been collected on over 4,900 cotton producing accessions planted at the CWN and in the field at College Station, TX. These images are in the process of being uploaded into the CottonGen database (www.cottongen.org) for pairing with descriptors for optimal use by the cotton community. The digital library or "virtual herbarium" created by the use of high resolution cameras to produce 'virtual' voucher specimens provides easy access to examine the morphological variation within the genus that was previously unattainable with classic herbarium specimens. It is hoped that the digital image library promotes standardization of descriptor data and image creation by cooperating groups and collections, thereby promoting a greater ability to characterize the diversity within *Gossypium*, address gaps in the U.S. and other collections and effectively share and backup germplasm between collections.

http://dx.doi.org/10.5772/58386

Agronomic Traits	Descriptor Name	Method of Observation	Descriptor State
Architecture	Plant Height (cm)	Plant height in centimeters, grown in greenhouse. Measured from pot soil surface to terminal.	ht. (cm)
	Growth Habit	General architectural arrangement of plant type grown in greenhouse.	Compact → spreading Intermediate → bushy
Physiological	Photoperiod	Response of plants flowering habit over a short day to long day growth duration in greenhouse as compared to day neutral upland varieties grown in Lubbock, Texas.	day neutral → strong photo dependent → weak
Retention	Square	Retention of squares that mature into bolls and are not shed due to insect or environmental conditions.	good → weak fair → none
	Boll	Retention of bolls grown to maturity in greenhouse and are not shed due to insect or environment.	good → weak fair → none
	Fiber	Retention of fiber in burr until harvested.	good → weak fair→ none
Morphological	Flower Score	Flower score of early, medium or late as determined by the greenhouse planting date. Lubbock, Texas	Early → medium → late
	Flower Duration	Length of time a plant will produce floral buds, determined by photoperiodic response of plants growing in greenhouse during the fall and winter months. Lubbock, Texas	short → medium → long
	1st Flower Date	Date of first flowers when grown in greenhouse in number of days after planting. Lubbock, Texas	number of days after planting
	Nodes to 1st Fruiting	Node of first sympodial branch to set fruit on plant growing in greenhouse. Lubbock, Texas	node number (cotyledon = 0)
Production	Productive-ness	Quality and quantity of mature fiber and seed produced from plants grown in greenhouse. Lubbock, Texas	most productive good → fair → poor
	Seed Index	The weight of 100 fuzzy seed in grams.	WT. (g)

Table 3. Agronomic trait characteristics documented from *Gossypium* species grown in greenhouse environment for phenotypic evaluation at Texas A&M AgriLife Research, Lubbock, TX, USA

Although the U.S. NCGC tries to set standards and methodologies for characterizing the germplasm collection through its internal efforts, it also recognizes and encourages cooperation from the research community in this task. Due to the volume of accessions available for characterization, the finite resources of the collection, and the impact of genotype x environment interaction on many phenotypic traits of interest, a unilateral effort to collect descriptor data is not considered desirable. Collaborative efforts within the research community offer an attractive way to collect relevant data and make it widely available. One such effort has been conducted by Texas A&M Agrilife, Lubbock, TX from 2005 until 2013. Seed of accessions from the U.S. NCGC at College Station, TX were obtained and planted in the greenhouse at Lubbock for seed increase. In conjunction with seed increases, phenotypic descriptors of various *Gossypium* species were recorded and documented using digital photography. Traits selected for digital imaging were based on previous descriptive data recorded using the GRIN guidelines and published taxonomic documents. [27,10] Additional documentation elements were expanded to include descriptor name, state, and method of evaluation in a greenhouse environment (Table 3). Digital images depicting characteristic and state were used as reference standards to help alleviate misinterpretation of the descriptor. This allowed for more decisive, objective, and consistent data collection. Qualitative data has been documented on a nominal, ordinal, or binary scale and quantitative data consist of continuous or discrete numerical values. Over 800 accessions have been regenerated, digitally documented and evaluated (Table 1). The descriptors used by the Texas A&M AgriLife Research and Extension Center did not encompass all aspects of trait documentation, but were intended to give a general observation of an accession's attribute, measurable trait, or characteristic.

5. Evaluation efforts

The screening and evaluation of the national collection for traits such as disease, insect, and environmental stress resistance are beyond the capacity and resources of the national collection to achieve, and necessitate research community participation. Despite this fact, the collection in recent years has tried to move from a passive supplier of germplasm resources to an active participant in germplasm disease and insect resistance screening and evaluation efforts. The collection has a long history of evaluation efforts by the research community for biotic and abiotic stress resistance. In fact the origins of the collection are intertwined with the entry of the boll weevil into the United States in the 1890's and the search for a source of host plant resistance to that pest [4]. Numerous evaluations have been conducted on the collection for phenotypic characteristics of agronomic importance. A sampling of evaluations includes investigations of seed protein [40], seed oil [41], seed gossypol [42], boll weevil resistance [43] and Cercospora leaf spot and Verticillium wilt resistance [44]. Prior to 2000, over 320 accessions of the collection had been screened for resistance to pink bollworm (*Pectinophora gossypiella* Saunders) [45], and 471 race stocks of *G. hirsutum* were screened for resistance to root knot nematode (*Meloidogyne incognita*) and resistance found in 18 lines [46]. As of 1986, over 200 accessions of the collection had been reported to carry resistance to one or more pests [47].

More recently, in 2009, eleven ongoing evaluations of collection germplasm for disease, insect, and nematode resistance were reported in a status report of U.S. cotton germplasm [14].

In an ongoing project, the Cotton Improvement Program at the Texas A&M AgriLife Research Center, Lubbock, TX began in 2005 to screen accessions from the working collection for resistance to the thrips (Thysanoptera: Thripidae) pest. Thrips were ranked as the number three pest of U. S. cotton in 2012, reducing yield by 0.374 percent and causing a loss of 123,947 bales [48]. In the panhandle and far west Texas, 860,476 acres were treated for pest thrips in 2012 at a cost of $1.28 per acre [48]. By 2013, 516 accessions from the active collection of the U.S. National Cotton Germplasm Collection had been screened (Table 4). Resistance to thrips was identified in *G. barbadense* accession TX110 (PI 163608) in the first year of screening [49]. A series of studies conducted through much of the 20th century identified, confirmed and characterized thrips resistance in *G. barbadense*. Studies in this progression include: the discovery of resistance in glabrous Egyptian cotton cultivars and the conclusion that resistance is most likely due to a thicker leaf epidermal layer on lower sides of leaves allowing cotton seedlings to tolerate more thrips feeding [50]; confirmation of this work [51]; further characterization of feeding by thrips and measurement of the protrusion of the mandible past the fused maxillae at 11 microns [52] and the identification of a resistant group of *G. barbadense* cottons with a lower leaf epidermal layer of 10-13 microns [53]. This series of studies was summarized by Bowman and McCarty [54] who investigated the heritability of the traits conferring resistance. Interspecific hybridization between resistant *G. barbadense* accession, TX110 and two unreleased elite lines from the Lubbock Texas A&M AgriLife Research Cotton Improvement Program was used to begin a cultivar development project. Selections for thrips resistance and day-neutral flowering habit were made in the segregating F_2 plots, and this process continued for five years. Resistance has been carried to the F_5 and F_6 generations in many individuals, and day-neutral flowering habit and favorable agronomic traits have been improved.

Species	Genome	Accessions tested
Gossypium hirsutum	AD1	473
Gossypium barbadense	AD2	25
Gossypium mustelinum	AD4	3
Gossypium darwinii	AD5	6
Gossypium herbaceum	A1	2
Gossypium arboreum	A2	4
Gossypium thurberi	D1	1
Gossypium harknesii	D2-2	1
Gossypium davidsonii	D3	1

Table 4. By species, number of cotton accessions from U.S. National Cotton Germplasm Collection screened for resistance to the Texas High Plains pest thrips complex at Texas A&M AgriLife Research in Lubbock, Texas, 2005-2013.

In another ongoing project funded by USAID and USDA to identify sources of resistance to Cotton Leaf Curl Virus (CLCuV), germplasm resources were made available through the U.S. NCGC. The ready availability of accessions from the collection, combined with winter nursery seed increase capabilities, GRIN database information and especially the recent addition of standardized descriptor data and digital images, made possible a rapid coordinated CLCuV screening program. CLCuV is a major threat to cotton production in Pakistan and parts of India and has been reported in cotton producing countries in Africa, as well as China and Uzbekistan. This project to identify sources of resistance to CLCuV, helps not only countries such as Pakistan where the virus is already a problem, but also makes resistant germplasm available, should CLCuV become a threat to cotton production in other countries. As part of the project, accessions from the collection were increased at the CWN in Tecoman, Mexico. At the CWN, the collection curator and staff collected descriptor data and digital images for all the accessions. Part of the seed was sent to Pakistan and screened for CLCuV and the rest returned to the collection. In Pakistan, the disease is endemic which allowed replicated screening at three locations. At each location, the screening nurseries included regularly spaced host rows of highly susceptible plants. Any plants identified as resistant were re-tested the following year. All the screening data is being made available for inclusion in the collection database. Previous screening tests had identified *G. arboreum* and *G. herbaceum* as potential sources of resistance, so 1,050 *G. arboreum* and 100 *G. herbaceum* were increased at the CWN and sent for screening. Transferring resistance from diploid *G. arboreum* or *G. herbaceum* into tetraploid *G. hirsutum* is extremely difficult, so the project expanded to evaluate *G. hirsutum*. The NPGS GRIN database was used to identify a subset of 920 *G. hirsutum* accessions with a range of morphologies and originating from diverse geographic regions. CLCuV screening identified 12 resistant *G. hirsutum* accessions originating from northeast Brazil, Central America and the Caribbean. Travel to Pakistan is difficult and the plots could only be evaluated by the USDA researchers once during the field season. However, descriptor data and digital images were e-mailed throughout the season from the Pakistani partners for each of the 12 accessions. These could be compared to the descriptor data and digital images made by the collection curator at the CWN. This Collection information proved essential as 11 of the 12 accessions were photoperiod sensitive and did not flower during the field season in Pakistan. Additional accessions from these areas, as well as other geographic regions, were selected using GRIN and are being screened in Pakistan in 2013. This project has served as a model for a germplasm evaluation effort that serves the germplasm collection as well as the research community. In addition to identifying resistant sources to CLCuV for future cotton improvement efforts, the project made possible the seed renewal of numerous accessions of the collection under controlled conditions and the characterization and digital imaging of these same accessions.

Another current effort involves evaluating germplasm resources to identify lines with physiological and morphological traits that can improve water use efficiency and tolerance to extreme temperature and drought. The decline of water in glaciers, reservoirs and aquifers in many regions, combined with climate change and the unpredictability of precipitation during the growing season, has stimulated efforts to identify germplasm resources that can minimize the elevated production risks associated with crop water deficits. Cultivars with extensive root systems or physiological adaptations to their aerial parts may offer a means to minimize the impact of periods of short-term or prolonged water stress on yield or quality. Plants vary in their physiological response to stress and their responses vary with the severity and duration of the limited water availability, extreme heat exposure, and other abiotic stresses [55-57]. Diversity in cotton for root architecture has been reported [58], as well as variation in root resistance expressed as the redistribution of water through the soil layer-profile by the root system (hydraulic lift) [59]. Untapped genetic variability for plant and root morphology-architecture types is present in germplasm resources but lacking in modern commercial cultivars [60,61]. However, methods of morphological or phenotypical characterization have progressed slowly in the last 30 years [62]. Currently, accessions from the NCGC are being used by the USDA-ARS Cropping Systems Research Laboratory, Lubbock, TX to initiate this phenotypical characterization. Specifically, drought responses are being examined in accessions of the Gossypium Diversity Reference Set, created for an ongoing diversity study being conducted by the USDA-ARS at College Station, Texas. Physiological and biochemical plants responses such as photosynthesis and CO_2 rates, stomata conductance, and osmotic adjustment will be examined and monitored under heat and/or low-temperature stress conditions. Also, a rapid bioassay is being used for monitoring plant stress based on the ability of a "source" leaf to provide sufficient energy for plant growth. Water-deficit stress reduces new growth and lessens the demand on the source leaves. [63,64]. In addition, plant mapping (plant height, nodes, and fruiting position), agronomic (seed cotton yield, seed index, number of bolls per plants, lint percentage, etc.), and fiber quality (length, strength, and fineness) data are used to monitor drought tolerance among cotton entries or accessions. Accessions are evaluated in field replicated plots under well-irrigated and water-deficit stress conditions, using a randomized complete block or incomplete block design with 3–4 replications using five plants as subsamples per replication, or two replications when seed availability from accessions of selected germplasm is limited [65].

In another project to screen the germplasm collection for drought tolerance, 400 accessions have been evaluated for variation in growth parameters by the Cotton Breeding Program at the Texas A&M AgriLife Research Center, Lubbock, TX. Measurements were obtained for the 400 accessions under non-stress conditions by growing plants in granular diatomaceous earth contained in 30 inch tubes made from 3 inch PVC pipe. Adequate water and fertilizer were applied, and day and night temperatures were maintained at 75-85°F and 67-69°F, respectively, to obtain maximum growth rates. After 20 days, plants were removed from the growth medium, washed, and taproot and shoot length were measured. Plants were then separated into roots and shoots, and dried at 140°F for 48 hours. Parameters obtained were: taproot length, shoot length, total root and shoot weights, and shoot to root ratio. All experiments were conducted using a RCB design with five blocks. Recognizing that in many regions declining water levels are associated with increased salinity in irrigation water, the Lubbock AgriLife research group evaluated 290 collection accessions for NaCl tolerance in a hydroponic system. Plants grown in hydroponic medium were evaluated continuously for a variety of salt injury indicators. Seedlings were exposed to increasing increments of salt (NaCl) solution at a consistent rate from 3,000 to 35,000 ppm until plants suffered near 100 percent mortality. Preliminary studies conducted in 2006-2009 show accession, TX 307 (PI 165390) to have significantly better growth when treated with NaCl using the hydroponic screening system. Seed from a plant selection of TX 307 was increased to use as a control in further salinity studies.

Efforts also are underway to develop remote sensing and high throughput phenotyping methodology to evaluate germplasm variation for response to drought and other environmental stresses. Remote sensing instruments measure and record responses to drought by infrared camera monitoring, sensors and thermometers for leaf and plant canopy measurements. Soil water content is monitored using neutron moisture gages and bucket rain gages. Several research groups are working to develop high throughput field based equipment to phenotype thousands of plots and/or accessions in the minimum amount of time. Equipped with sensors for measuring spectral reflectance, canopy temperature, and plant mapping imaging; a high throughput vehicle has the potential to assess the responses of hundreds of accessions to stress in a fairly short time [62]. Many of the above instruments are developed or under development. Knowledge being acquired will provide acutely needed means of conducting uniform evaluations of germplasm for valuable drought, heat, salt, and other environmental stresses.

6. Genotyping

Molecular tools provide the means to characterize underlying genetic diversity that is not measurable through classical phenotypic descriptors [66]. With the advance of DNA marker technologies, it is now possible to characterize *Gossypium* germplasm not only phenotypically at the levels of whole plants but also genotypically at the levels of whole genomes [67,68]. In general, cotton lags behind other major crops in genomic tools that are available for effective manipulation and exploitation of beneficial genes otherwise buried in *Gossypium* germplasm collections. The first molecular maps for cotton [69-70] were based on the cumbersome and expensive restriction fragment length polymorphism (RFLP) technology that requires large amounts of genomic DNA and generation of radioactive probes physically disseminated to the research community as plasmid or phage clones. Thus, RFLP markers were poorly suited for high-throughput genotyping experiments in germplasm characterization [67]. New DNA marker technologies were needed to coordinate the systematic characterization and the simultaneous comparison among various research efforts involved in cotton diversity analysis and genetic resource preservation.

Microsatellites of simple sequence repeat (SSR) markers, in contrast to RFLP markers, are abundant, co-dominant, and widely distributed throughout the genomes of higher plants. They are amenable to high-throughput assay via multiplex polymerase chain reaction (PCR) bins on automated sequencers [72]. Thus, SSR markers are portable and simple to use for germplasm characterization. Over the last decade, several thousand SSR markers have been developed for the tetraploid genome of cultivated cottons [73-76]. For various applications in cotton, SSR markers have been systematically characterized and genetically mapped in cotton genomes. High-density genetic maps were constructed based on an immortal recombinant inbred line (RIL) population that was developed from a cross between TM-1 and 3-79, the genetic standards for *Gossypium hirstum* and *G. barbadense,* respectively [73,75]. Using a balanced diversity panel of 12 cultivated and exotic cotton genotypes representing six *Gossypium* species [77, Table 5], a core set of 105 SSR markers has been developed for coordinated germplasm characterization [72]. This initial set of core SSR markers were carefully selected on the basis of criteria that included reproducible DNA amplification, ability to be multiplexed, reasonable polymorphism information content (PIC), representation of different marker sources, and uniform distribution across the tetraploid cotton genome. The initial core set has only two DNA markers proposed for each chromosome arm of the 26 tetraploid cotton chromosomes [67]. The core markers serve as the standard descriptors to characterize workable sets of *Gossypium* accessions across different gene pools or germplasm sources.

With the development of molecular markers, genetic diversity studies within *Gosssypium* have been pursued using accessions from the U.S. NCGC with varying objectives, including understanding the evolutionary process of interspecific gene flow within *G. aridum* [78], the genetic relationships of geographically diverse *G. arboreum* cultivars [79], and the utility of microsatellite primers developed in tetraploid species in the diploid *G. davidsonii* [80], to name a few examples. As cultivars possess the most readily accessible genetic variation for use in breeding programs, a number of diversity investigations have occurred using improved cotton cultivars [81-84]. Typically, many of these diversity studies have been limited in the scope of accessions investigated or the number of markers used [85,79,82]. There has been little standardization in these studies, as different groups of molecular markers were used for each group of accessions. Attempts to characterize larger genomic groups using a standardized marker set have been made in the germplasm collections of Uzbekistan [86,87] and France [88]. Recognizing the need to characterize the genetic diversity within the NCGC and the utility of markers in characterizing and managing collection diversity, the working collection at College Station, TX initiated research to characterize a major portion of the collection using the core SSR marker set described above. Objectives of this characterization included: determining the structure of genetic variability within the collection with the goal of identifying targets for further germplasm collecting and exchange efforts; identification of redundancies, misidentifications, unintended introgression, and gaps within the collection; and developing and validating a core marker set that could be used in comparative studies across collections and over time. The core marker set developed to accomplish this task was used to genotype and analyze a *Gossypium* Diversity Reference Set (GDRS) of 2,254 accessions (approximately 20% of the NCGC). The GDRS represented the range of diversity of *Gossypium,* including nine genomes (eight diploid and one tetraploid genome) and 33 species as represented in the collection (Table 6). DNA profiles of these accessions showed strengths and deficiencies of using the core set of 105 SSR markers.

When applied to the GDRS, the core marker set was most successful at revealing DNA profiles in the *G. hirsutum* and *G. barbadense* species. This was expected, since the SSRs used in the core set were developed from these two species. Many of the remaining species showed incomplete DNA profiles due to lack of PCR amplification or non-informative profiles due to the amplification of monomorphic DNA fragments. The current 105 marker core set was capable of discriminating tetraploid species, and discriminating between the diploid A genome and all

CMD>#	CMD name	Description
CMD01	TM-1	*G. hirsutum* (AD_1) genetic standard
CMD02	3-79	*G. barbadense* (AD_2) genetic standard
CMD03	Acala Maxxa	California Upland cotton (AD_1)
CMD04	DPL 458BR	Upland cotton (AD_1) with significant acreage
CMD05	Paymaster 1218BR	Upland cotton (AD_1) with significant acreage
CMD06	Fibermax 832	Upland cotton (AD_1) with significant acreage
CMD07	Stoneville 4892BR	Upland cotton (AD_1) with significant acreage
CMD08	Pima S-6	Pima (AD_2) germplasm breeding source
CMD09	*G. arboreum* (A_2-8)	A genome representative
CMD10	*G. raimondii* (D_5-3)	D genome representative
CMD11	*G. tomentosum* (AD_3)	Introgression breeding source
CMD12	*G. mustelinum* (AD_4)	Introgression breeding source

Table 5. A standardized panel of *Gossypium* germplasm diversity for cotton marker development (CMD) [12]

other diploid genomes. Within *G. hirsutum* and *G. barbadense,* the marker set revealed misclassification, introgression, and accession redundancy and uniqueness, and therefore will be a significant tool in maintaining collection integrity within the primary species. It was determined that detailed characterization efforts would continue to use those core SSR markers that were informative, but further characterization would require the addition of markers that were genome-or species-specific. In this ongoing research effort, diversity reference sets will be identified to represent a minimum of 25% of the accessions available for a given species, genome, or group within the NCGC. Currently, reference sets are being created for the A genome, D genome, and tertiary genomes. These Individual reference sets are being assembled to minimize similarity between accessions within the set, with priority being given to those accessions representing geographic, ecological, and morphological diversity; and differing degrees of human manipulation (i.e., wild species, semi-adapted landraces, or improved cultivars) that would be of interest in a diversity structure analysis. This approach will more readily illustrate the genetic diversity of the 10,000+ accessions in the collection and enhance the usage of this large collection by geneticists and breeders world-wide. The analyses of results from genotyping reference sets will be used to guide the development of smaller core collections for species and genomes. Marker information also will be used to prioritize regeneration efforts, identify redundancy and uniqueness in the collection, and monitor integrity of accessions through regeneration cycles. Coordinated characterization between collections using markers could enhance exchange efforts and allow mutual protection of holdings. Efforts are underway to organize a cooperative international effort to genotype cotton collections with a standard set of markers and a uniform distribution of species and ecotypes.

http://dx.doi.org/10.5772/58386

Genome	Species	Accessions number (%)	Accession total in NCGC
A	*G. arboreum*	145 (8.4%)	1729
	G. herbaceum	49 (25.3%)	194
AD	*G. barbadense*	430 (27.1%)	1584
	G. darwinii	4 (2.9%)	138
	G. hirsutum	1541 (24.5%)	6302
	G. mustelinum	7 (36.8%)	19
	G. tomentosum	2 (12.5%)	16
B	*G. anomalum*	5 (71.4%)	7
C	*G. nandewarense*	1 (16.7%)	6
	G. sturtianum	3 (42.9%)	7
D	*G. aridum*	4 (28.6%)	14
	G. armourianum	2 (20.0%)	10
	G. davidsonii	9 (29.0%)	31
	G. gossypioides	7 (100.0%)	7
	G. klotzschianum	1 (1.7%)	59
	G. laxum	1 (50.0%)	2
	G. lobatum	1 (25.0%)	4
	G. raimondii	4 (7.1%)	56
	G. thurberi	9 (24.3%)	37
	G. trilobum	6 (54.5%)	11
E	*G. areysianum*	1 (50.0%)	2
	G. somalense	2 (66.7%)	3
	G. stocksii	2 (50.0%)	4
F	*G. longicalyx*	4 (100.0%)	4
G	*G. australe*	3 (27.3%)	11
	G. bickii	4 (80.0%)	5
	G. nelsonii	3 (75.0%)	4
K	*G. costulatum*	1 (50.0%)	2
	G. exiguum	1 (100.0%)	1
	G. marchantii	1 (100.0%)	1
	G. nobile	1 (100.0%)	1
	G. populifolium	1 (25.0%)	4
	G. pulchellum	1 (100.0%)	1
Overall		2256 (22.0%)	10276

Table 6. Accessions in the *Gossypium* Diversity Reference Set (GDRS), by genome and species.

The low resolution of the 105 core marker set used in the U.S. collection offers a first glimpse at, or general survey of the cotton germplasm collection, but it does not provide detailed characterization of specific genomic regions that may harbor important genes of interest. The size and complexity of the cotton genomes require many more widely applicable DNA markers for more effective germplasm characterization and gene discovery [72-74]. While the growing collection of well characterized SSR markers offers an opportunity of expanding the current set with additional core markers to meet the demand, single nucleotide polymorphism (SNP) markers represent a promising DNA marker system [89]. SNP markers are co-dominant and more abundant in a given genome than SSR markers, and they offer a new opportunity for generating large numbers of intraspecific polymorphisms [90]. Current efforts to develop large numbers of cotton SNP markers are based on reduced genome representation [91] or other limited sequence resources [92]. A targeted genotyping by sequencing (GBS) approach, that is simple and cost-effective, is being explored to simultaneously discover and map SNP markers for traits of interest [93]. With the current efforts to develop whole genome sequence in cotton [94,95] including several members of germplasm standards and mapping parents, hundreds of thousands of SNP markers will be identified in the cotton genomes. These SNP loci will be validated and sorted out in various orthologs, homeologs and paralogs as often encountered in the allotetraploid cotton. Individual sets of core markers specific for each genome, species or land race will be developed from evenly distributed genomic and genic regions, and they will be arrayed in public SNP genotyping chips for high-throughput and more detailed characterization and exploitation of genetic diversity of *Gossypium* germplasm [93,96].

Presently, an investigation has been made of the diversity of upland cotton cultivars using a larger set of available SSR markers. Commercial *G. hirsutum* cultivars being the most accessible sources of genetic variation available to breeding and genetic improvement efforts, a cooperative effort involving the collection was undertaken to determine the variability available and the structure of diversity in this elite group using a broader set of molecular markers. A set of 193 upland cotton cultivars from 26 countries that include most cotton growing regions of the world were sampled from the national collection and elsewhere. These cultivars represent a wide spectrum of the genetic diversity found within the cultivated upland cotton. Due to strong contributions and influence of the U.S. cultivars to early breeding efforts in other countries, a special emphasis was placed upon representing U.S. cultivars in this study. When selecting U.S. cultivars, the following factors were taken into consideration: breeding program, pedigree (if known), geographic region, era of release, planting acreage and breeding value (*e.g.* as a common parent in breeding programs). The 130 cultivars from the U.S. represented more than 100 years of breeding history. Four hundred forty-eight SSR markers were selected based on their mapping positions in the G. *hirsutum* TM-1xG. *barbadense* 3-79 genetic map [76]. In addition, whenever possible, the physical positions of the selected SSR markers were also located based on the reference sequence of *G. raimondii* genome [95]. The genome-wide linkage disequilibrium (LD) between pairs of SSR marker loci was calculated using the software package JMP Genomics 6.0 (SAS Corporation, Cary, NC). Genetic similarities between all pairs of cultivars were calculated based on the Dice's coefficient [97] using the software package NTSYS-pc [98]. Neighbor-joining (NJ) trees were generated to view the phylogenic relationship among the cultivars.

The 448 selected SSR markers revealed a total of 1590 alleles belonging to 732 loci that were distributed across the whole cotton genome (Table 7). Of these 732 loci, 523 were polymorphic and 209 were monomorphic. One hundred thirty nine unique alleles were observed in 69 cultivars. Of the 130 U.S. cultivars, 94 had information on the years of their release, ranging from 1899 ('Mebane') to 2010 ('UA48') [99,100]. Using this information, an analysis of unique marker allele numbers contained in the cultivars clearly demonstrated that modern U.S. upland cotton has been gradually losing its genetic diversity during the past century. The pair-wise genetic similarity between all cultivars averaged 0.760 with a range from 0.640 ('Pak 4F CB 4025' and 'Paymaster HS200') to 0.993 ('Rowden' and 'DES 716'). These cultivars were assembled into 15 groups with sub-groups present in groups 4 and 6 based on the phylogenic tree (Table 8). A detailed phylogenic tree can be found in Fang et al. 2013 [81]. Molecular marker analysis revealed little relationship between the genetic make-up of cultivars and their countries of origin. Instead, the results from genetic diversity analysis and phylogenic grouping based on molecular markers were largely congruent with the breeding history and pedigree information of many cultivars [100,101].

The information obtained from this research may benefit cotton geneticists and breeders in a variety of ways. First, breeders could use a subset or a whole set of the markers to genotype their germplasm. Then, they would be able to compare their germplasm to the cultivars analyzed in this study based on the molecular profiles. Second, depending on their breeding objectives, breeders may choose cultivars from the list as the parents to make new crosses, or choose one cultivar to cross with their own favorite cultivar(s) based on their molecular profiles and phylogenic groups. Third, breeders may use the information to re-evaluate their breeding programs. Fourth, breeders or geneticists may use all or a subset of these cultivars as starting materials to conduct an association mapping study.

Chromosome (A sub-genome)	No. loci	Chromosome (D sub-genome)	No. loci
1	17	14	31
2	18	15	25
3	27	16	20
4	16	17	16
5	39	18	18
6	17	19	39
7	22	20	13
8	21	21	21
9	28	22	20
10	14	23	24
11	21	24	18
12	26	25	19
13	17	26	19
not mapped	166		
Total			732

Table 7. Chromosome distribution of 732 loci within cotton genome for 448 markers used to genotype 193 cultivars.

Group	No. cultivars	No. unique alleles	No. countries of origin	Description
1	5	6	5	Common factor unknown or not clear
2	8	3	3	Cultivars with Coker 100 in their pedigrees
3	10	8	1	Pee Dee germplasm
4	22	34	6	Cultivars from Pakistan, multi-adversity resistance breeding program and Paymaster program in Texas
5	15	4	5	Cultivars from S. America, and those with disease resistance
6	70	29	4	Commercial cultivars developed in the U.S., Australia and China
7	13	4	2	Acala type
8	4	7	3	Common factor unknown or not clear
9	6	1	2	Cultivars from Paymaster program in Texas high plain
10	4	0	3	Common factor unknown or not clear
11	6	14	2	Common factor unknown or not clear
12	3	1	3	Common factor unknown or not clear
13	3	11	2	Common factor unknown or not clear
14	3	1	2	Coker cultivars related to Coker 310
15	19	14	9	Cultivars from Africa, and Coker cultivars with wilt resistance

Table 8. Summary of phylogenic grouping of 191 cultivars

7. Germplasm databases

In this chapter we have tried to briefly describe the U.S. National Cotton Germplasm Collection and some of the current efforts made to preserve, characterize, and distribute its contents. However, the utility of the germplasm collection and its genetic resources is directly proportional to the knowledge of the genetic diversity within the collection, and the accessibility of that knowledge. Without the ability to disseminate information about the collection broadly to a community with free and easy access, the utility of the collection is greatly diminished. Currently, information about the collection can be accessed at two main database sources: GRIN-GLOBAL and CottonGen. GRIN-GLOBAL (http://distribution.grin-global.org/gringlobal/search.aspx)has been adequately described elsewhere and will not be described here. The following is a description of CottonGen and efforts to expand its contents and capabilities.

CottonGen (www.cottongen.org, [102,103]) is a curated and integrated web-based relational database providing centralized access to publicly available genomic, genetic and breeding data for cotton. Initiated in 2011, as the successor to CottonDB [102], CottonGen contains annotated whole genome sequences, genes, transcripts, markers, trait loci, genetic maps, taxonomy, germplasm, publications, data analysis tools, and communication resources for the cotton community. Annotated whole genome sequences of *Gossypium raimondii* are available with

http://dx.doi.org/10.5772/58386

aligned genetic markers, transcripts and protein homologs. These whole genome data can be accessed through genome pages, search tools and the genome browser GBrowse. Most of the published cotton genetic maps can be viewed and compared using the comparative map viewer CMap, and are searchable via map search tools. Search tools also exist for markers, QTLs, germplasm, publications, and trait evaluation data.

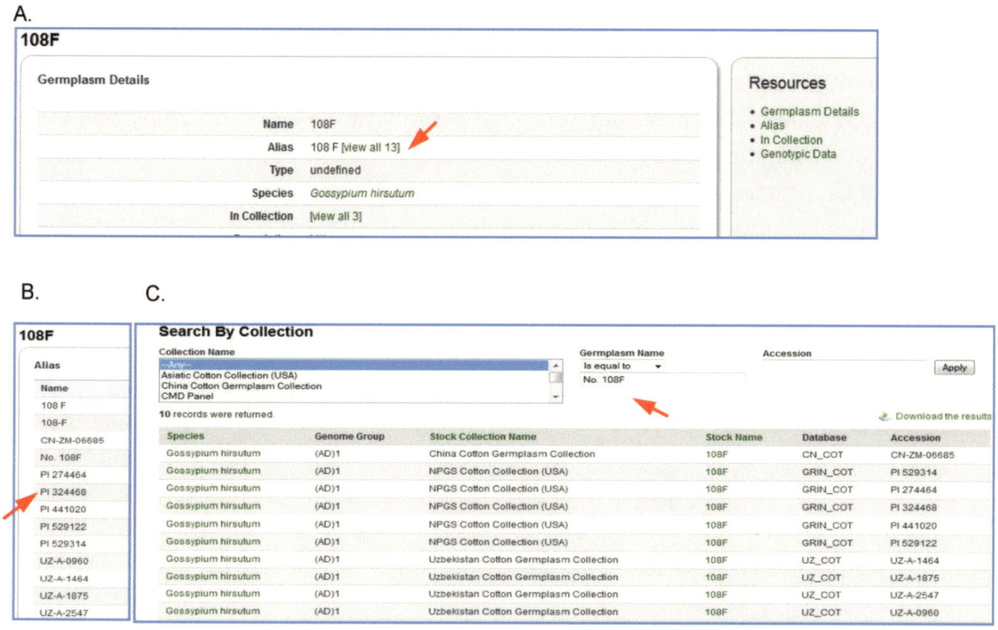

Figure 1. An example of how germplasm names can be used and displayed in CottonGen. A. The details page of germplasm '108F' which shows this germplasm individual has been recorded as 13 different names (aliases). B. lists the 13 names (aliases), some of them are the accessions from various germplasm collections or germplasm groups, such as 'PI 274464' which is an accession name used in GRIN. Other names show the others formats used for this germplasm, such '108 F' and 'No. 108F'. C. Any of the names in this germplasm aliases list can be used in the germplasm name search, such as 'No. 108F', the same result table will be displayed it matches any of the aliases or the standardized name.

A critical function of any community database is to provide data and information that is as accurate, unambiguous and non-redundant as possible. For germplasm pedigree and trait data, this can be particularly challenging as it involves identifying and rationalizing the many aliases used for accession names, and the different descriptors and measurement scales for the same trait. This is often compounded by a lack of standardization within and between collections due to data storage system restrictions, nomenclature differences, and unrecognized errors at the time of data entry. When these issues are resolved by the database curator, the curated data are integrated with other associated data and made accessible to scientists through easy-to-use interfaces to ensure utility to scientists.

The first step in the germplasm curation effort involved creating a validated list of unique cotton germplasm with unique IDs. A good starting point for this list was obtained from the

USDA-ARS GRIN [104] cotton collection PI numbers. In order to resolve the discrepancies, the apparently unique lines that could be identified from the passport data were given an unique "cdbgm" ID in CottonGen, and the accession numbers or names from different collections or germplasm groups (such as the CMD panel), and alternate names cross-referenced to these CottonGen unique IDs. The unique ID, germplasm names and aliases were then expanded to include other germplasm from the GRIN Cotton Crop Science Registration, GRIN Plant Variety Protection (PVP), pedigrees of 642 Upland and 20 Pima cultivars, plus 205 parents representing most of the cotton breeding lines and obsolete cultivars, (kindly provided by Dr. Bowman [100], the cotton germplasm collection of the China Cotton Research Institute, the Chinese Academy of Agricultural Sciences, and the cotton germplasm collection of Uzbekistan Center of Genomics and Bioinformatics, Academy of Sciences of Uzbekistan. As a result of curation efforts, CottonGen currently contains 14,959 assigned unique IDs connected to 53,645 corresponding aliases obtained from 14 collections for 49 *Gossypium* spp. Access and display of germplasm names (standardized and aliases) in CottonGen are shown in Figure 1.

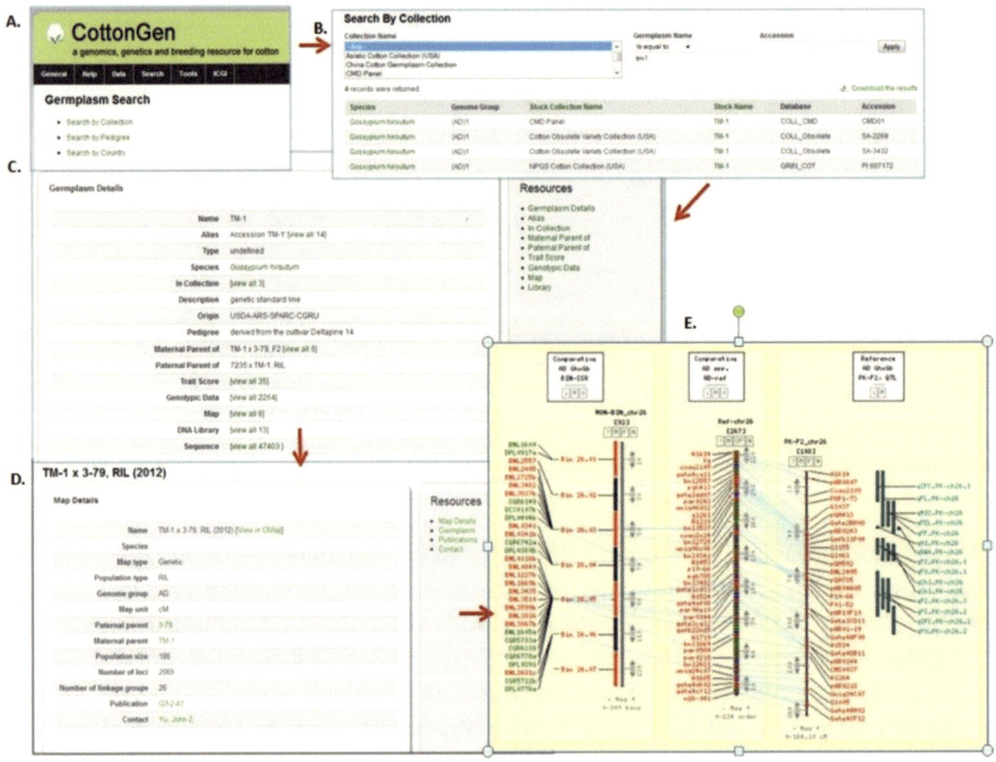

Figure 2. Germplasm search site in CottonGen. A. Multiple germplasm search sites are available based on the type of information users are interested in. B. An example search interface where users can view and search for germplasm and their collection center. C. Germplasm detail page with various tabs to show the detailed information. D. Map tab of the germplasm page shows all the maps for which the germplasm has been used. E. From the map page users can go to CMap for accessed to marker between and within maps, with hyperlinks to the markers detail page.

In addition to germplasm name (and aliases), germplasm data housed in CottonGen includes pedigrees, publicly available passport data, stock collection center information, associated maps, libraries and sequences. The trait evaluation database in CottonGen contains over 118,000 trait scores from 9,000 accessions. The *Gossypium* species summary page (http://www.cottongen.org/data/species) provides a list of species along with information such as genome group, haploid chromosome number, geographic origin, and number of accessions, sequences and DNA libraries per species. The species name in the table leads to individual species pages, which show more detail such as common name, images and other additional data such as functional analysis of the genes, both from the National Center for Biotechnology Information (NCBI) and whole genome sequences, which includes Kyoto Encyclopedia of Genes and Genomes (KEGG) [105] and Gene Ontology (GO) [106] analysis reports. The germplasm search page, accessible from http://www.cottongen.org/search/germplasm provides access to different types of searchable data (Figure 2). The search by collection page provides a list of germplasm along with stock collection center information. The search can be filtered by collection center name, germplasm name and/or accession name in the stock center. The search by pedigree page provides an interface to search germplasm by pedigree and the search germplasm by country page searches by the country of origin. From the germplasm search page, researchers can go to the germplasm details page, which shows all the detailed information such as pedigree, passport, collection center, image and associated genotypic and phenotypic data (Figure 2). Germplasm can also be searched based on their trait evaluation data. Both the qualitative trait evaluation search and quantitative trait evaluation search site allows the trait values of up to three trait descriptors to be specified to view the germplasm trait data. Data from all the search result sites can be downloaded in Excel files.

Among ongoing efforts of CottonGen is the development of a digital image library to store over 100,000 images provided by the USDA-ARS Research Project: "Genotypic and Phenotypic Analysis and Digital Imaging of Accessions in the US National Cotton Germplasm Collection". The associated phenotypic data from the same project will be stored in CottonGen as well. Provision of other germplasm data to CottonGen is actively encouraged.

8. Conclusion

The National Cotton Germplasm Collection is a complex amalgamation of several previously existing collections, which present challenges to its continued growth, preservation, characterization, and evaluation. Although habitat loss and international treaties have had significant impact on germplasm collection and exchange efforts, the NCGC continues to grow through mutually beneficial collecting efforts and germplasm exchanges with cooperating countries. Given finite and sometimes constricting resources; efficiency and effectiveness in preserving, characterizing, and evaluating the collection's contents becomes imperative. One means of increasing the efficiency and effectiveness of the collection has been to enlist the research community in characterizing and evaluating the collection. Currently there are dynamic cooperative efforts to evaluate the collection for drought, heat, and other environmental stresses associated with global climate change. Efforts to find resistance to biotic stresses within the collection continue, as do efforts to identify positive variation within the collection for agronomic and fiber quality characteristics. The development of genetic marker technology greatly increases the ability to investigate the genetic variation of the collection and offers needed means to manage the collection's contents through identification of redundancy, misclassification, introgression, and sources of unique variability within the collection. Cooperative efforts within the research community to characterize and evaluate the collection, while very effective, could be replicated at an international level with greater impact.

Author details

Richard G. Percy[1*], James E. Frelichowski[1], Mark D. Arnold[2], Todd B. Campbell[3], Jane K. Dever[2], David D. Fang[4], Lori L. Hinze[1], Dorrie Main[5], Jodi Scheffler[6], Monica A. Sheehan[2], Mauricio Ulloa[7], Jing Yu[5] and John Yu[1]

*Address all correspondence to: Richard.Percy@ars.usda.gov

1 USDA-ARS, College Station, TX, USA

2 Texas A&M AgriLife Research, Texas A&M Agrilife Research& Extension Center, Lubbock, TX, USA

3 USDA-ARS, Florence, SC, USA

4 USDA-ARS, New Orleans, LA, USA

5 Department of Horticulture, Washington State University, WA, USA

6 USDA-ARS, Stoneville, MS, USA

7 USDA-ARS, Lubbock, TX, USA

References

[1] Ware JO. Plant Breeding and the Cotton Industry. U.S.D.A. Yearbook; 1936.

[2] Mauer FM. The Cottons of Mexico, Guatemala, and Columbia. Suppl. 47, Bull. Appl. Bot. Genet. and Pl. Br. 1930.

[3] Percival AE, Wendel JF, Stewart JM. Taxonomy and Germplasm Resources. In: Smith CW and Cothren JT (eds.) Cotton: Origin, history, technology, and production. New York: John Wiley & Sons; 1999. p. 33-64.

[4] Smith CW, Cantrell RG, Moser HS, Oakley SR. History of Cultivar Development in the United States. In: Smith CW, Cothren JT (eds.) Cotton: Origin, history, technology, and production. New York: John Wiley & Sons; 1999. p99-172.

[5] SCSB. Preservation and Utilization of Germplasm in Cotton 1968-1980. Southern Cooperative Series Bulletin No. 256. 1981

[6] SCSB. Genetics and Cytology of Cotton 1956-67. Southern Cooperative Series Bulletin No. 139. 1968.

[7] SCSB. Genetics and Cytology of Cotton 1948-55. Southern Cooperative Series Bulletin No. 47. 1956.

[8] IBPGR. Descriptors for Cotton Species. International Board for Plant Genetic Resources Working Group, Rome, Italy. 1980.

[9] Beasley JO. Meiotic chromosome behavior in species, species hybrids, haploids and induced polyploids of *Gossypium*. Genetics 1942; 27 25-54.

[10] Percival AE. The National Collection of *Gossypium* Germplasm. Southern Cooperative Series Bulletin No. 321. 1987.

[11] Vertucci WE, Roos EE. Theoretical basis of protocols for seed storage. Plant Physiol. 1990;94 1019-1023.

[12] Cromarty AS, Ellis RH, Roberts EH. The design of seed storage facilities for genetic conservation. International Board for Plant Genetic Resources, Rome, Italy. 1982.

[13] Abdalla AM, Raddy OUK, El-Zik KM, Pepper AE. Genetic diversity and relationships of diploid and tetraploid cottons revealed using AFLP. Theor. Appl. Genet. 2001;102 222-229.

[14] Wallace TP, Bowman D, Campbell BT, Chee P, Gutierrez OA, Kohel RJ, McCarty J, Myers G, Percy R, Robinson F, Smith W, Stelly DM, Stewart JM, Thaxton P, Ulloa M, Weaver DB. Status of the USA cotton germplasm collection and crop vulnerability. Genet. Resour. Crop Evol. 2009;56 507-532.

[15] Xu Q, Zhang X, Nie N, Feng CD. Genetic diversity among cotton cultivars (*G. hirsutum* L.) resistant to Fusarium wilt as estimated by RAPD markers. Scientia Agricultura Sinica 2002;35(3) 272-276.

[16] Multani DS, and Lyon BR. Genetic fingerprinting of Australian cotton cultivars with RAPD markers. Genome 1995;38 1005-1008.

[17] Ulloa M., Brubaker C., Chee P. Cotton. In: Kole C. (ed.) Genome Mapping & Molecular Breeding. Vol. 6: Technical Crops. Heidelberg, Berlin, New York, Tokyo: Springer; 2007. p1-49.

[18] Ulloa M, Percy R, Hutmacher RB, Zhang J. The future of cotton breeding in the Western United States. J. Cot. Sci. 2009;4 246-255.

[19] Ulloa M, Abdurakhmonov IY, Perez-M C, Percy R, Stewart McDJ. Genetic diversity and population structure of cotton (*Gossypium* spp.) of the New World assessed by SSR markers. Botany 2013;91 251-259.

[20] Percival AE, Kohel RJ. Distribution, collection, and evaluation of *Gossypium*. Adv. Agron. 1990;44 225-256.

[21] USDA. The Regional Collection of *Gossypium* Germplasm. United States Department of Agriculture, Agriculture Research Service, ARS-H-2, Oct. 1974.

[22] Bretting, PK. The U.S. National Plant Germplasm System in an era of shifting international norms for germplasm exchange. In: KE Hummer. (ed.) Plant Gen. Resources, Proc. XXVII IHC-S1, Onternational Society of Horticultural Science. Acta. Hort. 760, ISHS. 2007.

[23] FAO. The Second Report on the State of the World's Plant Genetic Resources for Food and Agriculture. Rome. 2010. P370. Available from http://www.fao.org/agriculture/seed/sow2/ (accessed 10 September, 2013).

[24] Wallace TP, Bowman D, Campbell BT, Chee P, Gutierrez A, Kohel RJ, McCarty J, Meyers G, Percy R, Robinson F, Smith W, Stelly DM, Stewart JM, Thaxton P Ulloa M, Weaver DB. Status of the USA cotton germplasm collection and crop vulnerability. Gen. Res.Crop Evol. 2009;56 507-532.

[25] Campbell BT, Saha S, Percy R, Frelichowski J, Jenkins J N, Park W, Mayee CD, Gotmare V, Dessauw D, Giband M, Du X, Jia Y, Constable G, Dillon S, Abdurakhmonov I Y, Abdukarimov A, Rizaeva SM, Abdullaev A, Barroso PAV, Padua JG., Hoffmann LV, Podolnaya L. Status of the global cotton germplasm resources. Crop Sci. 2010;50 1161-1179.

[26] Ulloa M, Stewart JM, Garcia-C EA, Godoy-A A, Gaytán-M A, Acosta-N S. Cotton genetic resources in the western states of Mexico: in situ conservation status and germplasm collection for ex situ preservation. Genet. Resour. Crop Evol. 2006;53 (4) 653-668.

[27] Fryxell PA. The Natural History of the Cotton Tribe. College Station and London: Texas A&M University Press; 1979.

[28] Fryxell PA. A revised taxonomic interpretation of *Gossypium* L. (Malvaceae). Rheedea 1992;2 108-165.

[29] Fryxell PA, Craven LA, Stewart JM. A revision of *Gossypium* sect. *Grandicalyx* (Malvaceae), including the description of six new species. Systematic Botany 1992; 17 91-114.

[30] Grover CE, Grupp KK, Wanzek RJ, Wendel JF. Assessing the monophyly of polyploidy *Gossypium* species. Plant Syst. Evol. 2012;298 1177-1183.

[31] Schwendiman J, Percival AE, Belot JL. Cotton collecting on Caribbean Islands and South Florida. FAO/IBPGR Plant Genetic Resources Newsletter. 1986;66 20-5.

[32] Krapovickas A, Seijo G. *Gossypium ekmanianum* (Malvaceae), algodon Silvestre de la Republica Dominicana. Bonpl. 2008;17(1) 55-63.

[33] Anonymous. Descriptors for Cotton. AGP:IBPGR. 1980;10.

[34] Toll JA. Processing of germplasm, associated material and data. In: Guarino L, Ramanatha RV, Reid R, (eds.) Collecting Plant Genetic Diversity: Technical Guidelines. Rome, Italy: International Plant Genetic Resources Institute (IPGRI), Plant Production and Protection Division, FAO; 1995. p577-595.

[35] Mackay M, Alercia A. Processing of germplasm, associated material and data. In: Guarino L, Ramanatha RV, Goldberg E. (eds.) Collecting Plant Genetic Diversity: Technical Guidelines-2011 Update. Rome, Italy: Bioversity International; 2011. p1-4.

[36] Puzone L, Hazekamp T. Characterization and documentation of genetic resources utilizing multimedia databases. Proc. Workshop, Dec. 19-20, 1996, Naples, Italy: IPGR; 1998. p67.

[37] Mincione A, Filippone E, Monti LM. Construction of an image-based germplasm data base for *Phaseolus* spp. Euphytica. 1994;75 149-159.

[38] Smykalova I, Hampel D, Pavelek M. Determination of duplicates of accessions in a germplasm collection of flax/linseed by means of digital image analysis. Indust. Crops Prod. 2012;36 177-187.

[39] Dever JK, Sheehan MA. Update of cotton race-stock screening and phenotypic characterization. Proc.Beltwide Cotton Conf., 4-7, January 2011, Atlanta, GA. p718-719; 2011.

[40] Sheehan M A, Dever JK, Arnold MD. Phenotypic documentation of *Gossypium* species from the US Cotton Germplasm Collection, USDA-ARS, Using Digital Photography. Proc. Beltwide Cotton Conf., 4-7, January 2010, New Orleans, LA. p753-756; 2010.

[41] Kohel RJ, Glueck J, Rooney LW. Comparison of cotton germplasm collections for seed-protein content. Crop Sci. 1985;25 961-963.

[42] Kohel, RJ. Survey of *Gossypium hirsutum* L. germplasm collections for seed-oil percentage and seed characteristics. Agric. Res. Serv., U.S. Dept. of Agriculture, ARS-S-187; 1978.

[43] Dilday RH, Shaver TN. Survey of the regional *Gossypium hirsutum* L., primitive race collection for flowerbud gossypol. Agr. Res. Serv., U.S. Dept. of Agriculture, Publ. ARS-S-146; 1976.

[44] Jenkins JN, Parrott WL. Field evaluation of primitive races of Gossypium hirsutum L. for resistance to boll weevil. Technical Bulletin, Mississippi Agricultural and Forestry Experiment Station, 91; 1978.

[45] Jenkins JN, Parrott WL. Field evaluation of primitive races of Gossypium hirsutum L. for resistance to *Cercospora* leaf spot and *Verticillium* wilt. Miss. Agric. & For. Exp. Stat. Tech. Bull. 92; 1978.

[46] USDA. A laboratory evaluation of primitive cotton (*Gossypium hirsutum* L.) races for pink bollworn resistance. USDA. ARS W-30;1975. 9pp.

[47] Shepherd RL. New sources of resistance to root-knot nematodes among primitive cottons. Crop Sci. 1983;23 999-1002.

[48] Jenkins, JN. Host plant resistance: advances in cotton. In: Brown JM, Nelson TC. (eds.): proceedings of the Beltwide Cotton Conferences, 4-9 January 1986, Las Vegas, NV, USA. Memphis, TN: National Cotton Council; 1986.

[49] Williams, MR. Cotton insect losses 2012. In: Boyd S, Huffman M, Robertson B. (eds.): proceedings of the Beltwide Cotton Conferences, 7-10 January 2013, San Antonio, TX, USA. Memphis: National Cotton Council; 2013.

[50] Arnold MD, Gannaway JR, Sheehan MA. Screening obsolete race stocks and other wild cottons for thrips resistance at the Crops Genetic Research Facility at the Texas A&M Research and Extension Center at Lubbock, Texas. In: Boyd S, Huffman M, Richter D, Robertson B. (eds.): proceedings of the Beltwide Cotton Conferences, 9-12 January 2007, New Orleans, LA. Memphis: National Cotton Council; 2007.

[51] Wardle R, Simpson R. The biology of Thysanoptera with reference to the cotton plant. Annals of Applied Biology 1927;14 513-528.

[52] Watts, JG. A study of the biology of the flower thrips Frankliniella tritici (Fitch) with special reference to cotton. South Carolina Agricultural Experiment Station Bulletin 306. 1936; 46p.

[53] Painter RH. Insect Resistance in Crop Plants. New York: MacMillan Co.; 1951.

[54] Gawaad, AAA, El-Gayar FH, Soliman AS, Zaghlool OA. Studies on *Thrips tabaci* Lindeman, X. Mechanism of resistance to *Thrips tabaci* L. in cotton varieties. Zeitschrift fuer Angewandte Entomologie 1973;73 251-255.

[55] Bowman DT, McCarty, Jr. JC. Thrips (Thysanoptera: Thripidae) Tolerance in Cotton: Sources and Heritability. Journal of Entomological Science 1997;32:460-471.

[56] Turnbull MH, Whitehead D, Tissue DT, Schuster WS, Brown KJ, Griffin KL. Responses of leaf respiration to temperature and leaf characteristics in three deciduous tree species vary with site of water availability. Tree Physiol. 2001;21 571-578.

[57] Chinnusamy V, Schumaker K, Zhu JK. Molecular genetic perspectives on cross-talk and specificity in abiotic stress signalling in plants. J. Exp. Bot. 2004;55 225-236.

[58] Nixon PJ, Barker M, Boehm M, de Vries R, Komenda J. FtsH-mediated repair of the photosystem II complex in response to light stress. J. Exp. Bot. 2005;56 357-363.

[59] McMichael BL, Quisenberry JE. Genetic diversity for root-shoot relationships among cotton germplasm. J. Environ. Exptl. Bot. 1991;31 461-470.

[60] McMichael BL, Lascano RJ. Evaluation of hydraulic lift in cotton (Gossypium hirsutum L.) germplasm. J. Environ. Exptl. Bot. 2009;68 26-30.

[61] Ulloa M, Brubaker C, Chee P. Cotton. In: C. Kole (ed.) Genome Mapping & Molecular Breeding. Vol. 6. Heidelberg, Berlin, New York, Tokyo: Technical Crops, Springer; 1991. p1-49.

[62] Ulloa M, Abdurakhmonov IY, Perez-M C, Percy R, Stewart McDJ. Genetic diversity and population structure of cotton (*Gossypium* spp.) of the New World assessed by SSR markers. Botany 2013;91 251-259.

[63] White JW, Andrea-Sanchez P, Gore MA, Broson KF, Coffelt TA, Conley MM, Feldmann KA, French AN, Heun JT, Hunsaker DJ, Jenks MA, Kimball BA, Roth RL, Strand RJ, Thorp KR, Wall GW, Wang G. Field-based phenomics for plant genetics research. Field Crop Research 2012;133 101-112.

[64] Burke JJ. Evaluation of source leaf responses to water-deficit stresses in cotton using a novel stress bioassay. Plant Physiol. 2007;42 108-121.

[65] Burke JJ, Franks C, Burow GB, Xin Z.. Selection System for the Stay-Green Drought Tolerance Trait in Sorghum Germplasm. Agronomy Journal. 2010;102(4) 1118-1122.

[66] Burke JJ, Ulloa M. Initial characterization of a Stoneville 474 x Phytogen 72 recombinant inbred population. In: Boyd S, Huffman M, Robertson B. (eds.): proceedings of the Beltwide Cotton Conferences, 7-10 January 2013, San Antonio, TX, USA. Memphis: National Cotton Council.

[67] Tanksley SD, McCouch SR. Seed bank and molecular maps: Unlocking genetic potential from the wild. Science 1997;277 1063-1066.

[68] Kohel RJ, Yu JZ. Molecular characterization of *Gossypium* germplasm for cotton improvement, p 67-75. In Engels JMM, Rao VR, Brown AHD, Jackson MT (eds), Managing Plant Genetic Diversity, CAB International Publishing, Inc., Wallingford, UK. 2001. 512 pp.

[69] Abdurakhmonov IY, Buriev ZT, Shermatov SE, Abdullaev AA, Urmonov K, Kushanov F, Egamberdiev SS, Shapulatov U, Abdukarimov A, Saha S, Jenkins JN, Kohel RJ, Yu JZ, Pepper AE, Kumpatala S, Ulloa M. Genetic diversity in *Gossypium* genus. In: Çalişkan M.(ed.) Genetic Diversity in Plants. New York, NY: InTech; 2012. p313-338.

[70] Reinisch AJ, Dong J, Brubaker CL, Stelly DM, Wendel JF, Paterson AH. A detailed RFLP map of cotton, *Gossypium hirsutum* X *Gossypium barbadense*-chromosome organization and evolution in a disomic polyploid genome. Genetics 1994;138 829-847.

[71] Shappley ZW, Jenkins JN, Meredith WR, Mccarty JC. An RFLP linkage map of Upland cotton, *Gossypium hirsutum* L. Theoretical and Applied Genetics 1998;97 756-761.

[72] Yu JZ, Kohel RJ. Cotton genome research in the United States. In: Jenkins JN, Saha S. (eds.) Genetic improvement of cotton: Emerging technologies. Plymouth, UK: The Science Publishers, Inc; 2001. p103-121.

[73] Yu JZ, Fang DD, Kohel RJ, Ulloa M, Hinze LL, Percy RG, Zhang J, Chee P, Scheffler BE, Jones DC. Development of a core set of SSR markers for the characterization of *Gossypium* germplasm. Euphytica 2012;187 203-213.

[74] Blenda A, Scheffler J, Scheffler B, Palmer M, Lacape J-M, Yu JZ, Jesudurai C, Jung S, Muthukumar S, Yellambalase P, Ficklin S, Staton M, Eshelman R, Ulloa M, Saha S, Burr B, Liu S, Zhang T, Fang D, Pepper A, Kumpatla S, Jacobs J, Tomkins J, Cantrell R, Main D. CMD: A cotton microsatellite database resource for *Gossypium* genomics. BMC Genomics 2006;7 132. doi:10.1186/1471-2164-7-132.

[75] Yu JZ, Kohel RJ, Fang DD, Cho J, Van Deynze A, Ulloa M, Hoffman SM, Pepper AE, Stelly DM, Jenkins JN, Saha S, Kumpatla SP, Shah MR, Hugie WV, Percy RG. A high-density SSR and SNP genetic map of the tetraploid cotton genome. G3: Genes, Genomes, Genetics 2012;2 43-58.

[76] Blenda A, Fang DD, Rami JF, Garsmeur O, Luo F, Lacape JM. A high density consensus genetic map of tetraploid cotton that integrates multiple component maps through molecular marker redundancy check. PLoS ONE 2012;7(9) e45739. doi: 10.1371/journal.pone.0045739.

[77] Fang DD, Yu JZ. Addition of four-hundred fifty-five microsatellite marker loci to the high-density *Gossypium hirsutum* TM-1 x *G. barbadense* 3-79 genetic map. Journal of Cotton Science. 2012;16 229–248.

[78] Yu JZ. A standard panel of *Gossypium* genotypes established for systematic characterization of cotton microsatellite markers. Plant Breeding News Edition 2004;148 (1.07).

[79] Alvarez I, Wendel JF. Cryptic interspecific introgression and genetic differentiation within *Gossypium aridum* (Malvaceae) and its relatives. Evolution 2006; 60:505-517.

[80] Kantartzi SK, Ulloa M, Sacks E, Stewart JM. Assessing Genetic Diversity in *Gossypium arboreum* L. Cultivars using Genomic and EST-derived Microsatellites. Genetica 2009; 136:141-147.

[81] Kuester AP, Nason JD. Microsatellite Loci for *Gossypium davidsonii* (Malvaceae) and Other D-genome, Sonoran Desert Endemic Cotton Species. American Journal of Botany 2012; 99 91-93.

[82] Fang DD, Hinze LL, Percy RG, Li P, Deng D, Thyssen G. A Microsatellite-Based Genome-Wide Analysis of Genetic Diversity and Linkage Disequilibrium in Upland Cotton (*Gossypium hirsutum* L.) Cultivars from Major Cotton-Growing Countries. Euphytica 2013; 191 391-401.

[83] Hinze LL, Dever JK, Percy RG. Molecular Variation Among and Within Improved Cultivars in the U.S. Cotton Germplasm Collection. Crop Science 2012; 52 222-230.

[84] Kalivas A, Xanthopoulos F, Kehagia O, Tsaftaris AS. Agronomic Characterization, Genetic Diversity and Association Analysis of Cotton Cultivars using Simple Sequence Repeat Molecular Markers. Genetics and Molecular Research 2011; 10 208-217.

[85] Maleia MP, Filho PSV, Goncalves-Vidigal MC, Gonela A, Lacanallo GF, Moiana LD, Chamuene A, de Sousa LL, Darben LM. Genetic Divergence Among African and American Cotton (*Gossypium hirsutum* L. race latifolium H.) Cultivars and Inbred Lines Through Random Amplification of Polymorphic DNA (RAPD) Markers. African Journal of Biotechnology 2010; 9 8539-8548.

[86] Kebede H, Burow G, Dani RG, Allen RD. A-genome Cotton as a Source of Genetic Variability for Upland Cotton (*Gossypium hirsutum*). Genetic Resources and Crop Evolution 2007; 54 885-895.

[87] Abdurakhmonov IY, Kohel RJ, Yu JZ, Pepper AE, Abdullaev A, Kushanov FN, Salakhutdinov IB, Buriev ZT, Saha S, Scheffler B, Jenkins JN, Abdukarimov A. Molecular Diversity and Association Mapping of Fiber Quality Traits in Exotic *G. hirsutum* L. Germplasm. Genomics 2008; 92 478-487.

[88] Abdurakhmonov IY, Saha S, Jenkins JN, Buriev ZT, Shermatov SE, Scheffler BE, Pepper AE, Yu JZ, Kohel RJ, Abdukarimov A. Linkage Disequilibrium Based Association Mapping of Fiber Quality Traits in *G. hirsutum* L. Variety Germplasm. Genetica 2009; 136 401-417.

[89] Lacape J-M, Dessauw D, Rajab M, Noyer J-L, Hau B. Microsatellite Diversity in Tetraploid *Gossypium* Germplasm: Assembling a Highly Informative Genotyping Set of Cotton SSRs. Molecular Breeding 2007; 19 45-58.

[90] Van Deynze A, Stoffel K, Lee M, Kozik A, Wilkins TA, Cantrell RG, Yu JZ, Kohel RJ, Stelly DM. Sampling nucleotide diversity in cotton. BMC Plant Biology. 2009. 9:125.

[91] Byers RL, Harker DB, Yourstone SM, Maughan PJ, Udall JA. Development and mapping of SNP assays in allotetraploid cotton. Theoretical and Applied Genetics 2012; 124 1201-1214. doi: 10.1007/s00122-011-1780-8.

[92] Verma S, Young CJ, Pepper AE, McCormick R, Percy RG, Yu JZ. De novo SNP discovery and development of an interspecific cotton genome map using a simplified genotyping-by-sequencing (GBS) approach. Proceedings of the Research Conference on International Cotton Genome Initiative. 2012. Raleigh, NC.

[93] Hulse A, Hoegenauer K, Wang F, Stelly D, Ashrafi H, Van Deynze A, Zhang H, Saski C, Patterson AH, Schmutz J, Chen ZJ, Udall J, Yu JZ, Jones DC. Localization of allotetraploid *Gossypium* SNPs using physical mapping resources. Proceedings of the Research Conference on International Cotton Genome Initiative. 2012. Raleigh, NC.

[94] Yu JZ, Young CJ, Verma S, Percy RG, McCormick R, Pepper AE. Development of single nucleotide polymorphism markers via sequence-based genotyping in cotton (*Gossypium* spp). In: Proceedings of the International Conference on Plant and Animal Genomes, 11-16 January 2013, San Diego, CA.

[95] Wang K, Wang Z, Li F, Ye W, Wang J, Song G, Yue Z, Cong L, Shang H, Zhu S, Zou C, Li Q, Yuan Y, Lu C, Wei H, Gou C, Zheng Z, Yin Y, Zhang X, Liu K, Wang B, Song

C, Shi N, Kohel RJ, Percy RG, Yu JZ, Zhu Y-X, Wang J, Yu S. The draft genome of a diploid cotton *Gossypium raimondii*. Nature Genetics. 2012; 44(10) 1098-1104.

[96] Paterson AH, Wendel JF, Gundlach H, Guo H, Jenkins J, Jin D, Llewellyn D, Showmaker KC, Shu S, Udall J, Yoo M, Byers R, Chen W, Faigenboim AD, Duke MV, Gong L, Grimwood J, Grover C, Grupp K, Hu G, Lee T, Li J, Lin L, Liu T, Marler BS, Page JT, Roberts AW, Romanel E, Sanders WS, Szadkowski E, Tan X, Tang H, Xu C, Wang J, Wang Z, Zhang D, Zhang L, Ashrafi H, Bedon F, Bowers JE, Brubaker CL, Chee PW, Das S, Gingle AR, Haigler CH, Harker D, Hoffmann LV, Hovav R, Jones DC, Lemke C, Mansoor S, Rahman M, Rainville LN, Rambani A, Reddy UK, Rong J, Saranga Y, Scheffler BE, Scheffler JA, Stelly DM, Triplett BA, Van Deynze A, Vaslin MFS, Waghmare VN, Walford SA, Wright RJ, Zaki EA, Zhang T, Dennis ES, Mayer KFX, Peterson DG, Rokhsar DS, Wang X, Schmutz J. Repeated polyploidization of *Gossypium* genomes and the evolution of spinnable cotton fibres. Nature 2012; 492 423–427.

[97] Ganal MW, Durstewitz G, Polley A, Berard A, Buckler IV ES, Charcosset A, Clarke JD, Graner E, Mcmullen MD, Falque M. A large maize (*Zea Mays* L.) SNP genotyping array: development and germplasm genotyping, and genetic mapping to compare with the B73 reference genome. PLoS One. 2011. 6(12):e28334. DOI: 10.1371/journal.pone.0028334.

[98] Dice LR. Measures of the amount of ecologic association between species. Ecology 1945; 26 297-302.

[99] Rohlf FJ. NTSYSpc: Numerical taxonomy and multivariate analysis system, version 2.1. Exeter Software. Setauket, NY; 2000.

[100] Bourland FM, Jones DC. Registration of 'UA48' cotton cultivar. Journal of Plant Registrations 2010; 6 15-18.

[101] Bowman DT, Gutierrez OA, Percy RG, Calhoun DS, May OL. Pedigrees of upland and pima cotton cultivars released between 1970 and 2005. Mississippi State Univ, Mississippi State, MS Mississippi Agricultural and Forestry Experimental Station Bulletin # 1155:http://msucares.com/pubs/bulletins/b1155.pdf. 2007.

[102] May OL, Bowman DT, Calhoun DS. Genetic diversity of US upland cotton cultivars released between 1980 and 1990. Crop Science 1995; 35 1570-1574.

[103] Yu J, Jung S, Cheng C, Ficklin S, Lee T, Zheng P, Jones D, Percy R, Main D. CottonGen: an Integrated Genomics, Genetics and Breeding Database for the Cotton Research Community. In: Proceedings of the International Cotton Genome Initiative Research Conference, 9-12 October 2012, Raleigh, NC, United States. 2012.

[104] Main D., Yu J, Jung S, Cheng CH, Ficklin SP, Zheng P, Lee T, Jones D, Percy R. Update on CottonGen: An Integrated Genomics, Genetics and Breeding Database for the Cotton Research Community. In: Proceedings of the International Plant and Animal Conference, 12 January 2012, San Diego, CA, United States. 2012.

[105] Wiersema,J. H. Taxonomic information on cultivated plants in the USDA/ARS germplasm resources information network (GRIN). In: Tukey Jr, HB. (ed). Acta Horticulturae 413. International Society for Horticultural Science. Proceedings of the Second International Symposium on the Taxonomy of Cultivated Plants, 10-14 August 1994, Seattle, Washington, USA. Leuven. Belgium; 1995. ISBN 90 6605 967 2. Individual papers from this Acta are available to download from http://www.actahort.org/books/413/

[106] Kanehisa M, Goto S. KEGG: kyoto encyclopedia of genes and genomes. Nucleic Acids Research 2000; 28(1) 27-30.

[107] Harris M, Clark J, Ireland A, Lomax J, Ashburner M, Foulger R, Eilbeck K, Lewis S, Marshall B, Mungall C, *et al.* The Gene Ontology (GO) database and informatics resource. Nucleic Acids Research 2004; 32 D258–D261.

Chapter 8

The Diploid D Genome Cottons (*Gossypium* spp.) of the New World

Mauricio Ulloa

Additional information is available at the end of the chapter

http://dx.doi.org/10.5772/58387

1. Introduction

The genetic diversity of cotton (*Gossypium* spp.) is exclusively wide with diverse geographic and ecological niches [1]. The *Gossypium* genus belongs to the *Malvaceae* family. This genus contains more than 45 diploid species and five well-documented allotetraploid species [2-4]. Species of this genus are grouped into nine genomic types (x=n=13, 2n=26 diploid, and 4x=52 tetraploid) with the following designations: AD, A, B, C, D, E, F, G, and K [3]. Genomic designations are based on the similarities in chromosome size and structure, and the success of interspecific crosses. Based on their chromosomal uniformity, the diploid D genome species of the New World include 26 somatic chromosomes. Some hybrids within genomes are fertile and their chromosomes recombine during meiosis. However, hybrids across genomes are generally infertile and they have a few stable bivalents at meiosis as a result progeny-plant survival from interspecific crosses is sometime low [4]. The allotetraploid cottons [Upland, *G. hirsutum* (AD_1) and *G. barbadense* (AD_2)] of the New World dominate world natural-fiber production. And they can be described as large shrubs to trees [3,5]. An allotetraploid is a species that derived from the combination of two different genomes or doubling of genomes that are different. The At subgenome is probably best represented by a composite of two diploid genomes ([*G. herbaceum* L. (A_1) and *G. arboreum* L. (A_2)] from the Old World. These Asiatic species-progenitor cottons primarily produce fibers for non-industrial-textile consumption in India and Asia [4]. The Dt subgenome has a more complex genome (D) of the diploid species-progenitors from the New World. The D genome is comprised of formally reported 13 species [3,7-9] and several undescribed taxa e.g. US-72 [8-11]. Eleven of the 13 species of the New World reside in the country of Mexico (Fig. 1). Taxonomically, these species are recognized as the *Houzingenia* subgenus [5,7]. None of these D genome diploid species produce commercial fibers. These species of the D genome are not well known to public and private breeding programs around the world, and their utilization for cotton improvement has not been fully exploited. Some species of the D genome [*G. aridum* (D_4), *G. lobatum* (D_7), *G. laxum* (D_9), etc] with arborescent growth habits express unique flowering and fruiting habits (following defoliation in the dry season). And even though none of the D diploid species produce commercial fibers, the diploid D genome species of the New World harbor important genes for improving fiber quality, pest and disease resistance, and drought and salt tolerance in the modern cultivated Upland and Pima cottons.

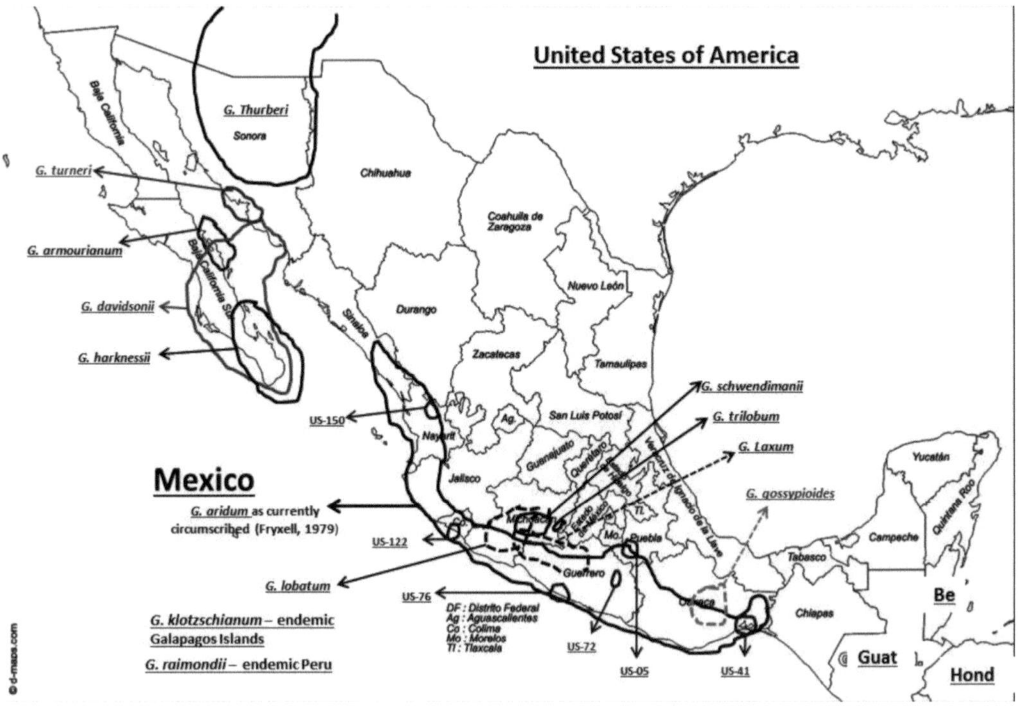

Figure 1. The country of Mexico, states, and approximate areas-boundaries of the diploid species of the D genome endemic to this country. The location of new taxa with US-XX (XX=number – Table 2) is indicated representing possible new species.

Even though Mexico's natural heritage of cotton genetic resources equals that of maize, until recently no national resources were dedicated to the preservation of this natural treasure [8]. The collection/exploration trips of these species have been difficult to document. Increasing human population and urbanization have severely reduced the survival of some of these species. *In situ* conservation of some of these species is threatened. New roads and population growth continue to increase. At this point, one species (*G. aridum* as formally reported) of the subsection *Erioxylum* appears not to be threatened, probably because of the great diversity (botanical and geographic) encompassed by this species. However, some of the most recent collected and non-described taxons (e.g., US-72) or ecotypes of the *G. aridum* species may be in the process of becoming extinct in the wild. In addition, the D_8 *G. trilobum* species is almost

http://dx.doi.org/10.5772/58387

extinct or already extinct. If *in situ* diversity of the Mexican cottons is severely eroded, the germplasm collections all over the world and the USDA Cotton Germplasm Collection will assume a highly significant role in the preservation of the diversity previously residing in Mexico's cotton species of the D genome.

Recently, the genome sequence of the best model, closest living ancestor relative of the allotetraploid cottons-of the Dt subgenome *(G. raimondii),* was published. This new information compiled with the ongoing next generation sequencing (NGS) projects around the world will provide insights into the evolution, population structure, genetic diversity, and utilization of this genetic resource. The next generation of genomic research will sequence characterize and locate genes that will help molecular breeders to identify differences among germplasm and breeding lines and to apply traditional genetic analyses to infer genes for marker assisted selection (MAS). In addition, the new sequence information obtained through NGS will be an important resource to improve the cotton crop through transgenic technology.

2. Classification of the D diploid species, distribution, and dissemination

The country of Mexico, besides being a part of the center of origin/diversity of *G. hirsutum,* also harbored 11 out of the 13 formally reported D species [3,7] and several non-described taxa of the New World diploid *Gossypium* species (one non-described taxon US-72,) [8-10]. The species of the *Houzingenia* subgenus are classified into six subsections: subsection *Houzingenia* Fryxell [*G. thurberi* Todaro (D_1) and *G. trilobum* (Mociño & Sessé ex DC.) Skovsted (D_8)]; subsection *Integrifolia* Todaro [*G. davidsonii* Kellogg ($D_{3\text{-}d}$) and *G. klotzschianum* Andersson ($D_{3\text{-}k}$)]; subsection *Caducibracteolata* Mauer [*G. armourianum* Kearney ($D_{2\text{-}1}$), *G. harknessii* Brandegee ($D_{2\text{-}2}$), and *G. turneri* Fryxell (D_{10})]; subsection *Erioxylum* Rose & Standley [*G. aridum* (D_4), *G. lobatum* (D_7), *G. laxum* (D_9), and *G. schwendimanii* Fryx. & Koch (D_{11})]; subsection *Selera* (Ulbrich) Fryxell [*G. gossypioides* (D_6)], and subsection *Austroamericana* Fryxell [*G. raimondii* Ulbrich (D_5)] [3,4,7]. Eleven of the 13 species of the subgenus *Houzingenia* are distributed in Mexico and extend northward into Arizona (Fig. 1). The other two D species have disjointed distributions; *G. raimondii* is endemic to Peru, while *G. klotzschianum* is found in the Galápagos Islands. The species of the D genome are not well known and utilized in public and private breeding programs around the world. Additional information about morphological characteristics and distribution of the species can be found in Fryxell monograph [12] and several other publications [8-9]. A supplemental information about recent collections [8-9] can be found at the USDA-ARS, SPA, CSRL, Plant Stress and Germplasm Development website (http://www.lbk.ars.usda.gov/psgd/index-cotton.aspx). Also, the Mexican Instituto Nacional de Investigaciones Forestales Agricolas y Pecuarias (INIFAP), Iguala Gro. Mex. nursery has provided us with the opportunity to further study some of these species *ex situ*. Table 1 provides information on 12 of the species during their *ex situ* preservation at the Iguala nursery in Mexico. Data from *G. klotzschianum* is missing from this table. Species planted at the nursery flower from September to January, while *in situ,* some of the populations from these species flower through March-April..

Species	Genome	Petal color	Filament color	Anther color	Leaf shape	Number of seed per capsule	Seed Size length mm	Seed width mm
G. aridum	D_4	Cherry	Purple	Purple	Cordate	14	7.3	1.7
G. armourianum	D_2	Yellow	White	Cherry	Ovate	13	6.0	1.7
G. davidsonii	$D_{3\text{-}d}$	Yellow	Yellow	Yellow	Cordate	14	4.8	1.8
G. gossypioides	D_6	Cherry	Purple	Purple	Palmate	9	5.0	1.8
G. harknessii	$D_{2\text{-}2}$	Yellow	Amarlla	Yellow	Cordate	7	6.6	4.3
G. laxum	D_9	Cherry	Purple	Purple	Lobed	6	8.8	1.6
G. lobatum	D_7	Cherry	Purple	Purple	Lobed	8	10	1.8
G. schwendimanii	D_{11}	Cherry	Purple	Purple	Cordate	7	10	2.5
G. raimondii	D_5	Yellow	Purple	Purple	Cordate	12	7.0	3.6
G. thurberi	D_1	Yellow	White	Yellow	Palmate	14	3.3	1.6
G. trilobum	D_8	Yellow	Yellow	Yellow	Lobed - Palmate	12	4.0	1.2
G. turneri	D_{10}	Yellow	Yellow	Yellow	Cordate	10	3.8	1.8

Table 1. Averages of flowers and seed characteristics taken on some of the *Gossypium* species of the D genome established in the permanent nursery at Iguala, Guerrero Mexico.

Gossypium aridum(**D_4**), as formally reported, is the most widely distributed wild *Gossypium* in Mexico [5,9]. The distribution of this species, non-described taxa (one non-described taxon US-72, [8-11]), and described ecotypes [8-9,11] of the New World extends from the northern state of Sinaloa to the southern state of Oaxaca (Fig. 1). The species and taxa/ecotypes can be described as medium to large trees from five to 18 m tall or larger. As expected from its wide range, this *Gossypium* species occupies a number of habitat niches (http://www.lbk.ars.usda.gov/psgd/index-cotton.aspx). Comparisons among specimens of on-site observations indicate extensive differences in leaf size, vestiture of the leaves, morphology in the lysigenous glands on the capsules, and period of flowering. Morphologically, the leaves of the ecotype from Oaxaca are the largest of the species, with a relatively dense but fine indumentum. Several populations of *G. aridum* that appear to be very similar in morphology are distributed along the coastal foothills of Jalisco, Colima, Guerrero, and possibly Michoacán. Figure 2 presents an accessions of a population collected from recent exploration/collection trips [8-9]. The elevation of these populations range from <60 m up to >1000 m. Generally, these populations have almost no leaf trichomes, and small mature capsules (Table 1). Also, flowering in the states of Sinaloa, Nayarit and Jalisco is delayed until March and April in these types, and their capsules do not mature until late April-May (Fig. 2). While the Coastal populations in the states of Colima, Guerrero, and Oaxaca mature their capsules in February and March. Well-documented populations of collected *G. aridum* have now been made from several regions representing different non-described taxa and ecotypes [9]. These collections will continue to allow for *ex situ* preservation, maintenance and evaluation. This will also allow common-garden comparisons of all populations.

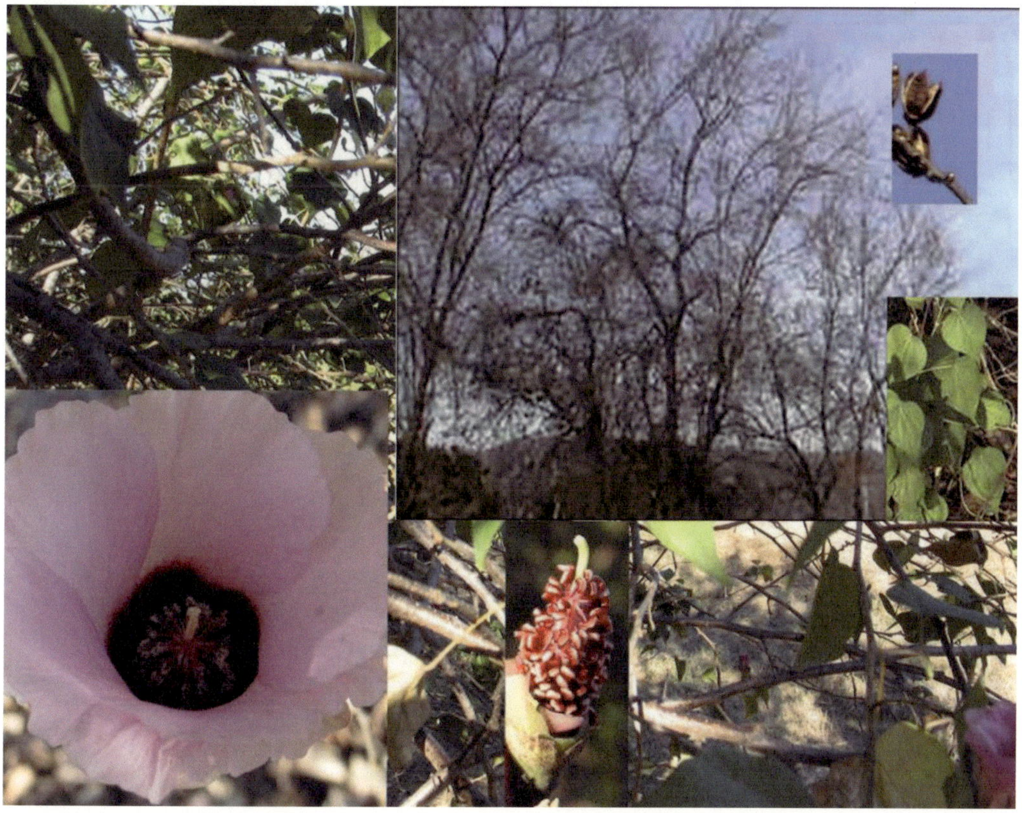

Figure 2. Habitat, trees, flower, capsule, and leaves of collected accessions of the *G. aridum* species.

For the most part, populations of *G. aridum* occur as a part of the native vegetation in deciduous woodlands. Different non-described taxa and ecotypes appear to thrive in areas where the woodland is disturbed, particularly along road banks where the canopy is opened. In the niches where they occur, some of these populations are usually found in abundance, although these locations may be separated by many kilometers. This species, as presently circumscribed, is very diverse (non-described taxa/ecotypes) and some of these populations do not appear to be threatened (Fig. 1).

Gossypium armourianum(**D_2**) is distributed from Baja California to the Gulf of California on the San Marcos Island (Fig. 1). This species can be described as a compact branched shrub of around one m tall. The species for the most part contains ovate leavesyellow flowers with withe filaments and cherry anthers. The seeds are contained in a capsule with three to four cells, and seeds averaging 6.0 x 1.7 mm with brownish tightly compressed fibers (Table 1; [12]).

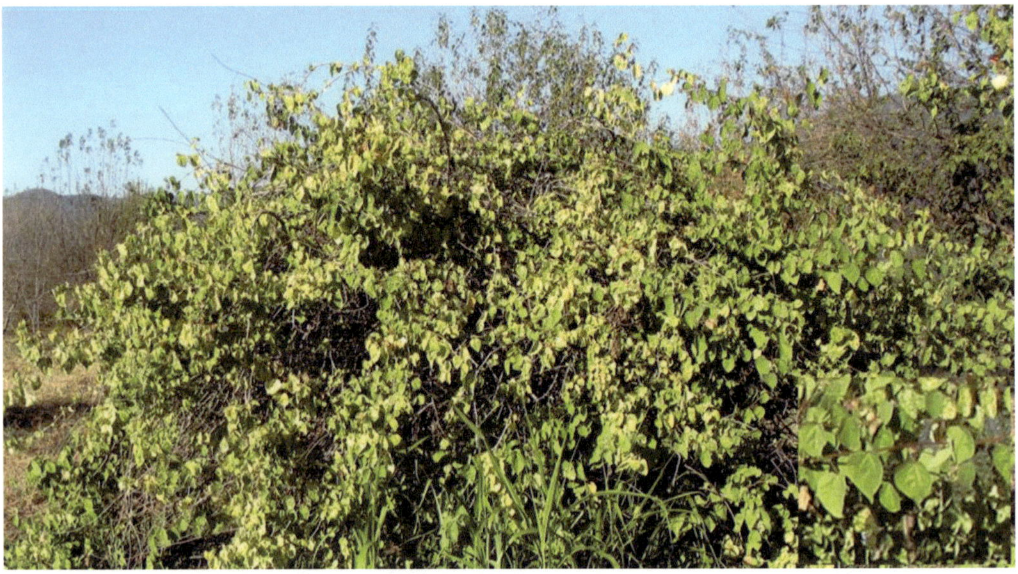

Figure 3. A two-year shrub of the species of *G. davidsonii*.

Gossypium davidsonii(**$D_{3\text{-}d}$**) is adapted to the desert environments of the southern Baja California peninsula and across the Gulf of California in the state of Sonora. This species is described as a branched shrub of one to two m tall and for the most part with cordate leaves. Figure 3 presents one of the accessions maintained at the Iguala nursery with cordate leaves. This species has flowers with yellow colored petals, filaments, and anthers. The seeds are contained in a capsule commonly with four cells and seeds averaging 4.8 x 1.8 mm with sparse compressed fibers (Table 1; [12]).

Gossypium gossypioides(**D_6**) is distributed in the central part of the state of Oaxaca and is adapted to a higher altitude than any other arborescent D *Gossypium* species, >1000 m. This species has been encountered only in the state of Oaxaca. It has been hypothesized that the distribution of *G. gossypioides* may be strongly influenced by elevation. One aspect of *G. gossypioides* that was recently reported is its deciduous habit as a drought escaping mechanism [8]. This species, like the other arborescent *Gossypium* species in the section *Erioxylum,* occurs in dry deciduous woodlands of Oaxaca and defoliates with the onset of the dry season. However, unlike the species of subsection *Erioxylum,* it flowers and fruits near the end of the wet season before defoliating. Fryxell [5] was unaware of the deciduous nature of the foliage similar to the other arborescent species of Mexico, which defoliated as a mechanism to escape drought. This species is comprised of small trees from three to seven m tall. Figure 4 presents one of the accessions (one year old) maintained at the Iguala nursery with flowers with light cherry color, and purple filaments and anthers. Also, this species as *G. raimondii* possess a unique petal mutation called reverse petal spot (pigment is present on adaxial and abaxial petal surfaces). *G. gossypioides* has been reported with cryptic repeated genomic recombination during speciation, with conflicting morphological, cytogenetic, and molecular evidence of its phylogenetic affinity to other New World cottons [13]. Figure 4 presents trees and mature capsules encountered at the natural habitat of this species. The seeds are contained in a capsule with three cells and seeds averaging 5.0 x 1.8 mm with grayish sparse compressed fibers (Table 1; [12]).

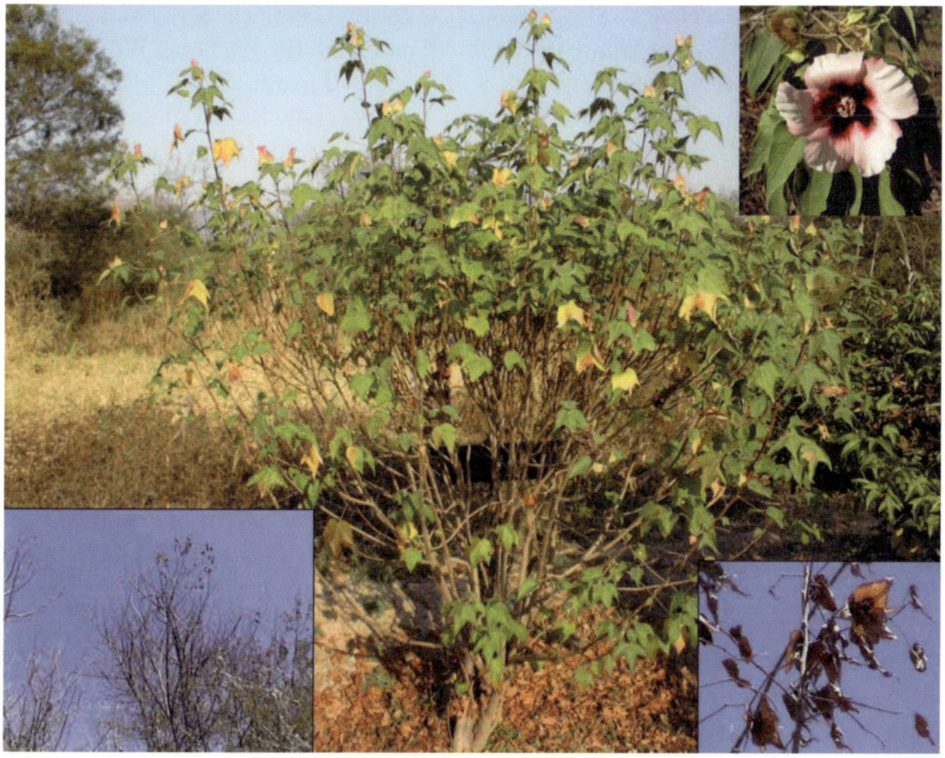

Figure 4. One year accession of the species *G. gossypioides* which was maintained at the Iguala Guerrero Mex. nursery with a flower, also, trees and mature capsules encountered at its natural habitat.

Gossypium harknessii(**$D_{2\text{-}2}$**) is adapted to the desert environments of Baja California in the Cape region and adjacent islands. This species is described as a shrub of around three m tall and for the most part with cordate leaves. Plants present flowers with yellow colored petals, filaments, and anthers. The seeds are contained in a capsule commonly with three-to four cells and seeds averaging 6.6 x 4.3 mm with grayish sparse compressed fibers (Table 1; [12]).

Gossypium klotzschianum(**$D_{3\text{-}k}$**) is one of the two species with disjointed distribution (not found in the country of Mexico) and is endemic to the Galápagos Islands. This species is described as a shrub up to four m tall and for the most part with petiolate-cordate leaves. Plants maintained at the Iguala nursery present flowers with yellow petals, filaments, and anthers.

The seeds are contained in a capsule commonly with four cells, ciliate on inner suture margins, and seeds averaging 5.0 x 2.5 mm with sparse inconspicuous fibers [12].

Gossypium laxum(**D_9**) is reported to be located in the Cañon del Zopilote in the central state of Guerrero, and, more recently, it was reported to be found in the state of Michoacan along the road between Huetamo and Nuevo Churumuco. The full range of *G. laxum* is yet to be determined, but it probably extends many kilometers along the Rio Balsas watershed east and west of Cañon del Zopilote. This taxon does well in areas of open sunlight, such as road cuts, like other members of subsection *Erioxylum*. However, it can also be found as part of natural deciduous woodland vegetation. Morphological diversity is not extensive among the accessions that have been collected so far. The collected accession (US-98, $D_{9\text{-}6\text{-}M}$, [9]) significantly extended the range of this species to the west. It is adapted to altitudes ranging from 200 to 900 m. Because some habitat sites of this species have generally been found not suitable for agriculture, *G. laxum* may be able to survive Mexico's demographic changes and does not seem to be threatened at present. This species is another arborescent *Gossypium* species of the subsection *Erioxylum* and comprises trees up to 10 m tall *in situ*. It flowers and produces fruits near the end of the wet season before defoliating. Plants of these populations present flowers with light cherry color, and purple filaments and anthers. US-98 accession presented flowers similar to *G. lobatum*. The seeds are contained in a capsule with three-to five-cells and seeds averaging 8.8 x 1.6 mm with densely pubescent fibers (Table 1; [12]).

Gossypium lobatum (D_7) is adapted to the environment of the central state of Michoacan. The collected accession (US-112, $D_{7\text{-}10\text{-}M}$, [9]) extended the range of this species to the west of the state. The distribution of this taxon is probably throughout the Rio Tepalcatepec watershed with an eastern extension along the Rio Balsas watershed. *G. lobatum* has unique features such as its distichous leaf insertion and tomentose calyces with prominent lobes, the characteristic from which its name is derived. While all accessions had distichous leaves, the calyces of the western accession-populations were less hairy and the lobes less prominent. It is unknown how much suitable habitat has already been destroyed. Overall the species does not appear to be threatened at present. It is adapted to altitude ranging from 200 to 400 m. This species is another arborescent *Gossypium* species of the subsection *Erioxylum* and comprises trees up to 10 m tall *in situ*. It flowers and fruits near the end of the wet season before defoliating. Plants of these populations present flowers with light cherry color, and purple filaments and anthers. The seeds are contained in a capsule with three-cells and seeds averaging 10.0 x 1.8 mm with densely pubescent fibers (Table 1; [2]).

Gossypium raimondii(**D_5**) is the other of the two D species that has disjointed distribution and is endemic to Peru. This species was originally described as a shrub two to three m tall. However, accessions planted at the Iguala nursery from seed provided by the USDA-ARS Cotton Germplasm Collection, College Station TX were able to produce shrub like trees up to 10 m tall. For the most part, accessions at the Iguala nursery present large cordate leaves, flowers with yellow petals, and purple filaments and anthers. The seeds are contained in a capsule commonly with four-cells, narrowly ovoid, and seeds averaging 7.0 x 3.6 mm with densely pubescent fibers [12]. *G. raimondii* is considered the closest living ancestor relative of the allotetraploid cottons (Dt subgenome) [4,12].

Gossypium schwendimanii **(D_{11})** is the most recently described *Gossypium* species of the D genome from Mexico [3,12]. This species was encountered for the first time at the Guerrero-Michoacán border near Infiernillo where a population of *G. aridum* was located only 2 km from "typical" *G. schwendimanii*. Collected accessions from this location showed some morphological features similar to *G. aridum* that suggested some introgression between the two species. Recently, *G. schwendimanii* [9] was collected from an area about 20 km south of *G. lobatum*. Seeds were collected from two additional populations of *G. schwendimanii* from the hills above the west side of Presa Infiernillo. Little morphological diversity was evident among the populations. The full natural distribution or native range of *G. schwendimanii* is unclear because of the limited information available on the species. One factor that has an impact on its genetic identity is its apparent sympatry with *G. aridum* and *G. lobatum* over parts of its range. It is adapted to altitude ranging from 200 to 400 m. This species is another arborescent *Gossypium* species of the subsection *Erioxylum* and comprises trees up to 10 m tall *in situ*. It flowers and produces fruits near the end of the wet season before defoliating. Plants of these populations present flowers with light cherry color, and purple filaments and anthers. The seeds are contained in a capsule with three-or four-cells and seed averaging 10.0 x 2.5 mm with densely pubescent fibers (Table 1; [9]).

Gossypium thurberi **(D_1)** is distributed from the state of Arizona, U.S.A to the state of Sonora, Mexico. This species can be described as a small tree or shrub of around 3 m tall. The species for the most part contains palmate leaves with flowers from white to yellow color, white filaments, and yellow anthers. The seeds are contained in a capsule with three-cells and seeds averaging 3.3 x 1.6 mm with blackish color and no fibers (Table 1; [12]).

Gossypium trilobum **(D_8)** is generally limited to moderately high elevations (1200 m) in western Mexico. This species belongs to section *Houzingenia* and is a sister species to *G. thurberi*, the most northerly (Sonora-Mex to Arizona-U.S.) distributed species of the *Gossypium*. Even though Fryxell [5] indicated that it was widely distributed from the state of Sinoloa to the state of Morelos, few if any collections have been made in the last 30 years in any of these locations. Based on the results of a survey made by Ulloa et al [8-9] special mention should be made of *G. trilobum*. In 2002-2004, sites were visited where herbarium specimens were collected in the past. In each of five widely separated locations represented by herbarium (MEXU) collections (sites in N and W México, Jalisco, Michoacán, and Morelos), *G. trilobum* plants or populations were unable to be located. Although the status of *G. trilobum* in remote areas is unknown, the results from the survey by Ulloa et al [8-9] confirmed that the distribution of this species has been severely eroded by agricultural and human-population pressures. For the most part, the habitat of this species has been replaced by intense and extensive agricultural production of guava (*Psidium* spp.) in the State of Michoacan, Mexico. At this point, *G. trilobum* species is almost extinct or is becoming extinct in the wild. This species can be described as a small tree or shrub of around 4 m tall. The species for the most part contains lobed-palmate leaves, and yellow flowers, filaments and anthers. The seeds are contained in a capsule with three-cells and seeds averaging 4.0 x 1.2 mm with blackish color and compressed pubescence (Table 1; [12]).

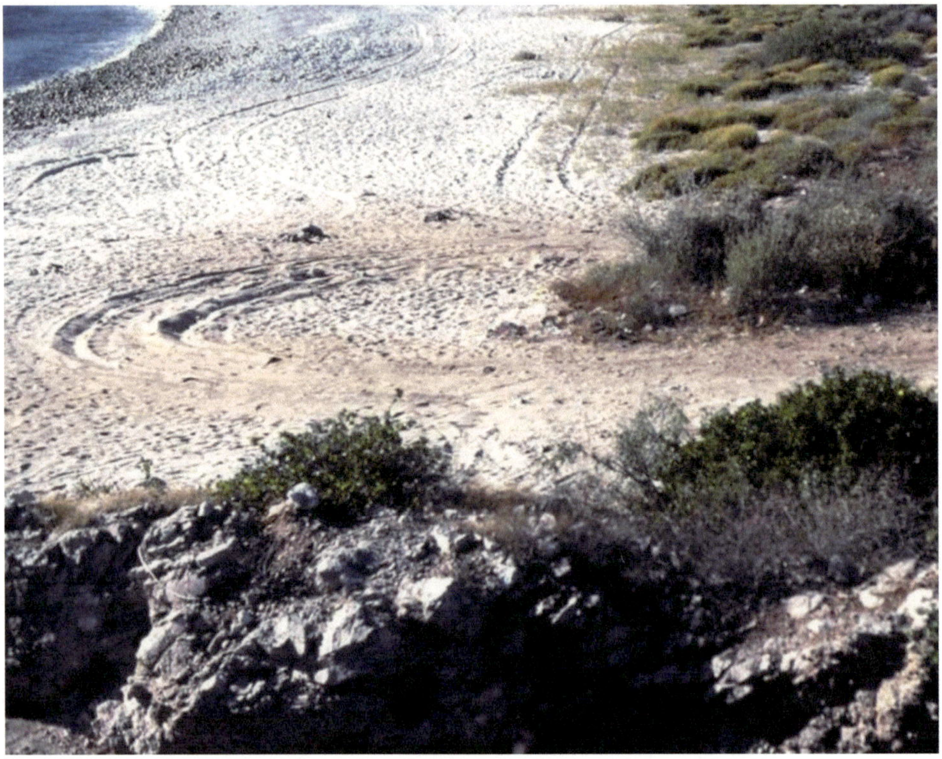

Figure 5. Shrubs of *G. turneri* in their natural habitat showing green vegetation after extended drought.

Gossypium turneri(**D_{10}**) is adapted to the coast of the state of Sonora Mpio. of Guaymas and primarily associated with soils of weathered igneous concentration (Fig. 1). On a long-term basis, *G. turneri* is well adapted to the sea-shore environments and sea level altitude in which it occurs. Based on a recent exploration (J.M. Stewart and M. Ulloa, 2004 expedition), the species has salt and drought resistance mechanisms that allow it to survive extended periods without rain. During this trip, the first *G. turneri* bush encountered was actually in the yard/sea-cliff. Although the species had a very small yield of seed the year when it was encountered because of drought, no evidence was seen of plants that died from the lack of water. Like most other *Gossypium,* in those areas where the species occurs, the plants are quite numerous. Unless unforeseen expansion of the resort industry occurs along the coastal region north of La Manga, the species habitat, in general, probably will not undergo rapid degradation. If resort construction should occur on the sea cliffs and adjoining valleys, then the species most likely would be lost in the wild. This species can be described as a shrub of around 1 m tall. Figure 5 presents shrubs in their natural habitat still showing green vegetation after extended drought. The species for the most part contains cordate leaves with yellow flowers, filaments and anthers. The seeds are contained in a capsule with three-to five-cells and seeds averaging 3.8 x 1.8 mm with blackish color and compressed pubescence (Table 1; [12]).

3. Collections/explorations and unclassified taxa

The gene pool of Upland/Acala *G. hirsutum* from the country of Mexico derived one of the primary sources for improvement of most of the Acala and Upland cotton growing in the world today. In addition, another cotton genetic resource of this country is the 11 formally reported D diploid *Gossypium* species and several unclassified taxa [8-11] of the Western Hemisphere. Mexico and its boundaries are the center of diversity of these endemic species. Some of these species and their genomes (US-72, D_4, D_7, D_9, D_{10}, and D_{11}) with arborescent or shrub growth habits express unique flowering and fruiting habits (following defoliation in the dry season) and salt and drought resistance mechanisms that allow them to survive extended periods without rain.

Because of the importance of the gene pool of *G. hirsutum* from Mexico, the collection/exploration trips of the D diploid species have been difficult to execute and document. Two of the greatest explorers and taxonomists of the *Gossypium* genus, and especially species from the country of Mexico, were Drs. Fryxell and Stewart. P.A. Fryxell made several collection-expeditions from 1968 to 1975 in the country, providing a larger number of specimens to several Herbariums (Herbarium Nacional de Mexico-MEXU and Herbarium Instituto de Ecologia A.C. Mexico-XAL) with clear and precise descriptions of habitat and location of collected accessions [5]. He also made the most recent taxonomic classification of *Gossypium* species [7]. A. E. Percival, J. M. Stewart (USDA), A. Hernandez and F. de Leon (INIFAP) made several collection-expeditions in 1984 throughout the states of the Yucatan Peninsula and in parts of the states of Tamaulipas, Veracruz, Tabasco, Oaxaca and Chiapas. Also, A. E. Percival (USDA-ARS), J. M. Stewart (Univ. of Arkansas), E.A. Garcia, and L. Peréz (INIFAP, Mexico) made additional collection-expeditions in 1990 in the state of Baja California Sur and parts of the states of Sonora and Sinaloa. As a result of their early efforts, a number of *Gossypium* accessions of the subgenus *Houzingenia* from various parts of Mexico were deposited in the USDA-ARS Cotton Germplasm Collection College Station, TX, USA. Also, during the 1980s, Dr. Lemeshev of the Academy of Science of Russia established a *Gossypium* nursery in Iguala City, state of Guerrero in the country of Mexico. Also, some or all of these species are catalogued in the germplasm collection of the Vavilov Institute in St. Petersburg and in several collections of Former Soviet Union countries (e.g., Uzbekistan) based on several collection-expeditions by the Universidad Autónoma de Guerrero Mexico and the Academy of Science of Russia in the states of Veracruz, Tabasco, Campeche, Yucatán, Chiapas, Guerrero, Oaxaca, Michoacán, Morelos, Colima, Sinaloa, Sonora and Baja California Sur between 1989 and 1993 by F. Talipov, C. Cataláio, F. Salgado and M. Bahena. This nursery was abandoned upon Dr. Lemeshev's return to Russia (Q. Obispo, personal communication; [8]).

Until recently no national resources were dedicated to the preservation of this natural treasure [8-9]. In 2002-2006, the United States Department of Agriculture – Agriculture Research Service (USDA-ARS) and the Mexican Instituto Nacional de Investigaciónes Forestales Agricolas y Pecuarias (INIFAP) sponsored joint *Gossypium* germplasm collection trips by U.S. and Mexican cotton scientists. As a result of these efforts, a significant number of *Gossypium* accessions of the subgenus *Houzingenia* from various parts of Mexico were collected (Table 2). Collected

No. of Accessions	Species	Genome	Entry ID
2	*G. hirsutum*	AD_1	TM-1 and Acala Maxxa
1	*G. barbadense*	AD_2	Pima 3-79
1	*G. tomentosum*	AD_3	G-tom
1	*G. mustelinum*	AD_4	G-must
1	*G. darwinii*	AD_5	G-darw
12	*G. herbaceum*	A_1	$A_{1\text{-}8\text{-}1}$, $A_{1\text{-}8\text{-}2}$, $A_{1\text{-}5}$, $A_{1\text{-}9}$, $A_{1\text{-}17}$, $A_{1\text{-}18}$, $A_{1\text{-}19}$, $A_{1\text{-}22}$, $A_{1\text{-}23}$, $A_{1\text{-}40}$, $A_{1\text{-}49}$, and $A_{1\text{-}52}$
11	*G. arboreum*	A_2	$A_{2\text{-}8}$, $A_{2\text{-}41}$, $A_{2\text{-}47}$, $A_{2\text{-}61}$, $A_{2\text{-}72}$, $A_{2\text{-}82}$, $A_{2\text{-}106}$, $A_{2\text{-}141}$, $A_{2\text{-}194}$, $A_{2\text{-}234}$, and $A_{2\text{-}241}$
7	*G. thurberi*	D_1	D_1, $D_{1\text{-}4}$, $D_{1\text{-}23}$,$D_{1\text{-}24}$, $D_{1\text{-}35}$, $D_{1\text{-}37}$, and $D_{1\text{-}35XD8\text{-}6}$
5	*G. armourianum*	D_2	$D_{2\text{-}1}$, $D_{2\text{-}2}$, $D_{2\text{-}q}$, $D_{2\text{-}w}$, and $D_{2\text{-}19XD2\text{-}17}$
5	*G. davidsonii*	D_3	$D_{3\text{-}1}$, $D_{3\text{-}2}$, $D_{3\text{-}23}$, $D_{3\text{-}26}$, and $D_{3\text{-}28}$
32	*G. aridum*	D_4	$D_{4\text{-}1\text{-}P}$ (US004), $D_{4\text{-}2\text{-}P}$ (US005), $D_{4\text{-}3\text{-}O}$ (US010), $D_{4\text{-}4\text{-}O}$ (US011), $D_{4\text{-}5\text{-}O}$ (US012), $D_{4\text{-}6\text{-}O}$ (US013), $D_{4\text{-}7\text{-}O}$ (US15), $D_{4\text{-}8\text{-}O}$ (US016), $D_{4\text{-}9\text{-}O}$ (US017), $D_{4\text{-}10\text{-}O}$ (US041), $D_{4\text{-}11\text{-}G}$ (US072), $D_{4\text{-}12\text{-}G}$ (US076), $D_{4\text{-}13\text{-}G}$ (US078), $D_{4\text{-}14\text{-}G}$ (US080), $D_{4\text{-}15\text{-}G}$ (US081), $D_{4\text{-}16\text{-}C}$ (US117), $D_{4\text{-}17\text{-}C}$ (US120), $D_{4\text{-}18\text{-}C}$ (US121), $D_{4\text{-}19\text{-}C}$ (US122), $D_{4\text{-}20\text{-}C}$ (US126), $D_{4\text{-}21\text{-}J}$ (US128), $D_{4\text{-}22\text{-}J}$ (US130), $D_{4\text{-}23\text{-}J}$ (US136), $D_{4\text{-}24\text{-}N}$ (US138), $D_{4\text{-}25\text{-}C}$ (D4-168a), $D_{4\text{-}26\text{-}C}$ (D4-168b), $D_{4\text{-}27\text{-}C}$ (D4-168c), $D_{4\text{-}28\text{-}N}$ (US147), $D_{4\text{-}29\text{-}N}$ (US148-a), $D_{4\text{-}30\text{-}N}$ (US148-b), $D_{4\text{-}31\text{-}N}$ (US149), and $D_{4\text{-}32\text{-}N}$ (US150)
3	*G. raimondii*	D_5	$D_{5\text{-}1}$, $D_{5\text{-}2}$, and $D_{5\text{-}3}$
2	*G. gossypioides*	D_6	$D_{6\text{-}1\text{-}O}$ (US043) and $D_{6\text{-}2\text{-}O}$ (US046)
10	*G. lobatum*	D_7	$D_{7\text{-}1\text{-}M}$ (US086), $D_{7\text{-}2\text{-}M}$ (US101), $D_{7\text{-}3\text{-}M}$ (US103), $D_{7\text{-}4\text{-}M}$ (US104), $D_{7\text{-}5\text{-}M}$ (US105), $D_{7\text{-}6\text{-}M}$ (US106), $D_{7\text{-}7\text{-}M}$ (US109), $D_{7\text{-}8\text{-}M}$ (US110), $D_{7\text{-}9\text{-}M}$ (US111), and $D_{7\text{-}10\text{-}M}$ (US112)
9	*G. trilobum*	D_8	$D_{8\text{-}1\text{-}M}$ (US160), $D_{8\text{-}2\text{-}M}$ (US162), $D_{8\text{-}3\text{-}M}$ (US163), $D_{8\text{-}A}$, $D_{8\text{-}B}$, $D_{8\text{-}1}$, $D_{8\text{-}6}$, $D_{8\text{-}10}$, and $D_{8\text{-}6XD1\text{-}35}$
5	*G. laxum*	D_9	$D_{9\text{-}1\text{-}G}$ (US065), $D_{9\text{-}2\text{-}G}$ (US066), $D_{9\text{-}4\text{-}G}$ (US068), $D_{9\text{-}5\text{-}G}$ (US070), and $D_{9\text{-}6\text{-}M}$ (US098)
1	*G. turneri*	D_{10}	$D_{10\text{-}1\text{-}S}$ (US156)
3	*G. shwendimanii*	D_{11}	$D_{11\text{-}1\text{-}M}$ (US083), $D_{11\text{-}2M}$ (US084), and $D_{11\text{-}3M}$ (US100)

[a]Letter at the end of the Entry ID indicating the state where the accession was collected: C=colima, G=Guerrero, J=Jalisco, N=Nayarit, M=Michoacan, O=Oaxaca, P = Puebla , and S = Sonora ecotypes. This table was published in the following article: Ulloa M, Abdurakhmonov IY, Perez-M C, Percy R, Stewart McDJ. Genetic diversity and population structure of cotton (*Gossypium* spp.) of the New World assessed by SSR markers. Botany 2013;91 251-259. License agreement was provided by the NRC Research Press – Copyright Clearance Center.

Table 2. Summary of the 111 accessions used to investigate genetic diversity and population structure of the New World cottons (*Gossypium* spp.).

http://dx.doi.org/10.5772/58387

accessions were placed in a nursery or botanical garden in Iguala, Guerrero, Mexico, including several accessions of each of the arborescent species for ex *situ* conservation. Today, Mexico maintains this *Gossypium* nursery in Iguala, Guerrero (C. Perez-Mendoza. *personal communication*). Since the first collection-expedition trips were made, the *in situ* survival of these diploid species has been threatened by increasing human population, modernization of agriculture and urbanization. If *in situ* diversity of the Mexican cottons is severely eroded, then current and additional accessions in all the germplasm collections all over the world and the USDA Cotton Germplasm Collection assume a highly significant role in the preservation of the diversity previously residing in Mexico's dooryard (*G. hirsutum*) and cotton species of the D genome.

As formally reported, *G. aridum* is the most widely distributed wild *Gossypium* species in Mexico [5,7]. However, recent additional collections (http://www.lbk.ars.usda.gov/psgd/index-cotton.aspx) and several studies [8-11] have reported and suggested non-described taxa and ecotypes that can be considered separate species. Morphological comparisons among specimens of on-site observations indicate extensive differences in leaf size, vestiture of the leaves, morphology in the lysigenous glands on the capsules, and period of flowering. Molecular comparisons have provided useful information in the geographical, taxonomical distribution, and evolutionary history of the New World D genome-species. Based on molecular data (see additional information in the section below), in addition to previously D_{4-11-G}, US-072 reported new taxon, five new collected accessions [D_{4-10-O} (US-41), D_{4-2-P} (US-05), D_{4-12-G} (US-76), D_{4-19-C} (US-122), and D_{4-32-N} (US-150)] from five different geographical sites (ecotypes) from the states of Oaxaca, Puebla, Guerrero, Colima, and Nayarit may be recognized as new species [8-9]. Subsequent observations on greenhouse plants and a return visit to the sites when the plants are beginning to flower will taxonomically confirm that these populations represent undescribed taxa (new species) belonging to subsection *Erioxylum*.

4. Molecular characterization of the D genomes

When traditional taxonomy based on morphology (plant canopy, plant height, leaf and capsule shapes, flowers and petal spots, seed size, etc) do not distinguish two species with intermediate phenotypes, molecular methods provide an alternative solution of resolving these not well defined morphological differences between two species [9,14-15]. Molecular markers such as amplified fragment-length polymorphism (AFLP) [10-11] and microsatellites or simple sequence repeats (SSR) have been used to reveal genetic diversity and to distinguish not well defined differences between species or wild relatives [9]. Molecular marker-gene methods have also been used, for example: internal transcribed spacer (ITS) of ribosomal DNA or ribosomal DNA fragment gene-comparisons [16-18], and fragments of chloroplast DNA [19], or repetitive DNA [20-22]. In addition, a few loci of the *Adh* gene [19,23-25], *FAD*2-1 gene [26], and *Ces A1* gene [27] provided insight into the characterization of the *Gossypium* species. Moreover, the phylogeny of the New World diploid *Gossypium* was analyzed based on three independent single-copy genes (*A1341, AdhC,* and *CesA1b*) [28]. These genes were used in previous studies [22-23], showing a high ratio of phylogenetical informative fragment data.

Even though phylogenetic relationships with these three single-copy genes among species of the D genome still remain unclear, the molecular data supported the recognition of a new D species (US-72) closely related to *G. laxum* [28]. Similar observations were obtained when molecular diversity and phylogenetic relationships were examined among 33 accessions of arborescent *Gossypium* including 23 of *G. aridum* with Random Amplified Polymorphic DNA (RAPD) and AFLP fragments [11].

In 2013 Ulloa et al [9] reported a study of genetic diversity and population structure of cottons (*Gossypium* spp.) of the New World (Table 2). In this study, the genetic diversity and population structure of 111 cotton accessions of *Gossypium* were assessed with SSR markers with wide genome coverage. The species represented five allotetraploids ($AD_1 - AD_5$ genomes), 23 Asiatic diploids of the Old World (A_1 and A_2 genomes), and 82 diploids of the New World subgenus *Houzingenia* ($D_1 - D_{11}$ genomes) species (Table 2).

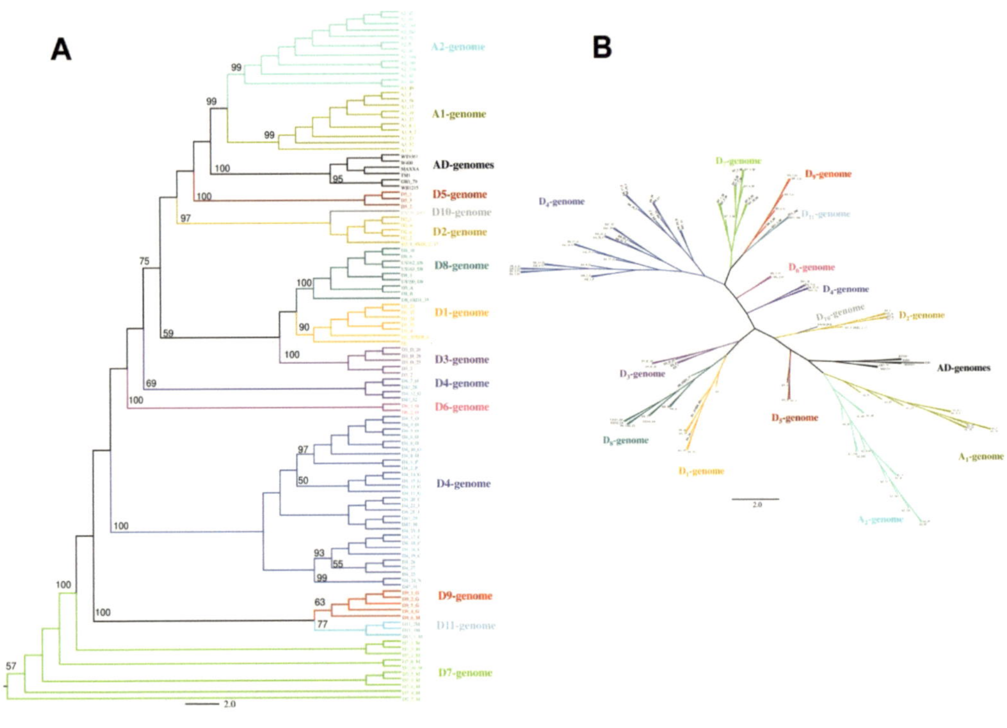

Figure 6. A) Phylogenetic neighbor-joining dendrogram arbitrarily rooted of 111 *Gossypium* accessions representing five allotetraploids ($AD_1 - AD_5$ genomes), 23 Asiatic diploids of the Old World (A_1 and A_2 genomes), and 82 diploids of the New World subgenus *Houzingenia* ($D_1 - D_{11}$ genomes). Phylogenetic tree developed based upon the proportion of alleles between accessions and B) Unrooted neighbor-joining dendrogram of the 111 *Gossypium* accessions. Branch lengths are shown with bootstrap values. Groups of cotton species and accessions specific to each ecotype are color-coded for simplicity. This figure was published in the following article: Ulloa M, Abdurakhmonov IY, Perez-M C, Percy R, Stewart McDJ. Genetic diversity and population structure of cotton (*Gossypium* spp.) of the New World assessed by SSR markers. Botany 2013;91 251-259. License agreement was provided by the NRC Research Press – Copyright Clearance Center.

The phylogenetic analysis grouped all species into distinct phylogenetic groups consistent with genomic origin (Fig. 6). Based on the Wright's F_{ST} index using AMOVA analyses [9] of the data sets for all-genomes and the diploid New World D-genomes accessions, the differentiation among the population groups of the different species was highly significant ($P \leq 0.0001$). A great deal of total genetic variance was attributed to the difference among and within groups, especially within the *G. aridum* population-groups or ecotypes (Table 2 and Fig. 6) [9]. The analysis clustered the diploids of the New World into six sections with the three bushy types [(*Houzingenia* (D_1 and D_8), *Integrifolia* ($D_{3\text{-d}}$), and *Caducibracteolata* ($D_{2\text{-}1}$, $D_{2\text{-}2}$, and D_{10})] and three arborescent types [*Erioxylum* (US-72, D_4, D_7, D_9, and D_{11}), *Selera* (D_6), and *Austroamericana* (D_5)]. The classification of the formally reported subgenus and species boundaries are well-understood [5,7]. These results are in agreement with other molecular studies [23-25,28]. Also, the statistical analysis of s*tructure* test was used in this study [through measurements of *ad hoc* (ΔK) quantity of Evanno statistics] to identify real number of K populations for the germplasm accessions (Table 2). The population structure analysis on this study shed light on the emergence and dispersion of the diploids of the New World and agreed with the hypothesis of a rapid radiation of the American diploid cotton linage that took place somewhere in southwestern Mexico, followed by a differentiation-speciation [9,23-25,28]. This radiation might have occurred before the separation of the Baja California peninsula (7-12 million years ago) from the mainland of the country of Mexico [9,28]. The population structure analyses [9] indicated that Baja California peninsula was colonized from two independent lineages, one from the subsection *Intergrifolia* (Q1, D_3-accessions) and the second from the subsection *Caducibracteata* (Q2, D_2-accessions) (Fig. 7). These two species (*G. harknessii*-D_2-accessions and *G. davidsonii*-D_3-accessions) are clearly distinguished by many morphological features: leaves, flowers, seed capsule, pubescence, etc.

The population structure analyses [9] with the geographic distribution and morphology of some of these species also supports the hypothesis that the New World D diploid species may derive from five major lineages (Q1-Q5) that eventually radiated and differentiated about 7-8 million years ago through the country of Mexico. Some species [*G. gossypioides* (D_6 genome), *G. laxum* (D_9 genome), *G. turneri* (D_{10} genome), and *G. schwendimanii* (D_{11} genome)] experienced a more recent differentiation event (Fig 7B). Interspecific gene flow has been recognized as an important evolutionary event in plants. It has also been suggested that improbable interspecific introgression and molecular differentiation may have occurred more often than predicted in angiosperm evolution [9-10,28]. Supra-specific coalescence of some alleles in these species may support the mixed sample-group of the D genome accessions (D_4, D_6, D_9, D_{10}, and D_{11}), experiencing more recent hybridization events.

The phylogenetic analysis grouped all species into distinct phylogenetic groups of the New World cottons (Fig. 8), consistent with genomic origin and classified species of the *Houzingenia* subgenus with the six subsections: subsection *Austroamericana* [*G. raimondii* (D_5)]; subsection *Caducibracteolata* [*G. armourianum* ($D_{2\text{-}1}$), *G. harknessii* ($D_{2\text{-}2}$), and *G. turneri* (D_{10})]; subsection *Houzingenia* [*G. thurberi* (D_1) and *G. trilobum* (D_8)]; subsection *Integrifolia* [*G. davidsonii* ($D_{3\text{-d}}$)]; subsection *Erioxylum* [*G. aridum* (D_4), *G. lobatum* (D_7), *G. laxum* (D_9), and *G. schwendimanii* (D_{11})]; and subsection *Selera* [*G. gossypioides* (D_6)] [3,4,7]. In addition, several non-described taxa of

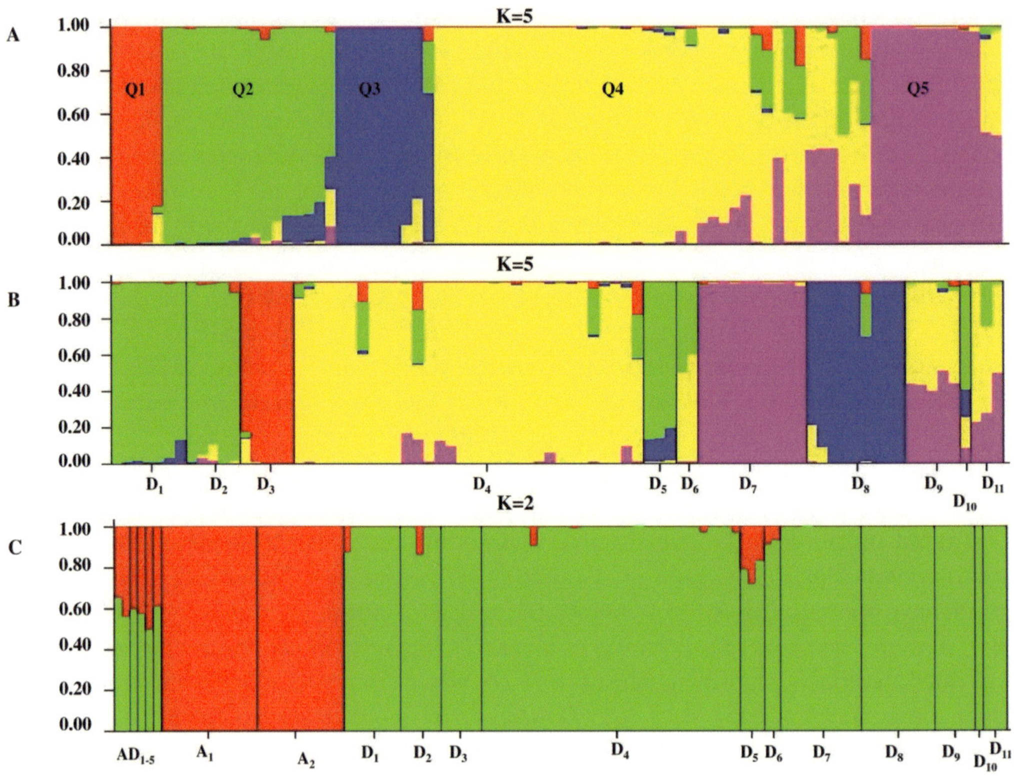

Figure 7. Population structure of cotton (*Gossypium* spp.) accessions: (A) Eighty-two D-genome cotton accessions (D_1 – D_{11}) population structure plots at K=5 grouped by Q-matrix, (B) grouped by genomic origins of the D-genome accessions, and C) 111 *Gossypium* accessions representing five allotetraploids (AD_1 – AD_5 genomes), 23 Asiatic diploids of the Old World (A_1 and A_2 genomes), and 82 diploids of the New World subgenus *Houzingenia* (D_1 – D_{11} genomes)-All-genome cotton accessions population structure plot at K=2, where Q1 (red) represents diploid A-genome accessions (A_1 and A_2), Q2 (green) represent diploid D-genomes (D_1 – D_{11}), and red and green represents the amalgamation of the tetraploid AD genomes (AD_1 – AD_5). This figure was published in the following article: Ulloa M, Abdurakhmonov IY, Perez-M C, Percy R, Stewart McDJ. Genetic diversity and population structure of cotton (*Gossypium* spp.) of the New World assessed by SSR markers. Botany 2013; 91 251-259. License agreement was provided by the NRC Research Press – Copyright Clearance Center.

the New World diploid *G. aridum* species were found to be distanced from their groups or ecotypes from the states of Nayarit, Guerrero, and Oaxaca (Fig. 8). As mentioned before, *G. gossypioides* has been reported with cryptic repeated genomic recombination during speciation, with conflicting morphological, cytogenetic, and molecular evidence of its phylogenetic affinity to other New World cottons [13]. It has been proposed that *G. gossypioides* might hybridize with an African A-genome and/or extinct taxon based on transfer of repetitive DNA [13]. In the neighbor-joining method, trees are constructed by linking together the two operational taxonomic units or in other words – leaves of the tree, or hypothetical taxonomic units that are the closest mutual "neighbors" [29-30]. The phylogenetic resolution of *G. gossypioides* has been found to be inconsistent because this species has been placed within the New World cotton of the D genome in a basal clade-position of the phylogenetic tree rather

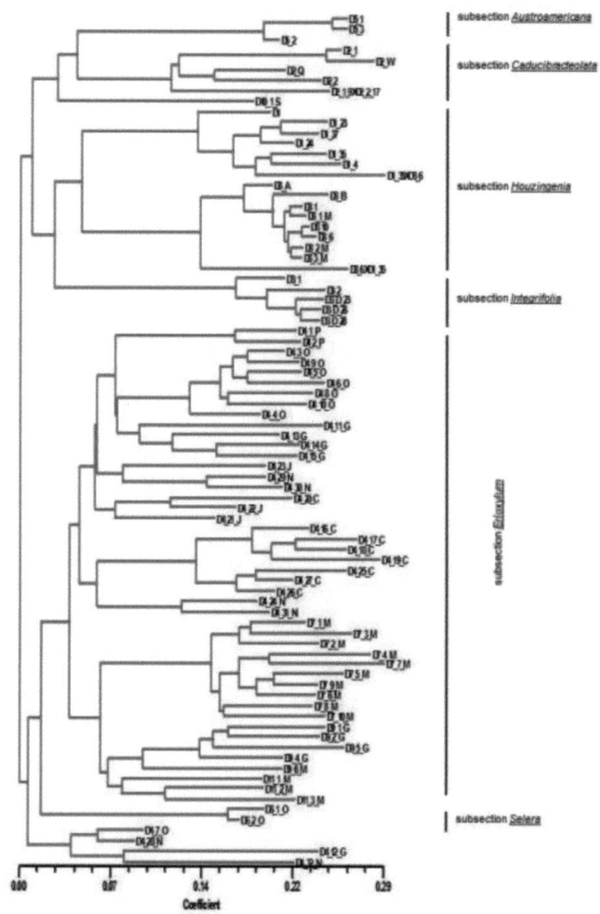

Figure 8. A) Phylogenetic neighbor-joining dendrogram using the midpoint rooted of the 82 diploids of the New World subgenus *Houzingenia* (D_1 – D_{11} genomes). Phylogenetic tree developed based upon the proportion of alleles between accessions.

than in the same clade with the previously proposed sister, *G. raimondii* [13]. This proposed relationship between these two species was based on phylogentic studies with chloroplast (cpDNA) genes. In Figure 8, *G. gossypioides* has been placed at the basal clade-position of the arborescent subsection *Erioxylum* while *G. raimondii* subsection *Austroamericana* shared a clade-position with species of the *Caducibracteolata* subsection. The clade-position of these two species may indicate two divergent evolutionary events through introgression or hybridization.

The arborescent subsection *Erioxylum* is among the most distinctive in the genus [31]. However, the sectional-levels of *G. aridum*, as formally reported [5-8], still remain unresolved. SSR markers have proved to be a powerful tool in elucidating genetic relationships and population structure of these accessions [9]. A proposed genetic distance (GD) minimum threshold of 0.20 [9] may be useful to define a new taxon, and a clear relationship among cotton species or genetically distant geographical accession-ecotypes of *G. aridum*. In addition to US-72 (newly identified taxon) [10,27], five newly collected accessions [$D_{4\text{-}10\text{-}O}$ (US-41), $D_{4\text{-}2\text{-}P}$ (US-05), $D_{4\text{-}12\text{-}G}$ (US-76), $D_{4\text{-}19\text{-}C}$ (US-122), and $D_{4\text{-}32\text{-}N}$ (US-150)] from five different ecotypes and states from the country of Mexico were proposed by Ulloa et al [9] to be recognized as new species based on GD. These collected accessions had the larger GD when compared with any other recognized *Gossypium* species of the D genome, GD > 0.28 and GD ≤ 0.41 [9]. Based on the most recent explorations/collections in the country of Mexico [8-9], the existing taxonomic classification of *Gossypium* of the D_4 diploid species made by Fryxell [31] and Fryxell et al [7] needs to be revised.

5. Evolution and review of beneficial genes of the D genomes

The evolution of the *Gossypium* genus started around 10-20 million years ago [32-33]. The initial step of this process might be started with the formation or origin of the American diploids or New World cottons, which may be estimated at around 6.7 million years ago. Following the formation of the diploid cottons was the allopolyploid formation that derived the New World tetraploid cottons around 1-2 million years ago [34], which included *G. hirsutum* and *G. barbadense* cottons. The origin of the allotetraploids is still not well understood. However, it is well established that the allotetraploids combine one genome derived from an A-genome ancestor and a second genome from a D-genome ancestor [9,33-36]. There is no evidence of any A-genome species in the New World, and there is no evidence of any D-genome species outside the New World. There has been considerable speculation over the years as to which D-genome species is the closest living relative of the ancestor of the Dt subgenome of the allotetraploid cottons. Based on molecular data, the best species model of the allotetraploid (AD) Dt subgenome is *G. raimondii*. However, recent discoveries through molecular data also revealed that *G. gossypioides* may be closer than originally thought to *G. raimondii* despite the geographical separation of these two species based on chloroplast (cpDNA) genes [13]. In terms of haploid nuclear DNA content or amounts (1C) the *Gossypium* genomes range from 1 to 3.8 pg=picograms (980 Mbp to 3425 Mbp). The D model genome is smaller with 2C amounts of 1 pg and a haploid length of 980 Mbp while the A-genome diploid nuclear genome contains about 3.8 pg of DNA (2C) and the length of a single copy of the genome is approximately 1860 Mbp. The genome size in the AD tetraploids for the most part is additive with 5.8 pg (2C) and with a haploid length of 3835 Mbp [35,37-40].

As previously established, each genomic designation (A, B, C, D...etc.) represents a functional group of chromosomes that share similar sizes and structures, as well as success of interspecific crosses. These designations also help breeders to find sources of genetic variability for the introgression of beneficial genes into elite cultivars and to determine rates of success of the introgression of these beneficial genes. Within the same designed genome, hybrid chromosomes recombine during meiosis and tend to be fertile. However, crosses made using genomes with different designation with similar basic chromosome number; hybrids are generally infertile with few stable bivalents at meiosis [39]. Breeders first turn to sources of genetic variability in the primary germplasm pool or within the same species, which includes wild or exotic and landrace germplasm of *G. hirsutum* and *G. barbadense* species. The elite public and private cultivars [*G. hirsutum* (Upland) and *G. barbadense* (Pima)] of these species contain a number of traits that originated in the primary germplasm pool e.g., the blight resistance genes [35], the nectariless trait from *G. tomentosum* [41], root-knot nematode resistance from landraces [42-43], resistance to Fusarium (*Fusarium oxysporum* f.sp. *vasinfectum* Atk. Sny & Hans) and Verticillium (*Verticillium dahlia* Kleb) wilt from landraces of *G. hirsutum* and from *G. darwinii* [44].

The diploid species of the A and D genome belong to the secondary germplasm pool and have contributed to improving Upland and Pima cultivars [4]. Bacterial blight resistance genes from species such as *G. arboreum*, *G. herbaceum* and *G. anomalum* have been introgressed into Upland cultivars [35]. Cytoplasm and restorer factors from *G. harknessii* [45] and *G. trilobum* [46] conditioning cytoplasmic male sterility, and D2 smoothness [47] have also been introgressed into Upland cultivars using these diploid species. Moreover, improvement of fiber quality characteristics or properties has been done via the triple hybrid (*G. hirsutum* x *G. arboreum* x *G. thurberi*) [48]. Introgression of high fiber strength and improvement of fiber quality parameters were obtained using progeny from these hybrid combinations. In addition, similar triple hybrid combinations that include *G. thurberi* [49] and *G. aridum* [50] have provided progeny that have been used to develop resistant germplasm and cultivars to root-knot nematode (*rkn*, *Meloidogyne incognita* Kofoid and White) and reniform nematode (Ren^{ari}, *Rotylenchulus reniformis* Linford and Oliveira). Resistance to several pests and diseases has been found in diploid cottons. However, in nature, the hybridization of diploid species with allotetraploid (Upland or Pima) species produces sterile hybrids because uneven genome or chromosome basic number and pairing during meiosis. One of the satisfactory mutagenic agents used by the breeders to induce doubling of chromosomes and balance chromosome paring on hybrids is colchicine. The difficulties of obtaining agronomically suitable introgressed progeny are high through this type of interspecific hybridization. The most successful method of introgression has been via hexaploid bridging.

Even though the *Gossypium* species of the D genome are not well known and utilized in cotton improvement and breeding, their significance as great reservoirs of important genes is starting to be noticed and documented. In a comparison quantitative trait loci (QTL) review-study [4], the Dt subgenome exhibits from 32% [4,51] to 57% [52] of QTLs on different chromosomes with QTL effects on different important traits for cotton improvements. These QTLs were located on different chromosomes of the Dt subgenome. And even though the species of the D genome does not produce spinnable fibers, the Dt subgenome of the tetraploid cotton was found to possess QTLs positively affecting fiber quality and morphological traits [53-55] and therefore harboring greater allelic diversity among tetraploid forms. Recently, based on the concept that some diploid species are tolerant to stress and may harbor important genes, a large number of genes were obtained from leaf and root tissues of the diploid *G. aridum* species. Plants of this species were subjected to various salt stresses to examine gene expression and to understand the salt tolerance mechanisms in *Gossypium* [56]. Most of the salt-regulated transcripts were found to be homologous to genes that are known to be associated with salt tolerance e.g., ethylene-responsive transcript factor, aquaporin PIP1, protein kinases (CBL-interacting and mitogen-activated) [56]. New transcriptome data from these plant tissue-species when eventually compared with available marker-QTL DNA sequence data and/or whole genome sequences will provide new insights into the evolution and expression of genes affecting important traits of cotton. QTL hotspots have been found affecting multiple fiber traits [32,51,57]. DNA sequences of marker-QTLs were found to be contributed by the D genome based on changes in expression of functionally diverse cotton genes [29]. Additional studies using the next generation sequencing (NGS) technology will provide additional information on these unique flowering and fruiting habits (following defoliation in the dry season), and salt and drought resistance mechanisms that allow the D genome species to survive extended periods without rain or stress conditions.

6. Future research of gene discovery and mining of the D genomes

The most widely cultivated cotton species in the world, which is known by various common names (e.g., Acala or Upland cotton, short staple cotton, Mocó cotton, and Cambodia cotton) is *G. hirsutum* [4-5,8,12]. Recent advances in genomics have provided considerable information regarding the discovery and expression of genes controlling important crop traits. In the future, the new generation of cotton breeders will have the opportunity to benefit from the vast information generated by NGS on genomic research. This information could be used to improve existing tools such as MAS for molecular breeding or to develop new tools to locate and characterize germplasm and cultivars or gene-sequences of DNA encoding proteins that controlled their expression of important traits, developmentally and temporally.

With the decrease in sequencing cost by NGS technology, it has been possible to obtain large numbers of base pairs of DNA sequences for identifying polymorphisms and directly mapping genes responsible for important traits through direct whole genome sequencing [58-59]. Molecular markers are being continuously developed, which will allow cotton geneticists to sample all regions of the cotton genome [4,9,32,60-61]. Plant breeders find molecular markers useful as a selection tool in monitoring alien genome introgression in cotton breeding programs [62-63]. Alien genome has the potential to increase genetic variability for economically valuable traits in cotton cultivars. The process of introgression of alien genes/genomes is not easy but clearly increases the amount of genetic diversity available for selection because it is likely that many useful alleles are to be found outside the current cultivated gene pools. Even when the inferred gene is yet to be located, sequenced, and characterized, molecular breeders could use these natural DNA sequence (SNP – single nucleotide polymorphism) to identify differences among germplasm and breeding lines, and applying traditional genetic analyses to infer genes for MAS. In addition, the efficacy of transgenic technology is entirely dependent on gene discovery. The functional genes identified with NGS would be important resources to improve the cotton crop through transgenic technology.

The understanding of the cotton genome is complex, especially the evolution and function of the major cultivated species, e.g., *G. hirsutum*. This complexity arises from the joint presence of the two subgenomes (At and Dt) in its nucleus [60]. The complete sequence of the allotetraploid genomes, including *G. hirsutum*, is still not completed. However, recently the genome sequence of the best model of the Dt subgenome *(G. raimondii)* was published [32,61]. *G. raimondii* was found to be 47% (around 350 Mb) of euchromatin, spanning 2,059 centiMorgan (cM) and 53% (around 390 Mb) of heterochromatin, spanning a repeat-rich of 186 cM. Transposable-elements accounted for 61% in which 53% were long-terminal-repeats (LTRs) retrotransposons. It was reported that the *G. raimondii* genome contains around 37, 505 assembled genes with 77,267 protein-coding annotated transcripts [31].

Increasing our knowledge and understanding of how cotton (*Gossypium* spp.) can sustain yield under drought and attack of pathogens is essential for sustained profitability and long-term survival of the cotton industry. Researchers and breeders are working to develop sources of germplasm that can improve water use efficiency (WUE), drought and extreme heat tolerance. An emergent concept from genomic studies is that different regulatory networks related to plant stress may be interconnected. For example, in most situations heat stress and drought stress are thought to be linked, and often resistance to pathogens is comprised by abiotic stress factors [64]. Improving cotton productivity in stress environments calls for the understanding of many traits involved in different system-level interactions. The integration of these plant responses and interactions with quantitative phenotypes is complex and requires the use of new approaches and technologies. These new NGS data and analyses will provide new information about the utility of the newly published *G. raimondii* genome sequence to target traits of interest in the allopolyploid species. When new NGS data of the future sequenced genomes and the genome saturation get combined with quantitative genetic analyses, cotton breeders finally will have the tools they need to identify the location of the genes (quantitative trait loci or QTLs) conditioning the expression of critical agronomic traits, such as yield, drought tolerance and water use efficiency [65-66]. If *in situ* diversity of the New World cottons is severely eroded, then current and additional accessions in International Collections and in the USDA Cotton Germplasm Collection assume a highly significant role in preservation of the diversity previously residing in these D genome species. The key to increasing genetic diversity among cultivated cottons is to continue collecting, evaluating and utilizing many different cotton germplasm, including diploid species of the *Gossypium* genus. The diploid D genome cottons (*Gossypium* spp.) of the New World are part of a great reservoir of important genes for improving fiber quality, pest and disease resistance, and drought and salt tolerance in the modern cultivated Upland/Acala (*G. hirsutum*) and Pima or Sea Island (*G. barbadense*) cottons.

Acknowledgements

In memory of Dr. James McD. Stewart. The author would like to thank Zack Quaintance, and Jazmine and Rebecca Ulloa for their time and efforts in helping to improve this chapter. The research contribution by the author of some of the information in this chapter was partially supported by a specific cooperative agreement between USDA-ARS and the Mexican agency INIFAP (ARIS Log Nos. 5303-21220-001-10S and 5303-2-F159). Mention of trade names or commercial products in this article is solely for the purpose of providing specific information and does not imply recommendation or endorsement by the U. S. Department of Agriculture. The U. S. Department of Agriculture is an equal opportunity provider and employer.

Author details

Mauricio Ulloa*

Address all correspondence to: Mauricio.Ulloa@ars.usda.gov

USDA-ARS, SPA, Cropping Systems Research Laboratory, Plant Stress and Germplasm Development, Lubbock, TX, USA

References

[1] Abdurakhmonov IY, Buriev ZT, Shermatov SE, Abdullaev AA, Urmonov K, Kushanov F, Egamberdiev SS, Shapulatov U, Abdukarimov A, Saha S, Jenkins JN, Kohel RJ, Yu JZ, Pepper AE, Kumpatala S, Ulloa M. Genetic diversity in *Gossypium* genus. In: Çalişkan M.(ed.) Genetic Diversity in Plants. New York, NY: InTech; 2012; p313-338.

[2] Fryxell PA. A revised taxonomic interpretation of *Gossypium* L. (Malvaceae). Rheedea 1992;2 108-165.

[3] Percival AE, Wendel JF, Stewart JM. Taxonomy and Germplasm Resources. In: Smith CW and Cothren JT (eds.) Cotton: Origin, history, technology, and production. New York: John Wiley & Sons; 1999; p. 33-64.

[4] Ulloa M, Brubaker C, Chee P. Cotton. In: Kole C. (ed.) Genome Mapping & Molecular Breeding. Vol. 6: Technical Crops. Heidelberg, Berlin, New York, Tokyo: Springer; 2007; p1-49.

[5] Fryxell PA. The Natural History of the Cotton Tribe. College Station and London: Texas A&M University Press; 1979.

[6] Kantartzi SK, Ulloa M, Sacks E, Stewart JM. Assessing Genetic Diversity in *Gossypium arboreum* L. Cultivars using Genomic and EST-derived Microsatellites. Genetica 2009; 136:141-147.

[7] Fryxell PA, Craven LA, Stewart JM. A revision of *Gossypium* sect.*Grandicalyx* (Malvaceae), including the description of six new species. Systematic Botany. 1992; 17:91-114.

[8] Ulloa, M, Stewart JM, Garcia-C EA, Godoy-A A, Gaytán-M A, Acosta-N S. Cotton genetic resources in the western states of Mexico: in situ conservation status and germplasm collection for ex situ preservation. Genet. Resour. Crop Evol; 2006. 53: 653-668.

[9] Ulloa M, Abdurakhmonov IY, Perez-M C, Percy R, Stewart McDJ. Genetic diversity and population structure of cotton (*Gossypium* spp.) of the New World assessed by SSR markers. Botany 2013; 91:251-259.

[10] Alvarez I, Wendel JF. Cryptic interspecific introgression and genetic differentiation within *Gossypium aridum* (Malvaceae) and its relatives. Evolution 2006; 60:505-517.

[11] Feng C, Ulloa M, Perez-M C, Stewart, JM. Distribution and molecular diversity of arborescent *Gossypium* species. Botany; 2011; 89:615-624

[12] Fryxell PA, Taxonomy and Germplasm Resources, In: Kohel RJ and Lewis CF (eds) Cotton. Agronomy No. 24, ASA, CSSA & SSSA. 1984; p. 27-58.

[13] Cronn RC, Small RL, Haselkorn T, Wendel JF. Duplicated genes evolve independently after polyploid formation in cotton. 2003; Evolution: 2475-2489.

[14] Ram SG, Thiruvengadam V, Vinod KK. Genetic diversity among cultivars, landraces and wild relatives of rice as revealed by microsatellite markers. J. Appl. Genet. 2007; 48:337-345.

[15] Vigouroux Y, Glaubitz JC, Matsuoka Y, Goodman MM, Sanchez GJ, Doebley J. Population structure and genetic diversity of New World maize races assessed by DNA microsatellites. Am. J. Bot. 2008; 95:1240-1253.

[16] Wendel JF, Schnabel A, Seelanan T. An unusual ribosomal DNA sequence from *Gossypium gossypioides* reveals ancient, cryptic intergenomic introgression. Mol. Phylogen. Evol. 1995; 4:298-313.

[17] Buckler ES, Ippolito A, Holtsford TP. The Evolution of ribosomal DNA: divergent paralogues and phylogenetic implications. Genetics. 1997; 145:821-832.

[18] Pillay M, Myers GO. Genetic diversity in cotton assessed by variation in ribosomal RNA genes and AFLP markers. Crop Sci. 1999; 39:1881-1886.

[19] Small RL, Ryburn JA, Cronn RC, Seelanan T, Wendel JF. The tortoise and the hare: Choosing between noncoding plastome and nuclear Adh sequences for phylogeny reconstruction of a recently diverged plant group. Am. J. Bot. 1998; 85:1301-1315.

[20] Zhao X, Si Y, Hanson RE, Crane CF, Price HJ, Stelly DM, Wendel JF, Paterson AH. Dispersed repetitive DNA has spread to new genomes since polyploidy formation in cotton. Genome Research. 1998; 8:479-492.

[21] Hanson RE, Zhao XP, Islam-Faridi MN, Paterson AH, Zwick MS, Crane CF, McKnight TD, Stelly DM, Price HJ. Evolution of interspersed repetitive elements in *Gossypium* (Malvaceae). Am. J. Bot. 1998; 85:1364-1368.

[22] Hanson RE, Islam-Faridi MH, Crane CF, Zwick MS, Czeschin DG, Wendel JF, McKnight TD, Price HJ, Stelly DM. Ty1-copia-retrotransposon behavior in a polyploid cotton. Chromosome Research 1999; 8:73-76.

[23] Cronn RC, Small RL, Wendel JF. Duplicated genes evolve independently after polyploid formation in cotton. Proc. Natl. Acad. Sci. 1999; 96:14406-14411.

[24] Small RL, Wendel JF. Phylogeny, duplication and intraspecific variation of Adh sequences in new world cotton (*Gossypium* L., Malvaceae). Mol. Phylogen. Evol. 2000a; 16:73-84.

[25] Small RL, Wendel JF. Copy number liability and evolutionary dynamics of the Adh gene family in diploid and tetraploid cotton (*Gossypium*). Genetics. 2000b; 155:1913-1926

[26] Liu Q, Brubaker CL, Green AG, Marshall DR, Sharp PJ. Singh S.P. Evolution of the FAD2-1 fatty acid desaturase 5′ UTR intron and the molecular systematics of *Gossypium* (Malvaceae). Am. J. Bot. 2001; 88:92-102.

[27] Wendel JF, Cronn RC, Johnston JS, Price HJ. Feast and famine in plant genomes. Genetica. 2002; 115:37-47.

[28] Álvarez I, Cronn R, Wendel JF. Phylogeny of the New World diploid cottons (*Gossypium* L., Malvaceae) based on sequences of three low-copy nuclear genes. Plant Systematics and Evolution. 2005; 252:199-214.

[29] Rohlf FJ. NTSYS pc: Numerical taxonomy system, Ver: 2.01. 2002; Exter publishing, Ltd. Setauket, NY.

[30] Saitou M, Nei N. The neighbor joining method: a new method for reconstructing phylogenetic trees. 1987; Mol Biol Evol 4: 406-425.

[31] Fryxell PA. A revised taxonomic interpretation of *Gossypium* L. (Malvaceae). Rheedea. 1992; 2: 108-165.

[32] Paterson AH, Wendel JF, Gundlach H, Guo H, Jenkins J, Jin D, Llewellyn D, Showmaker KC, Shu S, Udall J, Yoo M, Byers R, Chen W, Faigenboim AD, Duke MV, Gong L, Grimwood J, Grover C, Grupp K, Hu G, Lee T, Li J, Lin L, Liu T, Marler BS, Page JT, Roberts AW, Romanel E, Sanders WS, Szadkowski E, Tan X, Tang H, Xu C, Wang J, Wang Z, Zhang D, Zhang L, Ashrafi H, Bedon F, Bowers JE, Brubaker CL, Chee PW, Das S, Gingle AR, Haigler CH, Harker D, Hoffmann LV, Hovav R, Jones DC, Lemke C, Mansoor S, Rahman M, Rainville LN, Rambani A, Reddy UK, Rong J, Saranga Y, Scheffler BE, Scheffler JA, Stelly DM, Triplett BA, Van Deynze A, Vaslin MFS, Waghmare VN, Walford SA, Wright RJ, Zaki EA, Zhang T, Dennis ES, Mayer KFX, Peterson DG, Rokhsar DS, Wang X, Schmutz J. Repeated polyploidization of *Gossypium* genomes and the evolution of spinnable cotton fibres. Nature 2012; 492: 423–427.

[33] Wendel JF, Cronn RC. Polyploidy and the evolutionary history of cotton. Adv. Agro, Academic Press. 2003; 78:139-186.

[34] Senchina DS, Alvarez I, Cronn R, Liu B, Rong J, Noyes RD, Paterson AH, Wing RA, Wilkins TA, Wendel JF. Rate variation among nuclear genes and the age of polyploidy in *Gossypium*. Mol. Biol. Evol. 2003; 20:633-643.

[35] Endrizzi JE, Turcotte EL, Kohel RJ. Genetics, cytogenetics and evolution of *Gossypium*. Adv. Genet. 1985; 23:271-375.

[36] Brubaker CL, Bourland FM, Wendel JF. The origin and domestication of cotton. In Cotton: Origin, History, Technology and Production. Smith CW and Cothren JT (eds). Wiley, New York. 1999; p. 3-31.

[37] Edward GA, Endrizzi JE, Stein R. Genomic DNA content and chromosome organization in *Gossypium*. Chromosoma. 1974; 47:309-326.

[38] Bennett MD, Smith JB, Heslop-Harrison JS. Nuclear DNA amounts in angiosperms. Proc. R. Soc. Lond. B. 1982; 216:179-199.

[39] Stewart JM, Potential for crop improvement with exotic germplasm and genetic engineering. In Challenging the future: Proceedings of the World Cotton Research Conference. Constable GA and Forrester NW (eds). CSIRO Melbourne. 1995; p.313-327.

[40] Hendrix B, Stewart JM. Estimation of the nuclear DNA content of *Gossypium* species. Ann. Bot. 2005; 95:789-797.

[41] Meyer JR, Meyer VG. Origin and inheritance of nectariless cotton. Crop Sci. 1961; 1:167-169.

[42] Shepherd RL. Breeding root-knot-resistant *Gossypium hirsutum* L. using a resistant wild *G. barbadense* L. Crop Sci 1974; 14:687-691.

[43] Shepherd RL. Registration of Auburn 634. Crop Sci. 1982; 22:642.

[44] Bell AA. Cotton protection practices in the USA and world. Section B: Diseases. In: Kohel RJ, Lewis CF (eds) Cotton, Agronomy Monograph 24. ASSA, Madison, WI, USA. 1984; pp 288-309.

[45] Meyers VG. Male sterility from *Gossypium harknessii*. J Hered. 1975; 66:23-27.

[46] Stewart MJ. A new cytoplasmic male sterile and restorer. Proceedings Beltwide Cotton Conferences; USA. 1992; p610

[47] Meyer JR. Origin and inheritance of D2 smoothness in upland cotton. Crop Sci. 1957; 48:249-250.

[48] Harrell SC, Culp TW. Registration of Pee Dee 0259 and Pee Dee 2165 germplasm lines of cotton (Reg No GP39 and GP40). Crop Sci.1979; 19:418.

[49] Ulloa M, Wang C, Roberts PA. Gene action analysis by inheritance and quantitative trait loci mapping of resistance to root-knot nematodes in cotton. Plant Breeding. 2010; 129:541-550.

[50] Romano GB, Sacks EJ, Stetina SR, Robinson AF, Fang DD, Gutierrez OA, Scheffler JA. Identification and genomic location of a reniform nematode (*Rotylenchulus reniformis*) resistance locus (*Ren*^{aris}) introgressed from *Gossypium aridum* into upland cotton (*G. hirsutum*). Theor Appl Genet 2009; 120:139-150.

[51] Ulloa M. Saha S, Jenkins JN, Meredith WR Jr, McCarty JC, Stelly MD. Chromosomal assignment of RFLP linkage groups harboring important QTLs on an intraspecific cotton (*Gossypium hirsutum* L.) joinmap. J. Hered. 2005; 96132-144.

[52] Paterson AH, Saranga Y, Menz M, Jiang C, Wright RJ. QTL analysis of genotype x environmental interactions affecting cotton fiber quality. Theor Appl Genet. 2003; 106:384-396.

[53] Reinisch AJ, Dong JM, Brubaker CL, Wendel JF, Paterson AH. A detailed RFLP map of cotton, *Gossypium hirsutum x Gossypium barbadense*: chromosome organization and evolution in a disomic polyploid genome. Genetics. 1994; 138:829-847.

[54] Rong J-K, Abbey C, Bowers JE, Brubaker CL, Chang C, Chee PW, Delmonte TA, Ding XL, Garza JJ, Marler BS, Park C-H, Pierce GJ, Rainey KM, Rastogi VK, Schulze SR, Trolinder NL, Wendel JF, Wilkins TA, Williams-Coplin TD, Wing RA, Wright RJ, Zhao X, Zhu L, Paterson AH. A 3347-locus genetic recombination map of sequence-tagged sites reveals features of genome organization, transmission and evolution of cotton (*Gossypium*). Genetics. 2004; 166:389-417.

[55] Wright RJ, Thaxton P, El-Zik K, Peterson AH. D-subgenome bias of *Xcm* resistance genes in tetraploid *Gossypium* (cotton) suggest that polyploidy formation has created novel avenues for evolution. Genetics. 1998; 149:1978-1996.

[56] Xu P, Liu Z, Fan X, Gao J, Zhang X, Zhang X, Shen X. De novo transcriptome sequencing and comparative analysis of differentially expressed genes in *Gossypium aridum* under salt stress. Gene. 2013; 525:26-34.

[57] Rong J, Feltus FA, Waghmare VN, Pierce GJ, Chee PW, Draye X, Saranga Y, Wright RJ, Wilkins TA, May OL, Smith CW, Gannaway JR, Wendel JF, Paterson AH. Meta-analysis of polyploid cotton QTL shows unequal contributions of subgenomes to a complex network of genes and gene clusters implicated in lint fiber development. 2007; Genetics 176: 2577-2588.

[58] Abe A, Kosugi S, Yoshida K, Natsume S, Takagi H, Kanzaki H, Matsumura H, Mitsuoka C, Tamiru M, Innan H, Cano L, Kamoun S, Terauchi R.. Genome sequencing reveals agronomically important loci in rice using MutMap. Nat. Biotechnol. 2012; 30:174-178.

[59] Austin RS, Vidaurre D, Stamatiou G, Breit R, Provart NJ, Bonetta D, Zhang J, Fung P, Gong Y, Wang PW, McCourt P, Guttman DS. Next-generation mapping of Arabidopsis genes. Plant J. 2011; 67:715-725.

[60] Page JT, Huynh MD, Liechty ZS, Grupp K, Stelly D, Hulse AM, Ashrafi H, Van-Deynze A, Wendel JF, Udall JA. Insights into the evolution of the cotton diploids and polyploids from whole-genome re-sequencing. G3, 2013; 3: 1809-1818.

[61] Wang K, Wang Z, Li F, Ye W, Wang J, Song G, Yue Z, Cong L, Shang H, Zhu S, Zou C, Li Q, Yuan Y, Lu C, Wei H, Gou C, Zheng Z, Yin Y, Zhang X, Liu K, Wang B, Song C, Shi N, Kohel RJ, Percy RG, Yu JZ, Zhu Y-X, Wang J, Yu S. The draft genome of a diploid cotton *Gossypium raimondii*. Nature Genetics. 2012; 44(10) 1098-1104.

[62] Yu JZ, Kohel RJ, Fang DD, Cho J, Van Deynze A, Ulloa M, Hoffman SM, Pepper AE, Stelly DM, Jenkins JN, Saha S, Kumpatla SP, Shah MR, Hugie WV, Percy RG. A high-density SSR and SNP genetic map of the tetraploid cotton genome. G3: Genes, Genomes, Genetics 2012; 2:43-58.

[63] Ulloa M, Percy R, Hutmacher RB, Zhang J. The future of cotton breeding in the Western United States. J. Cot. Sci. 2009; 4 246-255.

[64] Zhang L, Li Y, Lu W, Meng F, Wu CA, Guo X. Cotton GhMKK5 affects disease resistance, induces HR-like cell death, and reduces the tolerance to salt and drought stress in transgenic *Nicotiana benthamiana*. J. Exp Bot. 2012; 63:3935-3951.

[65] Saranga Y, Menz M, Jiang C, Wright RJ, Yakir D, Paterson AH. Genomic Dissection of genotype x environment interactions conferring adaptation of cotton to arid conditions. Genome Res. 2001; 11:1988-1995.

[66] Burke JJ, Ulloa M. Initial characterization of a Stoneville 474 x Phytogen 72 recombinant inbred population. In: Boyd S, Huffman M, Robertson B. (eds.): Proceedings of the Beltwide Cotton Conferences, 7-10 January 2013, San Antonio, TX, USA. Memphis: National Cotton Council.

Chapter 9

Broadening the Genetic Base of Upland Cotton in U.S. Cultivars – Genetic Variation for Lint Yield and Fiber Quality in Germplasm Resources

Linghe Zeng

Additional information is available at the end of the chapter

http://dx.doi.org/10.5772/57606

1. Introduction

Global competition of cotton fibers has changed the U.S. cotton industry in the last decade from a mainly domestic consumer to exporter of cotton fibers in the world market. In 2012, the U.S. produced 17.3 million bales of cotton, 14.4 % of the world production. Only 3.4 million bales, 19.6 % of the total production, were used in the domestic textile industry with 13 million bales exported (USDA-FAS, 2013). Foreign customers demand stronger, longer and more uniform fibers, and less short fiber and impurity contents of raw fibers than domestic markets. Meanwhile, domestic surviving textile industries raised spinning speed by updating to modern high speed spinners in order to improve their competitive ability in the global market. Fiber quality standards were also raised in order to operate at maximum efficiency using the modern spinners. According to Estur (2004), the modern high-speed spinners require micronaire between 3.8 and 4.4, minimum 27.4 mm for 2.5% span length, 28 g/tex for strength, and 6 % for elongation, and maximum of 5 % short fiber content and 15/gram of seed coat fragments, and at least 83 % for length uniformity ratio. Currently, high yield U.S. cultivars of Upland cotton still lack sufficient fiber quality to fully meet these industry requirements. On the other hand, increasing lint yield in Upland cotton cultivars is always a top priority to keep profit for cotton growers. Increases of lint yield in U.S. cotton cultivars reached a plateau in the last two decades (Helms, 2000; Meredith, 2000; Gingle et al., 2006). Cotton yield peaked in the U.S. in 1992 and declined of an annual rate of 3.3 % in the next seven years (Helms, 2000). Furthermore, yearly fluctuation of yield increased 4 times from periods of 1960-1979 to 1980-1998 (Gingle et al., 2006). It is a great challenge for U.S. cotton breeders to simultaneously improve lint yield and fiber quality because of negative associations between yield traits and fiber quality (Miller and Rawlings, 1967; Smith and Goyle, 1997).

It is commonly accepted that the genetic base of Upland cotton cultivars in the U.S. is narrow (Bowman et al., 1996; Van Esbroeck and Bowman, 1998). The narrowed genetic base in commercial cotton cultivars of *G. hirsutum* was caused by using only a small number of introduced wild genotypes during domestication (Van Esbroeck and Bowman, 1998; Gingle et al., 2006), breeding practices for high yield and early maturity (May et al., 1995; May, 1999), the dominance of transgenic cultivars in recent years, and insufficient utilization of exotic germplasm resources in cotton breeding. The narrowed genetic base in Upland cotton cultivars is believed to be the cause for the limited success in breakup of the negative associations between lint yield and fiber quality. Introgression from exotic germplasm resources into cultivars may be the most effective approach to broaden the genetic base of Upland cotton. The word "exotic" was defined in Google Search as "strikingly different", "strikingly unusual", or "introduced from other region or country". The term exotic germplasm is defined in this chapter as the germplasm without commercial applicability before introgression of the germplasm which includes land races, wild species, and the induced mutation stocks. It is expected that the introgression of novel genes from exotic germplasm into cotton cultivars or breeding lines can increase genetic variation in the introgression populations for agronomic traits and fiber quality.

2. Genetic diversity in some cotton germplasm populations developed by public breeding programs in U.S.

Although many germplasm populations derived from interspecific crosses or race stocks have been used in cotton breeding, only a small portion of alleles in these germplasm were introgressed into the released cultivars due to the selection for regional adaption according to a survey by Van Esbroeck and Bowman (1998). Only 0.3% of the 668 released germplasm lines have been introgressed into successful cotton cultivars. However, most of the successful cultivars released between 1972 and 1996 have some exotic alleles in their pedigree according to this survey. For more successful introgression of exotic germplasm into cultivars, genetic variations of germplasm resources with exotic genetic backgrounds have to be explored.

In this section, the efforts on characterizing genetic diversity in the germplasm populations in a few U.S. public breeding programs were reviewed. There are different cotton breeding programs in U.S. that include both the private and public sectors. The germplasm developed in these programs constitutes the primary gene pool for breeding. Pee Dee and the New Mexico Acala germplasms are two historically important public breeding programs as highlighted by Bowman et al. (2006) in a description of U.S. cotton cultivars released between 1970 and 2005. Up to 50% of strength improvement in Upland cotton cultivars during 1980 and 2000 may have been attributed to alleles from Pee Dee and Acala germplasm populations (Bowman and Gutiérrez, 2003).

Although there is no a single reference that fully describes the Pee Dee germplasm due to the complex nature of this breeding program, there is a series of publications that reported germplasm lines derived from the program and evaluation of genetic variation in these germplasm resources (Culp and Harrell, 1973; Culp and Harrell, 1979a; Culp and Harrell, 1979b; Bowman and Gutiérrez, 2003; Campbell and Bauer, 2007; Campbell et al. 2009a; Campbell et al., 2009b; Campbell et al., 2011). As described by Culp and Harrell (1973) and Campbell et al. (2011), Pee Dee germplasm was introgressed from triple hybrid strains (*G. arboretum* L. × *G. thurberi* Todaro × *G. hirsutum* L.) since the 1940s and followed by 50 years of intercrosses among progenitor lines and crosses with commercial Upland cotton cultivars. Based on an evaluation of 82 released Pee Dee germplasm lines (Campbell et al., 2011), genetic variation for lint yield and fiber properties has been maintained in this germplasm population. Genetic similarity among these 82 lines ranged from 0.64 to 0.96 estimated by Simple Sequence Repeat (SSR) markers (Campbell et al., 2009b). The maintenance of genetic diversity in the Pee Dee germplasm after so many years of selection in breeding may be due to multiple breeding methods including random mating, backcrossing, and composite crossing in addition to pedigree selection applied during the breeding history (Culp and Harrell, 1973; Campbell et al., 2011).

Acala germplasm populations were developed by the New Mexico State University breeding programs. The history for the development of this germplasm has been described in detail by Smith et al. (1999). The series of Acala 1517 cultivars, commonly planted in the southwestern regions of U.S., were developed in this breeding program. Similar to Pee Dee germplasm, Acala germplasm also has genetic background of triple hybrids (*G. arboretum* L. × *G. thurberi* Todaro × *G. hirsutum* L.) (Smith et al., 1999). These germplasm populations are characterized by high fiber quality and Verticillium wilt tolerance and perform well in semiarid and hot regions in the southwestern of U.S. according to Zhang et al (2005a). Genetic diversity was maintained within Acala germplasm population. Genetic similarity ranged from 0.62 to 0.94 in 30 Acala cultivars estimated by SSR markers in this study. It was also concluded in this study that divergent germplasm introgressed in the Acala breeding program has contributed to the maintenance of genetic diversity in this germplasm and the genetic gain in the Acala cultivars.

Race stocks are another germplasm resource that can be utilized for introgression breeding. There are more than 2,000 primitive accessions in the cotton germplasm collection maintained by ARS at College Station, TX (Percival, 1987). However, utilization of these accessions has been limited due to their photoperiodic sensitivity which requires short days to flower and produce bolls. A group of U.S. public breeders have converted a large number of these accessions into the day-neutral lines by incorporating day-neutral genes in the primitive accessions through backcross breeding (McCarty et al., 1979; McCarty and Jenkins, 1992). Useful genetic variations for lint yield and fiber properties have been identified by evaluation of backcrossed progenies of 14 day-neutral accessions (McCarty et al., 1995) and F_2 bulks of crosses between 114 day-neutral accessions with Stoneville 474 and Sure-Grow 747 (McCarty et al., 2005). Twelve germplasm lines derived from converted day-neutral race stocks and introgression of wild species were evaluated and significant additive and dominant effects were identified for yield components and different fiber properties (Wu et al., 2010). Hinze et al. (2011) also identified significant variations for agronomic traits and fiber properties within four germplasm populations derived from non-photoperiodic race stocks. A study of genetic distance between four converted day-neutral lines and Delta and Pine 16 showed a wide range of genetic similarity in these germplasm lines, ranging from 0.37 to 0.65 (Zhong et al., 2002).

Species Polycross (SP) and JohnCotton (JC) germplasm populations were developed by U.S. breeders since the 1960s and 1970s. SP germplasm population was derived from multiple crosses among twelve cotton cultivars and strains of four tetraploid species: *G. barbadense* L., *G. tomentosum* Nutt., *G. mustelinum* Watt., and *G. darwinii* Watt. JC germplasm population was derived from multiple crosses between Acala 1517 type cultivars and *G. barbadense*. Both of these two germplasm populations underwent multiple generations of random mating and selfing. Significant genetic variations for lint yield and fiber properties have been identified in field evaluation of 260 SP lines (Zeng et al., 2007) and another evaluation of 200 JC lines (Zeng and Meredith, 2009a). A number of germplasm lines were selected and released from these two germplasm populations for desirable combinations between lint yield and fiber properties (Zeng and Meredith, 2009b; Zeng et al., 2010). Genetic similarity between 12 SP and JC lines and 4 Upland cultivars ranged from 0.44 to 0.99 (Zeng and Meredith, 2011).

In a few molecular studies of genetic distance among Upland cultivars (Gutiérrez et al., 2002; Rahman et al., 2002; Zhang et al., 2005b), genetic similarity ranged from 0.78 to 0.94 between pairs of cultivars in these studies. All the germplasm resources described above have larger genetic distance within the populations and from Upland cultivars. In a recent study of 193 Upland cotton cultivars collected from 26 countries using SSR markers, the pair-wise genetic similarity ranged from 0.64 to 0.99 (Fang et al., 2013). Only in this study, the genetic diversity was comparable to the germplasm populations described above. These studies are consistent with the argument that genetic diversity is maintained in the Pee Dee, New Mexico Acala, Day-neutral converted race stocks, SP, and JC germplasm.

3. Gene action and combining ability for lint yield and fiber quality in germplasm resources

Lint yield is determined by bolls per square meter, seeds per boll, and lint per seed (Worley et al., 1974; Worley et al., 1976). Although the yield component, bolls per square meter, is an inherited trait, it is highly depended on plant density, and environmental effects on this component are large (Meredith and Bridge, 1973). Lint yield is determined by seed cotton yield and lint percentage, and a number of within boll yield components contributing to lint yield including seeds per boll, lint per seed, lint weight per unit seed surface area, fibers per seed, and fibers per unit seed surface area (Worley et al., 1976; Coyle and Smith, 1997). Fiber quality

http://dx.doi.org/10.5772/57606

is a series of fiber properties which determine the spinnability of fibers and the efficiency of the high speed spinners in the modern textile industries. In a typical breeders' analysis, the measurements of fiber quality include micronaire, elongation, fiber strength, fiber length, short fiber content, and fineness. The neppiness traits including fiber neps, seed coat neps, and motes are getting more attention from breeders in recent years because of their severe affects in textile processing during spinning and dying (Jacobsen et al., 2001). While both lint yield and fiber quality are important traits to improve in Upland cotton cultivars, negative associations usually exist between them. For example, the potential of fiber productivity is highly related to fiber length and thickness of cell walls because longer fibers and thicker cell walls resulted from increased cellulose amount in the fibers (Kohel, 1999). However, the increase of fiber productivity by increasing cell wall thickness will be antagonistic with fineness, an important fiber property in fiber spinning. Determination of gene actions and combining ability for different attributes of yield and fiber quality in germplasm populations can be of help in understanding introgression and is useful information for breaking or reducing the negative associations among fiber traits.

Genetic variations of quantitative traits for yield and fiber quality are the main focus in this section which discusses the differences of gene actions and combining ability among germplasm resources. For variations related to morphological phenotypes or other taxonomic characteristics, readers can refer to the reports by Percy and Kohel (1999) and Lubbers and Chee (2009). A few recent studies of gene actions in genetic populations derived from different types of germplasm resources are summarized in Table 1. The general low additive gene action for lint yield and most fiber properties in these germplasm populations except for the populations derived from crosses among tetraploid species suggests non-efficiency of early selection for lint yield in the populations. High additive gene action in yield components and fiber strength suggests early selection efficiency for these traits in these germplasm populations. In five genetic populations developed by diallel crosses among Upland cotton cultivars, as reviewed by Meredith (1984), gene actions for yield traits and fiber properties were generally partial dominant. In order to compare gene action in these five genetic populations, the degree of dominance was estimated in the same way as described by Meredith (1984) as the ratios of dominant component to additive component with values less than 1 indicating partial dominance and values equal or larger than 1 indicating complete or over-dominance. As shown in Table 1, gene action in the introgression populations was either completely dominant or over-dominant for yield traits except for lint percentage among different germplasm resources. For fiber properties, gene actions were generally partially dominant for micronaire and fiber strength while over-dominant for fiber length, short fiber content, and fineness. A reduction of heterosis values from obsolete cultivars to the modern cultivars due to increased additive genes in breeding practice has been observed previously (Campbell et al., 2008). The increase of dominance gene action in the genetic populations derived from wild cotton and interspecific crosses indicates that the adding of non-additive genes by introgression from wild cotton may be an effective approach to promote heterosis.

Traits	**V_A** [†]	**V_D**	**$(V_D/V_A)^{1/2}$** [‡]	**Germplasm type**	**Sources**
Lint yield	0.06**	0.25**	2.0	Primitive accession derived F2, F3	McCarty et al. (2004)
	0.08**	0.12**	1.2	Upland cotton cultivars and breeding lines	Jenkins et al. (2009)
	0.38**	0.31**	0.90	Wild tetraploid species derived F2	Zeng and Wu (2012)
	0.01	0.06**	2.5	Chromosome substitution lines of TM-1 introgressed from *G. barbadense*	Saha et al (2010)
	0.250**	0.28**	1.1	Cultivars and race stock derived F2	Cheatham et al (2003)
Lint %	0.35**	0.11**	0.56	Primitive accession derived F2, F3	McCarty et al. (2004)
	0.33**	0.22**	0.82	Upland cotton cultivars and breeding lines	Jenkins et al. (2009)
	0.54**	0.10**	0.44	Chromosome substitution lines of TM-1 introgressed from *G. barbadense*	Saha et al (2010)
	0.49**	0.32**	0.81	Wild tetraploid species derived F2	Zeng and Wu (2012)
	0.81**	0.11*	0.37	Cultivars and race stock derived F2	Cheatham et al (2003)
Boll wt	0.18**	0.34**	1.4	Primitive accession derived F2, F3	McCarty et al (2004)
	0.27**	0.32**	1.1	Upland cotton cultivars and breeding lines	Jenkins et al. (2009)
	0.17**	0.00	0.00	Chromosome substitution lines of TM-1 introgressed from *G. barbadense*	Saha et al (2010)
	0.35**	0.31**	0.94	Wild tetraploid species derived F2	Zeng and Wu (2012)
	0.23**	0.29**	1.1	Cultivars and race stock derived F2	Cheatham et al (2003)
Seed index	0.39**	0.33**	0.92	Wild tetraploid species derived F2	Zeng and Wu (2012)
Lint index	0.44**	0.32**	0.85	Wild tetraploid species derived F2	Zeng and Wu (2012)
Seeds $boll^{-1}$	0.23**	0.36**	1.3	Wild tetraploid species derived F2	Zeng and Wu (2012)

http://dx.doi.org/10.5772/57606

Traits	V_A †	V_D	$(V_D/V_A)^{1/2‡}$	Germplasm type	Sources
MIC‡	0.14**	0.02*	0.37	Primitive accession derived F2, F3	McCarty et al (2004)
	0.27**	0.15**	0.75	Upland cotton cultivars and breeding lines	Jenkins et al. (2009)
	0.04**	0.60**	3.9	Cultivars and race stock derived F2	Cheatham et al (2003)
	0.07**	0.33**	2.2	Wild tetraploid species derived F2	Zeng et al (2013)
T1	0.19**	0.15**	0.89	Primitive accession derived F2, F3	McCarty et al (2004)
	0.57**	0.12**	0.46	Upland cotton cultivars and breeding lines	Jenkins et al. (2009)
	0.26**	0.31**	1.1	Wild tetraploid species derived F2	Zeng et al (2013)
	0.47**	0.01**	0.14	Cultivars and race stock derived F2	Cheatham et al (2003)
SL1	0.10**	0.18**	1.3	Primitive accession derived F2, F3	McCarty et al (2004)
	0.09**	0.18**	1.4	Wild tetraploid species derived F2	Zeng et al (2013)
	0.07**	0.24**	1.8	Cultivars and race stock derived F2	Cheatham et al (2003)
Short fiber	0.06**	0.41**	2.6	Wild tetraploid species derived F2	Zeng et al (2013)
Fineness	0.12**	0.39**	1.8	Wild tetraploid species derived F2	Zeng et al (2013)

*, ** Significant at < 0.05 and 0.01, respectively.

† V_A, additive variance component; V_D, dominance variance component; V_{AE}, additive by environment; V_{DE}, dominant by environment. All components were expressed as the ratio to V_P, the phenotypic variance.

‡ $(V_D/V_A)^{1/2}$ was calculated as described by Meredith (1984): V_A was set to 100; the dominant component (V_D) was converted to $V_D/V_A \times 100$.

§MIC, micronaire; T1, fiber strength; SL1, 50% span length.

Table 1. Variance components in different germplasm resources of Upland cotton.

Determination of general combining ability for lint yield and fiber quality in germplasm lines can identify parents with potential of simultaneous improvement of lint yield and fiber quality. In reality, a parent with good general combining ability (GCA) in fiber quality usually had negative GCA in yield components or vice versa. In review of the previous studies since 1990s, a line with all desirable combinations between lint yield and fiber properties has not been reported. However, a number of studies reported by the U.S. cotton breeders have identified cultivars or germplasm lines with good lint yield and one or a few desirable fiber properties in the half diallel mating design. Green and Culp (1990) detected PD 3249 having positive GCA for lint yield (79 kg ha^{-1}), strength (2.5 kN m kg^{-1}), and 2.5% span length (0.20 mm) in crosses among five cultivars. Coyle and Smith (1997) detected Deltapine 90 having positive GCA for lint percentage (1.1-1.2 %) and strength (2-10 kN m kg^{-1}) in crosses among four cultivars and two germplasm lines. Jenkins et al (2009) reported positive predicted GCA in Acala Ultima, FM 966, and PSC 355 for lint yield (8-84 kg ha^{-1}), strength (3.6-29 kN m kg^{-1}), and uniformity ratio (0.32-0.71%) in crosses among 10 cultivars and one breeding line. Zeng et al. (2011) identified five germplasm lines, SP156, SP224, SP192, SP205, and JC65, having positive GCA for lint yield and favorable GCA for a few fiber properties including strength, elongation, short fiber content, and fineness in crosses among four cultivars and twelve exotic germplasm lines by a North Carolina Design II mating design. These germplasm lines can be used as parents in breeding for simultaneous improvement of lint yield and fiber quality.

4. Genetic associations among yield traits and fiber properties in different breeding programs

Negative associations between lint yield and fiber quality is the main obstacle for simultaneous genetic improvement of yield and fiber quality. Genotypic correlations between lint yield and fiber properties in different genetic populations developed by some old and modern breeding programs are summarized in Table 2. In general, unfavorable correlations were identified for lint yield vs. strength, lint yield vs. span length, and lint yield vs. fineness. The highly unfavorable association between lint yield and fineness identified in studies by Miller and Rowlings (1967) and Zeng et al. (2007) are expected since the thickness of fiber walls relates to the total amount of cellulose in fiber production. Since fineness is an important property in textile industry, the breakup of this unfavorable association would be critical in future breeding. The genetic improvement of lint yield may be achieved by selection of within-boll yield components and a balance between lint weight per unit seed surface area and fibers per unit seed surface area. In contrast, the correlations of lint yield with elongation and short fiber content were generally favorable or not significant in these germplasm resources which indicated the possibility for simultaneous improvement of these traits.

Although general negative association between lint yield and fiber strength and between lint yield and span lengths have been reported, low negative correlations were identified in studies of Percy et al. (2006), Zeng et al. (2007), and Hinze et al. (2011) compared with studies in the old breeding programs. The low correlations in these genetic populations indicated the possible recombinants with breakup of the negative associations. The genetic populations described by Percy et al. (2006) and Zeng et al. (2007) were introgressed populations from interspecific crosses. It is possible that the novel genes introgressed from wild germplasm increased recombination among parental chromosomes and therefore increased the chance to breakup negative associations.

An elaborate explanation of interrelationships among fiber traits based on phenotypes has been difficult in the previous studies. The limited success in the past was mainly due to the confounding relationships of some fiber traits with other traits. Sometimes a correlation

http://dx.doi.org/10.5772/57606

Lint yield vs. fiber properties	r values	Germplasm types	Sources
Strength	-0.35 (0.16)†	6 generations mixed intermating of	Miller and Rowlings
Elongation	0.37 (0.25)	Empire 10 × TH131-5	(1967)
Fineness	0.46 (0.19)		
Strength	-0.38 (0.19)	2 generations random mating of	Meredith and Bridge
50% span length	-0.28 (0.23)	ST7A × PD165	(1971)
2.5 % span length	-0.67 (0.19)		
Elongation	00.15 (0.20)		
Strength	0.09	Introgressed recombinant inbred	Percy et al. (2006)
50% span length	0.06	population	
2.5% span length	-0.08		
Strength	-0.19***	A mixed intermating population	Zeng et al. (2007)
Elongation	0.03	(Species Polycross, SP)	
50% span length	0.02		
2.5% span length	0.06		
Short fiber content	-0.11**		
Strength	-0.53***	A mixed intermating population	Zeng and Meredith
Elongation	-0.17*	(John Cotton, JC)	(2009a)
50% span length	-0.26**		
2.5% span length	-0.11*		
Short fiber content	-0.08		
Fineness	0.57***		
Strength	-0.19*	21 F2 populations	Hinze et al. (2011)
UHM length	-0.46***		
Elongation	0.58***		
Uniformity	0.08		

*, **, *** Significant at $P < 0.05$, $P < 0.01$, $P < 0.001$, respectively.

† Values of standard variation were shown in parenthesis when the significance probability was not reported.

Table 2. Genetic associations between lint yield and fiber properties in the old and modern breeding programs.

between two traits appears unfavorable. However, it doesn't necessarily mean an unfavorable linkage of genes controlling the traits, but simply resulted from confounding effects from other traits. The relationships among maturity, short fiber content, and fineness in our previous studies can be an example to demonstrate how a relation between two traits is superimposed by relations among other traits. In a study of 200 germplasm lines from JohnCotton (JC) germplasm (Zeng and Meredith, 2009a), short fiber content was negatively correlated with fineness (r=-0.41). However, this relation was superimposed by their relations with maturity ratio, r=-0.77 for maturity ratio vs. short fiber content and r=0.81 for maturity ratio vs. fineness. This suggests that when fibers were more mature, short fiber content became less and fibers became coarser. In another study of 45 F_2 populations derived from crosses between five cultivars and nine SP and JC germplasm lines (Zeng et al., 2013), nearly zero additive correlation was observed between short fiber content and fineness which confirmed a lack of genetic mechanism underlying the phenotypic relationships between the two traits in these populations.

5. Conclusions and perspectives

Germplasm populations with novel genes from exotic resources heve been developed from different breeding programs. Molecular marker data showed genetic variation within these germplasm populations which indicated their usefulness in breeding for continuing genetic improvement of lint yield and fiber quality. Although useful genetic variations in different attributes related to lint yield and fiber quality exist in different germplasm populations, limited success has been reported in the identification of parents with desirable combination between lint yield and fiber properties. It is a challenge for U.S. cotton breeders to further broaden the genetic base of Upland cotton in the future to assist in a more successful breakup of linkages between lint yield and fiber quality.

There are a few approaches that should be considered in order to improve utilization of exotic germplasm resources and their introgression into Upland cotton cultivars for simultaneous genetic improvement of lint yield and fiber quality. (A) Genome-wide characterization of genetic diversity in different germplasm resources. There are a total of 5164 accessions of *G. hirsutum*, 1337 accessions of *G. barbadense*, and 25 accessions of *G. tomentosum*, *G. mustelinum*, and *G. darwinii* as primary gene pool, 1952 accessions for A, B, D, and F genome species as secondary gene pool, and 82 accessions for C, G, K, and E genome species as tertiary gene pool available at the National Plant Germplasm System of USDA-ARS (GRIN, 2013). These accessions have served as primary germplasm resources in cotton breeding worldwide, but most of these resources have yet to be utilized for genetic improvement of cotton cultivars. A genome-wide characterization of genetic diversity in these germplasm will undoubtedly improve their utilization in breeding. An establishment of a core set of these germplasm accessions according to the molecular characterization will definitely help their further utilization. (B) Elaboration of the complex interrelationships between yield traits and fiber properties. Because yield traits and fiber properties are often interrelated, the explanation of their interrelationships based on phenotypes would be difficult. Identification of molecular markers closely associated with these traits and determination of their genome location can help elaborate these interrelationships at the genome level and improve our understanding of the mechanisms underlying unfavorable associations between lint yield and fiber properties. (C) Use of alien chromosome substitution lines in introgression breeding. One of the major obstacles hindering utilization of exotic germplasm is the linkage between beneficial genes and unfavorable genes from the wild un-adapted germplasm during introgression. A group of U.S. scientists have developed an approach with a set of chromosome substitution lines to introgress beneficial genes from primary gene pools of *Gossypium* tetraploid species into Upland cotton (Stelly et al., 2005; Saha et al., 2011; Saha et al., 2013). The major advantage of

http://dx.doi.org/10.5772/57606

this approach for introgression breeding is the reduction of likelihood for undesirable associations by increasing recombination in the substituted alien chromosomes or chromosome segments (Saha et al., 2013). (D) Application of appropriate breeding methods such as random mating to maintain genetic diversity in germplasm populations or facilitate introgression of novel genes from wild germplasm resources to Upland cotton. Random mating may improve genetic variation in cotton germplasm populations and increase occurrence of recombinants and further improve opportunities to break up unfavorable associations between lint yield and fiber quality. A recent germplasm population, RMBUP-C4, was developed from crosses between three cultivars and 18 chromosome substitution lines followed by 4 cycles of random mating to introgress *G. barbadense* alleles into Upland cotton germplasm (Jenkins et al., 2013). This germplasm was released and available for cotton breeders worldwide in introgression breeding.

Author details

Linghe Zeng*

Address all correspondence to: linghe.zeng@ars.usda.gov

USDA-ARS, Crop Genetics Research Unit, Stoneville, USA

References

[1] Bowman, D.T., O.L. May, and D.S. Calhoun. 1996. Genetic base of upland cotton cultivars released between 1970 and 1990. Crop Sci. 36:577-581.

[2] Bowman, D.T., and O.A. Gutiérrez. 2003. Sources of fiber strength in the U.S. upland cotton crop from 1980 to 2000. The Journal of Cotton Sci. 7:164-169.

[3] Bowman, D.T., O.A.Gutierrez, R.G. Percy, D.S. Calhoun, O.L. May. 2006. Pedigrees of upland cotton and pima cotton cultivars released between 1970 and 2005. Bull. 1017. Miss. Agric. and For. Exp. Stn., Mississippi, MS.

[4] Campbell, B.T., and P.J. Bauer. 2007. Genetic variation for yield and fiber quality response to supplemental irrigation within the Pee Dee upland cotton germplasm collection. Crop Sci. 47:591-599.

[5] Campbell, B.T., D.T. Bowman, and D.B. Weaver. 2008. Heterotic effects in topcrosses of modern and obsolete cotton cultivars. Crop Sci. 48:593-600.

[6] Campbell, B.T., O.L. May, and D.C. Jones. 2009a. Registration of PD 99035 germplasm line of cotton. Journal of Plant Registrations 3:73-76.

[7] Campbell, B.T., V.E. Williams, and W. Park. 2009b. Using molecular markers and field performance data to characterize the Pee Dee cotton germplasm resources. Euphytica 169:285-301.

[8] Campbell, B.T., P.W. Chee, E. Lubbers, D.T. Bowman, W.R. Meredith, Jr., J. Johnson, and D.E. Fraser. 2011. Genetic improvement of the Pee Dee cotton germplasm collection following seventy years of plant breeding. Crop Sci. 51:955-968.

[9] Cheatham, C.L., J.N. Jenkins, J.C. McCarty, Jr., C.E. Watson, and J. Wu. 2003. Genetic variances and combining ability of crosses of American cultivars, Australian cultivars, and wild cottons. J. Cotton Sci. 7:16-22.

[10] Coyle, G.G., and C.W. Smith. 1997. Combining ability for within boll yield components in cotton, *Gossypium hirsutum* L. Crop Sci. 37:1118-1122.

[11] Culp, T.W., and D.C. Harrell. 1973. Breeding methods for improving yield and fiber quality of upland cotton (Gossypium hirsutum L.). Crop Sci. 13:686-689.

[12] Culp, T.W., and D.C. Harrell. 1979a. Registration of SC-1 cotton. Crop Sci. 19:410.

[13] Culp, T.W., and D.C. Harrell. 1979b. Registration of Pee Dee 4461 cotton germplasm. Crop Sci. 19:753.

[14] Estur, G. 2004. Quality requirements on export markets for U.S. cotton. International cotton advisory committee. Washington DC. Available at: http://www. icac.org/cotton_info/speeches/estur/2004/quality_reqs_us_exp.pdf. Accessed 11 April 2013.

[15] Fang, D., L.L. Hinze, R.G. Percy, P. Li, D. Deng, and G. Thyssen. 2013. A microsatellite-based genome-wide analysis of genetic diversity and linkage disequilibrium in Upland cotton (*Gossypium hirsutum* L.) cultivars from major cotton-growing countries. Euphytica 191:391- 401.

[16] Gingle, A.R., Yang, H., Chee, P.W., May, O.L., Rong, J., Bowman, D.T., Lubbers, E.L., Day,J.L. and Paterson, A.H. 2006. An integrated web resource for cotton. Crop Science 46:1998- 2007.

[17] Green, C.C, and T.W. Culp. 1990. Simultaneous improvement of yield, fiber quality, and yarn strength in Upland cotton. Crop Sci. 30:66-69.

[18] GRIN, 2013. Germplasm resources information network of USDA-ARS. Available at

[19] Gutiérrez, O.A., S. Basu, S. Saha, J.N. Jenkins, D.B. Shoemaker, C.L. Cheatham, and J.C. McCarty, Jr. 2002. Genetic distance among selected cotton genotypes and its relationship with F2 performance. Crop Sci. 42:1841-1847.

[20] Helms, A.B. 2000. Yield study report. *In* P. Dugger and D. Richter (ed.) Proc. Beltwide Cotton Prod. Conf., San Antonio, TX. 4-9 Jan. 2000. Natl. Cotton Council, Memphis, TN.

[21] Hinze, L.L., B.T. Campbell, and R.J. Kohel. 2011. Performance and combining ability in cotton (*Gossypium hirsutum* L.) populations with diverse parents. Euphytica 181:115-125.

[22] Jenkins, N.J., J.C. McCarty, Jr., J. Wu, and O.A. Gutierrez. 2009. Genetic variance components and genetic effects among eleven diverse upland cotton lines and their F2 hybrids. Euphytica 167:397-408.

[23] Jenkins, N.J., J.C. McCarty,Jr., O.A. Gutiérrez, R.W. Hayes, and D.C. Jones. 2013. Registration of RMBUP-C4, a random-mated population with Gossypium barbadense L. alleles introgressed into Upland cotton germplasm. J. Plant Regis. 7:224-228.

[24] Jacobsen, K.R., Y.L. Grossman, Y.L. Hsieh, R.E. Plant, W.F. Labor, and J.A. Jernstedt. 2001. Neps, seed coat fragments, and non-seed impurities in processed cotton. J. Cotton Sci. 5:53- 67.

[25] Kohel, R.J. 1999. Cotton germplasm resources and the potential for improved fiber productivity and quality. p. 167-182. *In* A.S. Basra (ed.) Cotton Fibers: Developmental biology, quality improvement, and textile processing. Food Products Press, New York.

[26] Lubbers, E.L., and P.W. Chee. 2009. The worldwide gene pool of G. hirsutum and its improvement. p. 23-52. *In* A.H. Paterson (ed.) Genetics and genomics of cotton. Springer, New York.

[27] May, O.L., D.T. Bowman, and D.S. Calhoun. 1995. Genetic diversity of U.S. upland cotton cultivars released between 1980 and 1990. Crop Sci. 35:1570-1574.

[28] May, O.L. 1999. Genetic variation in fiber quality. p. 183-229. *In* A.S. Basra (ed.) Cotton fibers: Developmental biology, quality improvement, and textile processing. Food Product Press, New York.

[29] McCarty, J.C., Jr., J.N. Jenkins, W.L. Parrott, and R.G. Creech. 1979. The conversion of photoperiodic primitive race stocks of cotton to day-neutral stocks. Miss. Agric. and Forestry Exp. Stn. Res. Rep. 4 (19):4.

[30] McCarty, J.C. Jr., and J.N. Jenkins. 1992. Characteristics of 79 day-neutral primitive race accessions. Miss. Agric. and Forestry Exp. Stn. Tech. Bull. 184.

[31] McCarty, J.C., Jr., J.N. Jenkins, and B. Tang. 1995. Primitive cotton germplasm: Variation for yield and fiber traits. Miss. Agric. and Forestry Exp. Stn. Tech. Bull. 202.

[32] McCarty, J.C., Jr., J.N. Jenkins, and J. Wu. 2004. Primitive accession derived germplasm by cultivar crosses as sources for cotton improvement: I. Phenotypic values and variance components. Crop Sci. 44:1226-1230.

[33] McCarty, J.C., Jr., J.N. Jenkins, and J. Wu. 2005. Potential of primitive accessions for cotton improvement. Miss. Agric. and Forestry Exp. Stn. Tech. Bull. 1141.

[34] Meredith, W.R., Jr., and R.R. Bridge. 1971. Breakup of linkage blocks in cotton, *Gossypium hirsutum* L. Crop Sci. 11:695-698.

[35] Meredith, W.R., Jr., and R.R. Bridge. 1973. Yield, yield components and fiber property variation of cotton. (Gossypium hirsutum L.) within and among environments. Crop Sci. 13:307-312.

[36] Meredith, W.R., Jr. 1984. Quantitative genetics. p. 131-150. *In* R.J. Kohel and C.F. Lewis (ed.) Cotton. ASA, CSSA, and SSSA, Madison, WI.

[37] Meredith, W.R. Jr. 2000. Cotton yield progress –Why has it reached a plateau? Better Crops 84:6-9.

[38] Miller, P.A., and J.O. Rawlings. 1967. Breakup of initial linkage blocks through intermating in a cotton breeding program. Crop Sci. 7:199-204.

[39] Percival, A.E. 1987. The national collection of Gossypium germplasm. So. Coop. Series Bull. 321.

[40] Percy, R.G., R.G. Cantrell, and J. Zhang. 2006. Genetic variation for agronomic and fiber properties in an introgressed recombinant inbred population of cotton. Crop Sci. 46:1311- 1317.

[41] Percy, R.G., and R.J. Kohel. 1999. Qualitative genetics. p. 319-360. *In* C.W. Smith and J.T. Cothren (ed.) Cotton: Origin, history, technology, and production. John Wiley & Sons, Inc., New York.

[42] Rahman, M., D. Hussain, and Y. Zafar. 2002. Estimation of genetic divergence among elite cotton cultivars-genotypes by DNA fingerprinting technology. Crop Sci. 42:2137-2144.

[43] Saha, S., J. Wu, J.N. Jenkins, J.C. McCarty, R. Hayes, and D.M. Stelly. 2010. Genetic dissection of chromosome substitution lines of cotton to discover novel Gossypium barbadense L. alleles for improvement of agronomic traits. Theor. Appli. Genet. 120:1193-1205.

[44] Saha, S., D.M. Stelly, D.A. Raska, J.Wu, J.N. Jenkins, J.C. McCarty, A. Makamov, V. Gotmare, I.Y. Abdurakhmonov, and B.T. Campbell. 2011. Chromosome substitution lines: concept, development and utilization in the genetic improvement of Upland cotton. P. 107-128. *In* I.Y. Abdurakhmonov (ed.) Plant breeding. InTech. Slavka Krautzeka 83/A. Open Access Publisher, Croatia.

[45] Saha, S., J. Wu, J.N. Jenkins, J.C. McCarty, and D.M. Stelly. 2013. Interspecific chromosomal effects on agronomic traits in *Gossypium hirsutum* by AD analysis using intermated *G. barbadense* chromosome substitution lines. Theor. Appl. Genet. 126:109-117.

[46] Smith, C.W., and G.G. Goyle. 1997. Association of fiber quality parameters and within boll yield components in upland cotton. Crop Sci. 37:1775-1779.

[47] Smith, C.W., R.G. Cantrell, H.S. Moser, and S.R. Oakley. 1999. History of cultivar development in the United States. p. 99-171. *In* C.W. Smith and J.T. Cothren (ed.) Cotton – Origin, history, technology, and production. John Wiley & Sons, Inc. New York.

[48] Stelly, D.M, S. Saha, D.A. Raska, J.N. Jenkins, J.C. McCarty, and O.A. Gutierrez. 2005. Registration of 17 Upland (Gossypium hirsutum) germplasm lines disomic for different G. barbadense chromosome or arm substitutions. Crop Sci. 45:2663-2665.

[49] USDA-FSA, 2013. Cotton: World markets and trade. Available at http://usda01.library.cornell.edu/usda/current/cotton-market/cotton-market-04-10-2013.pdf Accessed on 10 April 2013.

[50] Van Esbroeck, G. and D.T. Bowman, 1998. Cotton germplasm diversity and its importance to cultivar development. J. Cotton Sci. 2:121-129.

[51] Worley, S., T.W. Culp, and D.C. Harrell. 1974. The relative contribution of yield components to lint yield of upland cotton, Gossypium hirsutum L. Euphytica 23:399-403.

[52] Worley, S., Jr., H.H. Ramey, Jr., D.C. Harrell, and T.W. Culp. 1976. Ontogenetic model of cotton yield. Crop Sci. 16:30-34.

[53] Wu, J., J.C. McCarty, J.N. Jenkins, and W.R. Meredith. 2010. Breeding potential of introgressions into upland cotton: genetic effects and heterosis. Plant Breeding 129:526-532.

[54] Zeng, L., W.R. Meredith, D.L. Boykin, and E. Taliercio. 2007. Evaluation of an exotic germplasm population derived from multiple crosses among *Gossypium* tetraploid species. Journal of Cotton Sci. 11:118-127.

[55] Zeng, L., and W.R. Meredith, Jr. 2009a. Associations among lint yield, yield components, and fiber properties in an introgressed population of cotton. Crop Sci. 49:1647-1654.

[56] Zeng, L., and W.R. Meredith, Jr. 2009b. Registration of five exotic germplasm lines of cotton derived from multiple crosses among Gossypium tetraploid species. J. Plant Regis. 3:77-80.

[57] Zeng, L., W.R. Meredith, Jr., and B.T. Campbell. 2010. Registration of four exotic germplasm lines derived from an introgressed population of cotton. J. Plant Regis. 4:240-243.

[58] Zeng, L., and W.R. Meredith, Jr. 2011. Relationship between SSR-based genetic distance and cotton F_2 hybrid performance for lint yield and fiber properties. Crop Sci. 51:2362-2370.

[59] Zeng, L., W.R. Meredith, and D.L. Boykin. 2011. Germplasm potential for continuing improvement of fiber quality in Upland cotton: Combing ability for lint yield and fiber quality. Crop Sci. 51:60-68.

[60] Zeng, L., and J. Wu. 2012. Germplasm for genetic improvement of lint yield in Upland cotton: genetic analysis of lint yield and yield components. Euphytica 187:247-261.

[61] Zeng, L., J. Wu, and E. Bechere. 2013. Genetic effects and genetic values of fiber properties in F2 and F3 hybrids between germplasm lines and high yield cultivars. Euphytica 190:459- 469.

[62] Zhang, J.F., Y. Liu, H. Adragna, and E. Hughs. 2005a. Genetic improvement of New Mexico Acala cotton germplasm and their genetic diversity. Crop Sci. 45:2363-2373.

[63] Zhang, J.F., Y. Liu, R.G. Cantrell, and E. Hughs. 2005b. Molecular marker diversity and field performance in commercial cotton cultivars evaluated in the southwestern USA. Crop Sci. 45:1483-1490.

[64] Zhong, M., J.C. McCarty, J.N. Jenkins, and S. Saha. 2002. Assessment of day-neutral backcross populations of cotton using AFLP markers. J. Cotton Sci. 6:97-103.

Chapter 10

Cytogenetic Collection of Uzbekistan

Marina Sanamyan, Julia Petlyakova,
Emma Rakhmatullina and Elnora Sharipova

Additional information is available at the end of the chapter

http://dx.doi.org/10.5772/58589

1. Introduction

The genetic improvement of cotton demands the use of cytogenetic stocks for molecular mapping of QTLs and introgression of beneficaila genes from wild and unadapted germplasms in Upland cotton. Development of the collection of cotton cytogenetic lines with translocations and chromosome deficiencies are necessary to fulfill these goals. During long-term studies the series of translocations and monosome stocks were developed in the USA, which provide chromosome identification and localization of marker genes on chromosomes. As the result, totally, 63 translocations were accumulated over a period of more than 20 years in USA [1-2]. The 62 heterozygous translocations were transferred to homozygous state and identified. Twenty reciprocal translocations of the cytogenetic tester set of *G. hirsutum* were selected and cytologically characterized [3,4]. This tester set of the translocations marks 25 of the 26 chromosomes of *G. hirsutum*, with chromosome 26 being identified by elimination.

Cultivated allotetraploid cotton, *G. hirsutum* (2n=52), is tolerant to the loss of individual chromosomes or their arms. During long-term investigations a big number of monosomic plants of different origin were isolated in the USA [5-9]. The majority of monosomes were found for chromosomes 2, 4 and 6 of the A-genome [10]. Unfortunately, the complete series of 26 monosomic lines in cotton have not been recovered yet. The monosomes for 15 of the 26 nonhomological chromosomes of *G. hirsutum* were identified [2]. Therefore the development of one or more deficiencies which would involve a part and/or all of these chromosomes has been high priority [11]. Use of the new molecular cytogenetic methods – meiotic fluorescence in situ hybridization (FISH) was identifed a new cotton monosome of chromosome 23 [12]. Recently, another new monosome for chromosome 21 in cotton was reported [13]. During the last years the monosomic stocks were used for chromosome assignment genetic and molecular markers to specific chromosomes [14-21].

Use of F_1 hypoaneuploid hybrids resulting from the crosses of *G. hirsutum* aneuploids (2n-1 or 2n-1/2) and *G. barbadense* L. species (2n) in molecular-genetic analyses has facilitated the localization of different molecular markers on specific cotton chromosomes [22-25]. However, some loci were not assigned using the aneuploids due to the lack of a full set of cotton aneuploids [e.g. 21, 25-27]. In the last decade chromosome-deficient stocks of *G. hirsutum* have been used for the development of chromosome substitution lines for *G. barbadense, G. tomentosum* and *G. mustelinum* chromosomes or chromosomes segment(s) [28-29].

In Uzbekistan the investigations to induce chromosome aberrations and to develop new translocation and chromosome deficient stocks were conducted during more than 30 years [30-43]. As the result 94 primary and 22 tertiary monosomics, 20 monotelodisomics, 4 mono-isodisomics, 235 reciprocal translocations as heterozygotes, 33 homozygous translocation stocks, 4 haploids and 31 desynaptic plants were discovered (Table 1). Here we report cytogenetic and morphological characteristics of the new cotton translocation and monosomic lines. We also report the results of identification of some of the lines by means translocation test.

Origin	Number of plants							
	Translocation as heterozygote	Translocation as homozygote	Primary monosomic	Tertiary monosomic	Monotelo-disomic	Monoiso-disomic	Haploid	Desy-naptic
Combine treatment	23	13						
Neutron irradiation	72	14	10	9	1		1	11
Irradiation of pollen	140	6	65	13	10	3	2	20
Desynapsis			17					
Translocation			2					
Progeny of monosomic					9	1	1	
Totals	235	33	94	22	20	4	4	31

Table 1. The origin of the different aberrations in cotton *G.hirsutum* L.

2. Materials and methods

Inbred cotton lines L-458, L-461, L-500 and L-501 (*Gossypium hirsutum L.)* from the Genetic Collection of the National University of Uzbekistan were used for producing cytogenetic stock series. Three types of radiations were applied – combined treatment of colchicine and gamma rays (A) of the seeds, irradiation of seeds by thermal neutrons (B) and pollen gamma irradiation rays (C). The seeds of the hybrids F_0 (L-500 x L-461) were treated with 0.1% aqueous colchicines solution for 2 h, washed with water and irradiated with CO^{60} gamma-radiation at 50 and 100 Gy. The seeds used in this study were of the M_0 generation.

The irradiation of pollen by gamma rays was carried out in Institute of Silk research. The flowers of cotton line L-458 were emasculated a day before flowering and enclosed in parchment bags to prevent accidental crosspollination and in flowering stage the flowers with mature pollen were collected and irradiated with 10, 15, 20 and 25 Gy gamma radiation (Co^{60}). The irradiated pollen used to pollinate the emasculated flowers.

The neutron irradiation of cotton line L-458 seeds was carried out at the biological channel of the WW-SM reactor using doses of 15, 25, 27 and 35 Gy (Institute of Nuclear Physics of the Academy Sciences of the Republik of Uzbekistan, Tashkent). The seeds of M_0 generation were grown in same field condition. The M_1 plants were studied and used to raised the M_2 generation. The M_2 plants were grown in a field and investigated for chromosomal aberrations using cytological techniques.

The primary monosomics from our collection were numbered from Mo1 to Mo94 in the order of their detection. Transmission of the monosomics was studied in selfing and outcrossing progenies of monosomic plants both in the greenhouse and in the field. Translocation and monosomic lines were identified. Hybrids between translocation and monosomic lines were analyzed to identify 2n and 2n-1 translocation heterozygotes, respectively. Meiotic chromosomes were studied using the standard acetocarmine-squash technique [30].

3. Cytological analysis

The chromosome pairing at metaphase I of meiosis was studied. The calyx and corolla were removed and floral buds were fixed overnight in 96% alcohol and acetic acid (7:3). Buds were kept at room temperature for 3 days, immersed in fresh fixative and stored in a refrigerator. They were examined for meiotic associations in the pollen mother cells (PMCs) using iron acetocarmine squash technique [30]. The analysis of chromosomal changes was carried out on the basis of M I associations at the first meiosis. The development of PMCs was examined at the tetrad stage for each plant. The meiotic index was calculated as the percentage of tetrads whereas pollen fertility was estimated by acetocarmine staining.

4. Results

4.1. Reciprocal translocations

Reciprocal translocations were formed as segmental interchanges among two or more nonhomologous chromosomes. The exposure of seeds to three types of irradiation has resulted in the induction of translocations in 235 cotton plants [31, 32, 34, 37]. After different treatment of irradiation translocation plants were obtained in the M_1, M_2 and M_3 generations (Tables 2). They included exchanges between two different pairs chromosomes, translocations among three pair chromosomes and complex exchanges. Three types of the irradiation treatment were characterized by differences of the frequency and spectrum of the translocations. The treatment of seeds with combined colchicines and gamma-rays resulted 25 disomic plants with two or more translocations in the M_1 generation, with two, or even four multivalent configurations per PMCs in different plants. The unaffected plants from M_2 generation, a further 22 disomic plant with a number multivalents were detected. Progeny from different branches and bolls of one and the same parents was kept separate. Some of the parents were chimeras and as it was expected and subsequently confirmed, that different bolls from one and the same parent would give different result. From the meiosis, M_3 progenies were only recovered in which there was just one multivalent per PMC. Therefore, 23 translocations obtained in the M_3 generation were listed in the Table 1. In comparison to the single irradiation the combined irradiation treatment was most effective for producing the highest number of single as well as complex translocations in a number of meiocytes.

Treatment	Dose of irradiation (Gy)	Number of translocation heterozygotes			Translocation lines
		M_1	M_2	M_3	
Combined treatment of seeds by colchicine and gamma-rays	50	19	19	19	Tr1-Tr11, Tr25, Tr26
	100	6	3	4	0
Subtotal		25	22	23	13
Irradiation of seeds by thermal neutrons	1,3	1	0	0	0
	15	8	11	-	Tr17-Tr19, Tr22, Tr27, Tr30
	25	9	7	-	Tr20, Tr21
	27	7	8	10	Tr15, Tr16, Tr28, Tr31, Tr33
	35	6	5	-	Tr29
Subtotal		31	31	10	14
Irradiation of pollen by gamma-rays	10	3	9	13	0
	15	9	13	7	Tr12
	20	16	20	12	Tr13, Tr14
	25	25	10	3	Tr23, Tr24, Tr32
Subtotal		53	52	35	6

Table 2. The origin of the reciprocal translocations in cotton *G. hirsutum* L.

Irradiation of seeds by thermal neutrons induced 31 translocations in the M_1, 31 plants with interchanges in the M_2 and 10 - in M_3 generation (Table 2). Only four plants were recorded with complex translocations per PMC in the M_1 generation (Figure 1). Other translocations involved to two nonhomologous chromosomes (Figure 2) and four – of three chromosomes. Moreover, the concurrent appearance of the two chromosomal aberrations causing and inducing chromosomal deficiencies and rearrangements, was also detected. The highest number of the chromosome changes occurred from the thermal neutron and unique chromosomal aberrations such as complex of the interchanges on PMS, multiple translocations involving up to three nonhomological chromosomes.

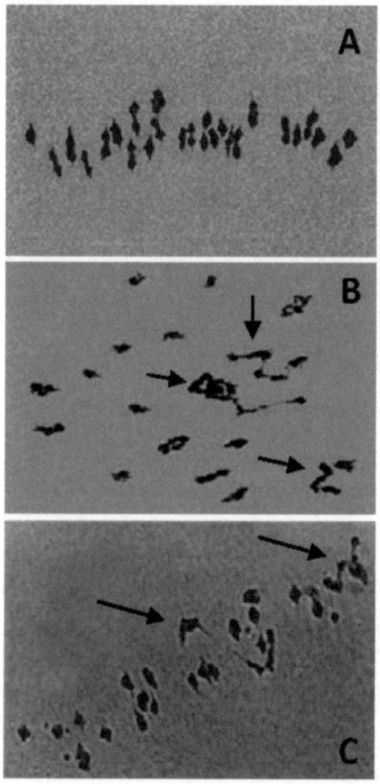

Figure 1. Meiotic configurations in translocation heterozygotes in cotton *G. hirsutum* obtained after irradiation of the seeds by thermal neutrons in M_1. (A) Meiotic metaphase I cell showing 26 bivalents in control plant. (B) Meiotic metaphase I cell showing 19 bivalents and 2 quadrivalents and 1 hexavalent in plant 364/10. (C) Meiotic metaphase I cell showing 21 bivalents and 1 quadrivalent and 1 hexavalent in plant 364/10. The arrows point to the quadrivalents and hexavalent. Note that the background of figures was cleaned using Adobe Photoshop CSS extended version 12

Moreover, such rare mutations induced have not been observed earlier in experiments with other treatments. Such rare mutations were cluster fruiting habit for translocation (Tr18-Figure 10 C, F), reduced stigma (Mo62-Figure 18 C), cytoplasmic mutation virescent simultaneous with translocation (Tr28), unique desinaptic plant, pollen semisterility in homozygous stock (Tr21). It is also notable that one of the translocation plant $1475/30_4$ had also a clear phenotypic character with cytoplasmatic mutation of yellow-green color of the leaf. This finding indicates the simultaneous appearance of chlorophyll deficiency and the chromosome translocation in a single plant. These specific mutations were not frequent, but they were specific for the thermal neutron irradiation and very important for cotton genetics as new genetic markers.

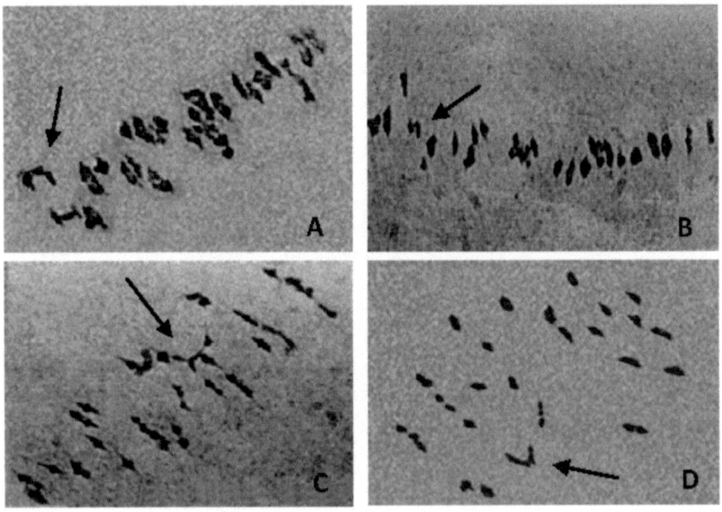

Figure 2. Meiotic configurations in translocation heterozygotes in cotton *G. hirsutum* obtained after irradiation of the seeds by thermal neutrons in M_3. Meiotic metaphase I cells showing 24 bivalents and 1 quadrivalent: in plant 1475/7_1-13 (A and B); (C) 1474/15_4-6; (D) 361/4-$b1_3$. The arrows point to the quadrivalents. Note that the background of figures was cleaned using Adobe Photoshop CSS extended version 12.

A similar analysis of chromosome aberrations showed that gamma-irradiation of pollen resulted in 53 translocations in the M_1 out of 331 studied plants, 52 plants with interchanges in the M_2 out of 348 Studied plants and 35 - in the M_3 generation out of 211 studied plants (Table 2). All translocations were involving of two nonhomologous chromosomes formed quadrivalent associations (Figure 3). Three translocations were involving of three chromosomes formed hexavalent associations. There were no PMCs with more than one multivalent among translocation plants after pollen irradiation. The greatest number of translocation plants with medium and high frequency (58.14%) was found in experiments with irradiation at 20 and 25 Gy. In comparison to the other irradiation the gamma-irradiation of pollen was the most effective for producing more different deficiencies.

Comparison of the mean frequency of multivalent per cell between translocations obtained in the M_1, M_2 and M_3 generations after irradiation suggests that the highest number (26,42%) of interchanges with a high average number of multivalent at the MI of meiosis occurred in the M_1 generation. M_2 and M_3 progenies had more normal karyotypes than that seen in the M_1 plants and translocations with a high frequency of multivalent were uncommen in next generations. Those translocations, integrated into this collection from homozygous translocation lines.

Among 235 translocations, 224 involved two chromosomes but only 11 involved three nonhomologous chromosomes. Different types of multivalent configurations were found with

http://dx.doi.org/10.5772/58589

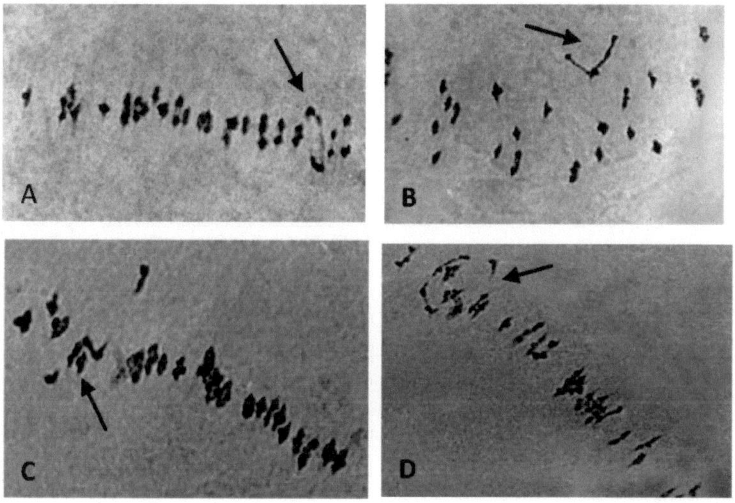

Figure 3. Meiotic configurations in translocation heterozygotes in cotton *G. hirsutum* obtained after pollen irradiation in M_2 and M_3. Meiotic metaphase I cells showing 24 bivalents and 1 quadrivalent in plant (A) $1069/10_1$; (B) $1568/21_{10}$; (C) $188/4_4$-3; (D) $187/3_{10}$-12. The arrows point to the quadrivalents. Note that the background of figures was cleaned using Adobe Photoshop CSS extended version 12.

alternate and adjacent orientations. The translocations were characterized by different frequencies of the multivalents at the MI of meiosis. Translocations with the large translocated chromosome segments are of greatest interest for tagging cotton chromosomes and developing new homozygous translocation lines. Electron microscopy of synaptonemal complexes at the pachytene stage revealed more cells with heterozygous chromosomal rearrangements than light microscopy at meiotic MI by a factor of 1.8 [44]. Those results indicate that the different frequencies of multivalents in heterozygotes for translocations at MI result from partial desynapsis and segregation of translocation multivalents into two "heteromorph " bivalents, which cannot be distinguished from normal bivalents at meiotic MI by light microscopy.

The analyses of tetrads were carried out in 201 translocations. Most of the translocations (76.41%) exhibited a high meiotic index (90-100%) when compared with the control (94.52±0.26). However, 20.51% translocations were characterized by a reduction in meiotic index (to 80.0%) and an increase in the percentage of tetrads with micronuclei when compared with the control (1.29±0.13%). Six translocations were characterized with a low meiotic index (from 52.15±1.99 to 79.37±1.32%) and number of abnormal tetrads containing micronuclei (from 16.53±1.48 to 3.66±0.53%).

The distribution of pollen fertility for 189 translocations is summarized in Figure 4. Pollen fertility was estimated by acetocarmine staining. Although the acetocarmine-based pollen fertility considered relatively insensitive method, it is widely used for preliminary screening of pollen quality in plants. The pollen fertility of translocations varied significantly from high fertility (70-100%) for 113 translocations, to semi-sterility (40-69.9%) for 35 translocations, and to low fertility (to 39.9%) for 23 translocations when compared with the control (96.99±0.44%).

In 19 translocations, pollen fertility varied between flowers of one and the same plant and 11 translocations were characterized by pollen sterility. On the whole, the high frequency of abortive pollen grains in flowers was typical for 48.5% of the translocations studied.

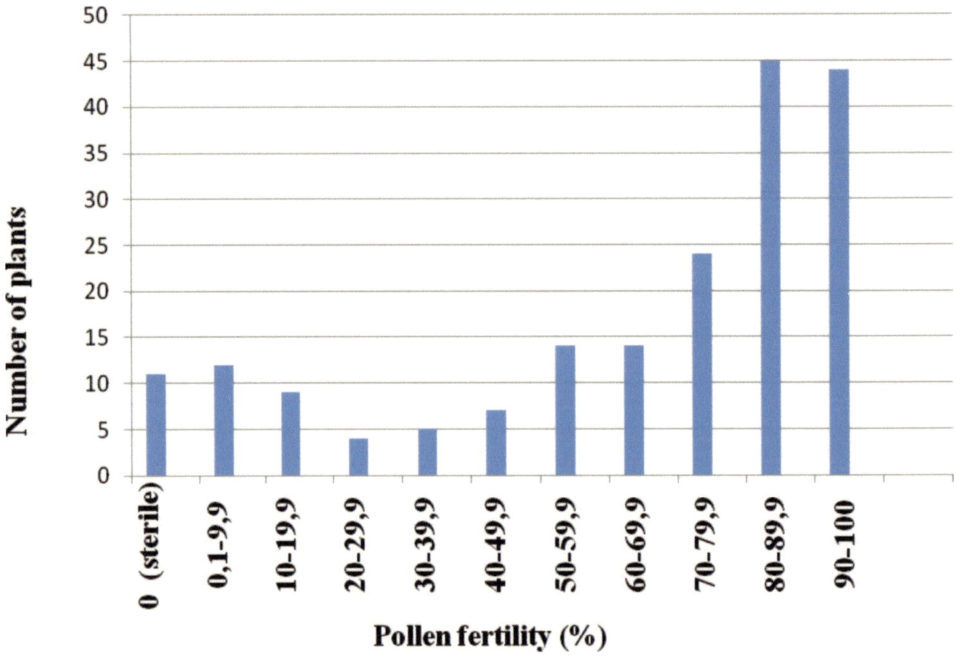

Note: the remaining 19 translocations were not included in the histogram due to their varied pollen fertility level in different flowers and 4 plants were complex interchanges.

Figure 4. Percentage distribution of pollen fertility for 189 reciprocal translocations in cotton

This broad variability of pollen fertility in the plants with interchromosomal exchanges hampers using this trait as a marker of heterozygosity for exchanges in cotton, in contrast to species of *Pisum, Zea, Sorghum*, and *Petunia*. Heterozygosity for translocations in these species is always accompanied by half-sterile pollen because of equal probabilities of ring-shaped and zigzag-shaped quadrivalent orientation. In addition, the detection of complete male and female sterility in some cotton translocants suggested that exactly the translocations were responsible for their sterility so far as these translocation plants did not produce any seed sets from self-pollination and intercrossing. Apparently, short translocated segments involved vital chromosome domains, whose rearrangements induced to abortive gametes.

Different techniques have been employed for isolating plants homozygous for the translocations [45]. Common methods have been used in maize and barley [46]. To identify homozygous, self the plants with normal pollen crossed to a standard normal line. If the normal being tested were homozygous for the translocation, all the F_1 hybrid plants should be partially sterile. A technique for quick isolation of translocation homozygotes that not require of the

http://dx.doi.org/10.5772/58589

analysis pollen fertility into account was also worked out. This character has been varied in the cotton translocation heterozygotes from high up to pollen sterility and cannot be used the marker characteristic. Such techniques allowed us to isolate the number of different translocation homozygotes in progeny of one and the same parent containing two or more interchanges per PMC.

Translocations have been confirmed as homozygous after cytogenetic studies from self-pollination progenies of the heterozygotes according to the scheme (Figure 5). Heterozygotes were selfed and progeny from each plant was examined at the metaphase I of meiosis. The plant that exhibited normal pairing were backcrossed to the control line L-458 in order to identify the plants homozygous for the translocations and the F_1BC_1 progeny was examined at the metaphase I of meiosis for the presence of multivalents. F_1BC_1 plants with multivalents pointed out homozygous for the translocation under consideration. As a result 33 new homozygous translocation stocks were isolated among those, 13 new translocation stocks of cotton (Tr1-Tr11, Tr25 and Tr26) were obtained in the combined treatment of seeds with colchicine and γ-rays hybrid progeny L-500 x L-461, one stock (Tr12) – in the pollen γ-irradiation hybrid progeny L-461 x L-501, while the others-from irradiation of seeds by thermal neutrons highly inbred line L-458.

In the progeny of the translocation heterozygotes, the deviations were found from the 1:2:3 ratio with a deficit of different types of plants. The latter can be explained by time limitation of examining plants or low viability by some types of progeny. So, it was not possible to establish one translocation (1020_1-9) in the homozygous condition because only heterozygotes and normal plants detected in progeny. Probably, it can be attributed to localization of the breakpoints in the region of the chromosome, which cannot be reconstructed. As it was discussed earlier for 28 of the 34 translocation lines in barley, homozygous plants were available, although one translocation – C 951 was not identified in the homozygous condition [47].

Translocation lines from our collection were numbered from Tr1 to Tr33 in the order of their detection. Thirty one translocations were simple reciprocal interchanges, involving only two nonhomologous chromosomes, whereas the two remaining (Tr2 and Tr20) were interchanges involving three non-homologous chromosomes. Translocation lines were characterized by normal pairing at metaphase I of meiosis with 26 bivalents and high meiotic index (from 90.73±0.33 for Tr24 to 98.05±0.19 for Tr22). The pollen fertility was also high (from 90.06±0.77% for Tr15 to 98.28±0.18 for Tr18) with the exception of Tr21 that was distinguished with a essential decrease in pollen fertility (to 66.01±1.28%). For the first time such semisterility of the pollen was detected in the cotton plants homozygous for the translocation. Such differences can be explained by heterogeneous translocations.

Subgenome assignment of the translocation was carried out with using hybrid DD-subgenome (F_1 *G. thurberi x G. raimondii).* Three types of modal configurations are expected at metaphase I of meiosis in the triploid hybrids [48]. Translocations being involving two A-subgenome chromosomes will have not A homoeologues in the triploid hybrid and showed modal chromosome configurations – 13 (DD) bivalents and 13 (A) univalents; translocations being involving two DD-subgenome chromosomes – 11 (DD) bivalents and 13 (A) univalents and one (DDDD) quadrivalent; translocations being involving AD-subgenome chromosomes – 12 (DD) bivalents and 12 (A) univalents and one (ADD) trivalent. Tests involved many translocation lines but results were obtained for 5 lines only.

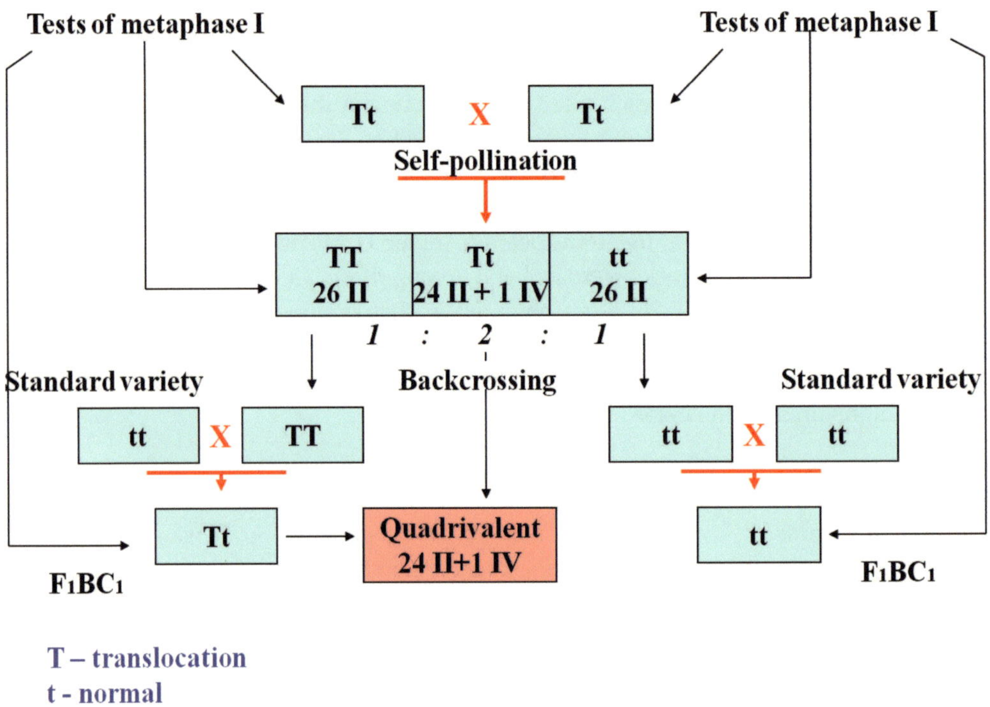

Figure 5. Scheme of the technique used for the isolation of translocation homozygous lines (further explanations noted in the text)

Translocation lines Tr1, Tr7, Tr8 and Tr16 had AA-subgenome location translocated chromosomes because their triploid hybrids shown modal configurations 13 DD-bivalents and 13-A univalents (Figure 6). Translocation line Tr2 is interchange which involves three non-homologous chromosomes. Their triploid hybrid characterized 11 univalents and 12 bivalents and one quadrivalent that pointed out on two A-subgenome and one D-subgenome location chromosomes.

Identification of translocation homozygotes from our collection was carried out using double translocation heterozygotes obtained after intercrossing translocation plants [1]. Modal chromosome configurations at metaphase I of meiosis – 21 bivalents (II)+1 quadrivalent (IV)+1 hexavalent (VI) and 22 bivalents (II)+2 quadrivalents (IV) showed the involvement the different chromosomes, modal chromosome configurations – 22 bivalents (II)+1 oktavalent (VIII) and 23 bivalents (II)+1 hexavalent (VI) indicated the chromosome in common and modal chromosome configurations – 26 bivalents (II) indicated the involvement of the same arms of the two homological chromosomes. It is important to note that translocation lines Tr2 and Tr20 showed multivalents in hybrids because of involving the translocations among three non-homologous chromosomes. With respect to the crosses between translocation lines Tr7, Tr8 and Tr9 in which the M_1 parent plant was formed of several quadrivalents in the same meiocyte, three types were present in homozygote giving rise to the three translocation lines. The data indicated that Tr7 and Tr8 involved the same two non-homological chromosomes, but Tr7 and Tr8 on the one hand and Tr9 on the other hand are different chromosomes.

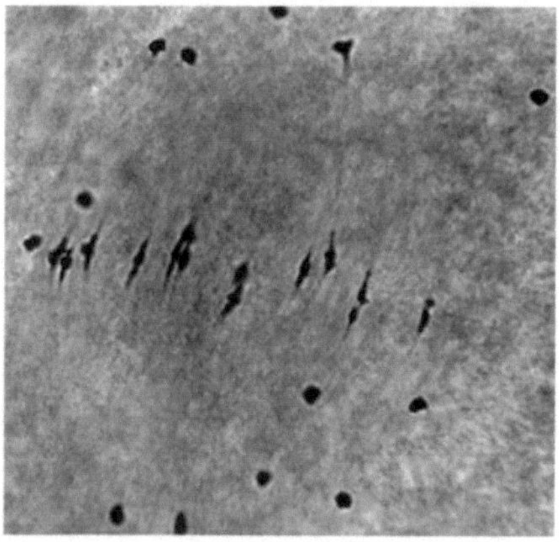

Figure 6. Meiotic configuration in hybrid from crossing the translocation line Tr 16 and hybrid F_1 (*G. thurberi x G. raimondii*). Meiotic metaphase I cells showing 13 univalents and 13 bivalents. Note that the background of figures was cleaned using Adobe Photoshop CSS extended version 12.

The differences were found between translocation stocks both in the number of hybrids and the number of common chromosomes in the translocations in our investigation. Thus, the translocation lines Tr7, Tr8, Tr14, Tr16 and Tr27 showed more common chromosomes, whereas other lines-Tr1, Tr18, Tr20, Tr21, Tr23 and Tr26 showed uncommon ones. From these data it is observed that chromosomes in the translocations Tr7, Tr8, Tr14, Tr16 and Tr27 were more frequently involved in chromosome translocations, but chromosomes from the translocations lines-Tr1, Tr18, Tr20, Tr21, Tr23 and Tr26 were less frequently involved in translocations (Figure 7). On the base of rare occurrence the chromosomes in common in the hybrid involved Tr1 and Tr20 translocation stocks (two and one, respectively) it was shown that these stocks have translocated chromosomes that were rare involving into interchanges. Thus, when Tr1 stock was crossed with Tr2 and Tr20 the ring consisting of 8 chromosomes was observed in both hybrids showing that Tr1 stock has interchanged chromosomes in common with Tr2 and Tr20 stocks. However, the crosses between Tr2 and Tr20 stock detected two rings consisting of six chromosomes that pointed out the involvement unique chromosome pair in Tr1 and Tr20. Preliminary chromosome numeration in the interchanges pointed out the involvement about 50% chromosome set into reciprocal translocations in 27 studied translocation stock from our collection.

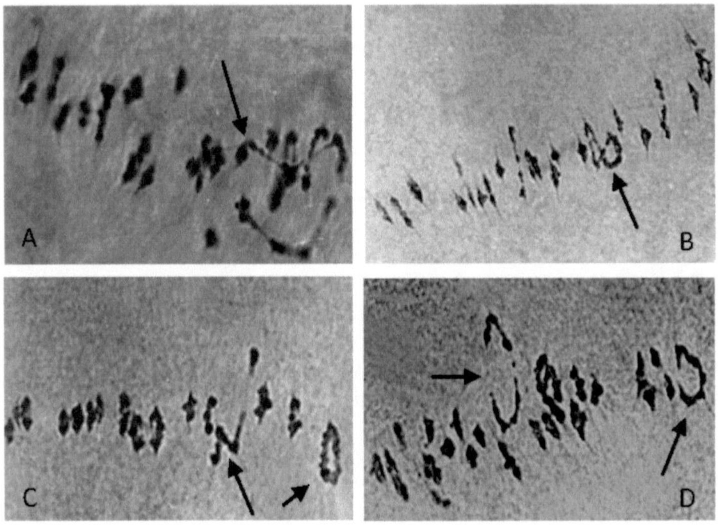

Figure 7. "Critical configurations" of the chromosomes at the meiotic metaphase I cells in cotton F_1 plants from crosses the different translocation lines: (A) Tr2 x Tr16 (22 II+1 VIII); (B) Tr8 x Tr6 (23 II+1 VI); (C) Tr1 x Tr23 (22 II+2 IV); (D) Tr15 x Tr10 (22 II+2 IV). The arrows point to the quadrivalents, hexavalent and oktavalent. Note that the background of figures was cleaned using Adobe Photoshop CSS extended version 12.

Moreover, translocation lines are different in morphological characters. 13 new translocation stocks of cotton *G. hirsutum* (Tr1-Tr11, Tr25 and Tr26) were obtained from the hybrid progeny (L-500 x L-461) after combine treatment, where two parent lines (L-500 and L-461) distinguished by leaf shape. 6 translocation lines (Tr1, Tr2, Tr4, Tr6, Tr9 and Tr26) have leaves palmate, such as 7 lines (Tr3, Tr5, Tr7, Tr8, Tr10, Tr11 and Tr25) – lanceolate (super okra) (Fig. 8). Moreover, translocation line Tr10 be showed dense growth and bract type "frego" (Fig. 8 and 10 B). Line Tr12 have compact grow, small round leaves and small spherical boll (Figure 8).

The other 19 translocation lines were obtained by the irradiation of the seeds line L-458 of the thermal neutrons (Figure 9).

The line Tr18 was characterized by compact grow, a dense stem pubescence, cluster flowers and bolls and absent of stigma protrusion over the staminate column (Fig.10 A, C, D, F). The line Tr23 differed by dense stem of pubescence. Tr28 line demonstrated yellow color of the leaf resulted from simultaneous cytoplasmic mutation type virescent. Moreover, Tr28 line showed difference in absence of external nectarines (Fig 10 E). Thus, it was shown that chromosome translocations had a specific influence in plant morphology and that some of translocations distinguished unique marker characters (Figure 10).

Final conclusions cannot be drawn without further cytogenetical studies to identify the chromosomes involved in the translocations. It is quite evident that translocation stocks of our collection may be used for marking cotton chromosome, for the identification of the monosomes and other chromosomal aberrations.

http://dx.doi.org/10.5772/58589

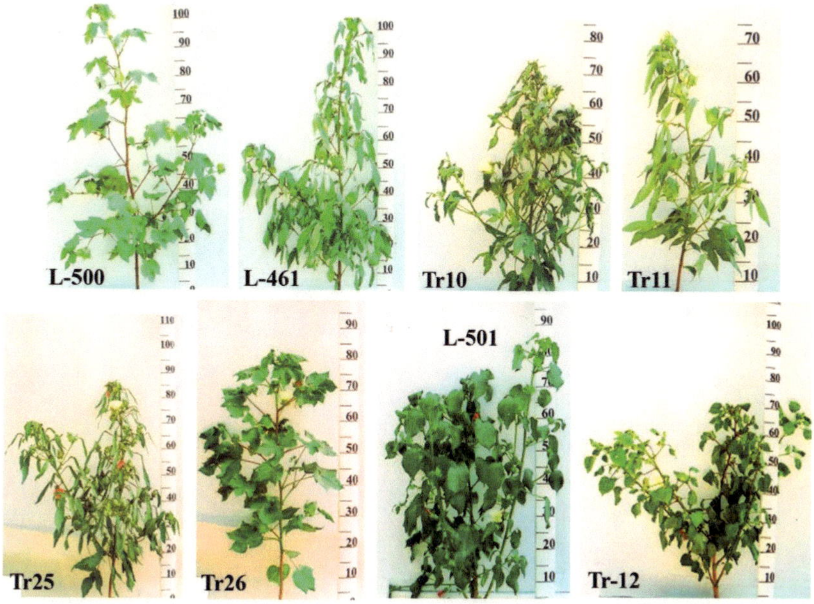

Figure 8. Some examples of morphology of cotton translocation lines (Tr10, Tr11, Tr25, Tr26, Tr12) compared to original parental lines (L-500, L-461, L-501).

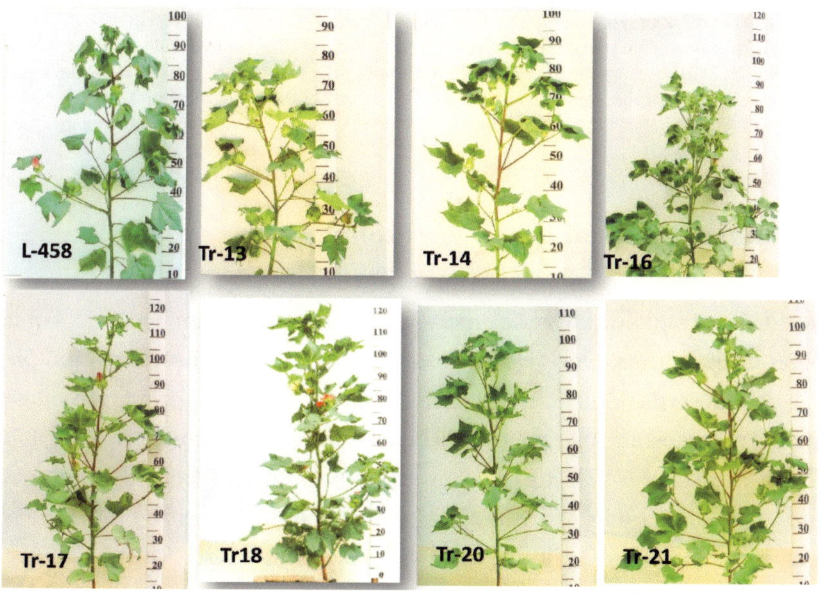

Figure 9. Some examples of morphology of cotton translocation lines (Tr13, Tr14, Tr16, Tr17, Tr18, Tr20, Tr21) compared to original parental line (L-458).

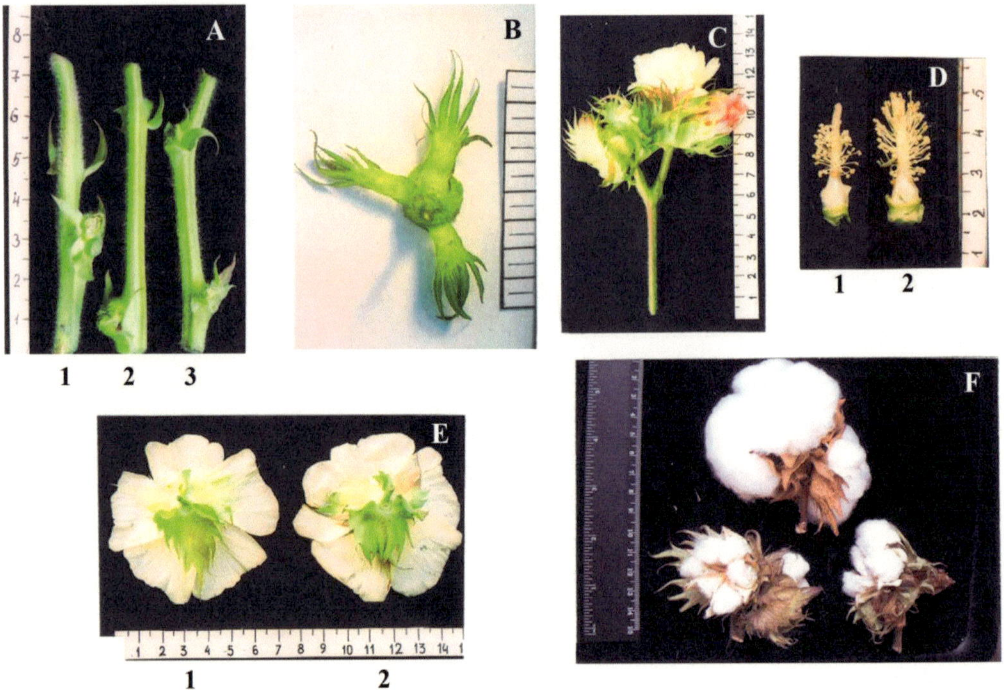

Figure 10. Some unique morphologic characters of the translocation lines: (A) a dense stem pubescence of the translocation lines Tr18 (1) and Tr23 (3) in comparison with parental line L-458 (2); (B) bract type "frego" of the translocation line Tr10; (C) cluster flowers in translocation line Tr18; (D) absent of stigma protrusion over the staminate column in translocation line Tr18 (2) in comparison with parental line L-458 (1); (E) absence of external nectarines in translocation line Tr28 (1) in comparison with parental line L-458 (2); (F) cluster bolls in translocation line Tr18.

5. Primary monosomics of the *G. hirsutum* L.

The cultivated allotetraploid cotton, *G. hirsutum* (2n=52), was tolerant to the loss of individual chromosomes or their arms. One of chromosome missing in monosomic cotton plant which has only 51 chromosoms. Meiotic metaphase I analysis of cotton primary monosomics are revealed modal chromosome pairing with 25 bivalents and univalent. Between 1987 and 2010, we developed a total of 94 *G. hirsutum* primary monosomics from the common genetic background of the highly inbred line L-458 after irradiation of seeds by thermal neutrons or pollen gamma-irradiation directly in M_1, M_2 and M_3 generations. Most of them (75 of 94) observed from the two irradiation types directly in M_1, M_2 and M_3 generations. The remaining 19 monosomic plants resulted from chromosome aberrant progenies (desynapsis and interchanges). Most of the primary monosomics (34) were induced in the M_1 generation as a result of pollen γ-irradiation by doses of 10, 15, 20 and 25 Gy (Table 3).

Treatment	Dose of irradiation (Gy)	Number of primary monosomics			Monosomic lines
		M_1	M_2	M_3	
Irradiation of seeds by thermal neutrons	1,3	0	0	0	-
	15	3	1	0	Mo58, Mo59, Mo60, Mo74
	25	0	1	0	-
	27	0	1	2	Mo1
	35	1	2	0	Mo56, Mo62
Total		4	5	2	7
Irradiation of pollen by gamma-rays	10	5	4	3	Mo10, Mo39, Mo40, Mo41, Mo50, Mo81, Mo82
	15	4	9	1	Mo3, Mo31, Mo53, Mo78
	20	11	8	4	Mo4, Mo7, Mo11, Mo22, Mo27, Mo28, Mo34, Mo35, Mo36, Mo66, Mo75, Mo90
	25	14	3	0	Mo9, Mo13, Mo15, Mo16, Mo17, Mo19, Mo38, Mo46, Mo48, Mo76, Mo77
Totals		34	24	7	34

Table 3. The origin of the cotton primary monosomics *G. hirsutum* L.

Seven of the monosomic plants had simultaneously independent chromosome interchanges so far as these shown both quadrivalent and univalent in MI meiosis. More than 70% of M_1 primary monosomics (25 of 34), were induced by high doses of pollen irradiation (20 – 25 Gy) (Table 3). The number of monosomics detected declined in subsequent generations (24 and 7, respectively), and one M_3 monosomic (Mo54) also displayed heterozygous translocation (Figure 11). A specific feature of the pollination with irradiated pollen of cotton was a lot of genomic mutations such as chromosome deficiencies, chromosome arm deficiencies (22.51%) in comparison with the neutron irradiation (16.85%). The latter resulted from elimination of whole chromosomes, chromosome arms, or even the complete paternal genome and yielded monosomic, monotelodisomic, and haploid plants.

Similar analysis of cotton plants from seed irradiation with thermal neutrons at doses of 15, 25, 27 and 35 Gy revealed fewer primary monosomics. After irradiation only 11 plants from three generations out of 335 studied plants were detected, moreover four of them were also interchanged heterozygotes. In M_1 generation there were only 4 chromosome deficient plants, 3 of them from the dose of 15 Gy and one from the 35 Gy. Similarly 5 monosomic plants were isolated in M_2 generation in all 4 doses, and two monosomic plants were identified from M_3 (Figure 12).

An addition to traditional radiation-induced cotton monosomics, we used the desynaptic effect which have been found to be a useful source of aneuploidy in other crops. Although desynaptic plants in different crops are usually sterile or show extremely low fertility, the desynaptic

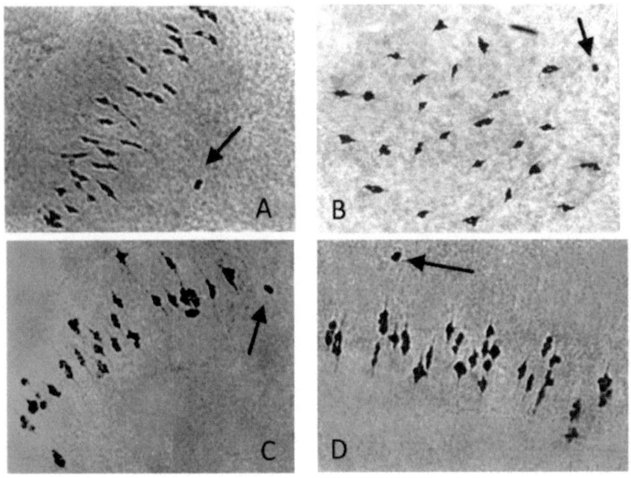

Figure 11. Meiotic configurations in primary monosomics in cotton *G. hirsutum* obtained after pollen irradiation in M_1 and M_2. Meiotic metaphase I cells showing 25 bivalents and 1 univalent in plant (A) 1596/5; (B) 161/1; (C) 199/4_2 ; (D) 186/12_5.. Note that the background of figures was cleaned using Adobe Photoshop CSS extended version 12.

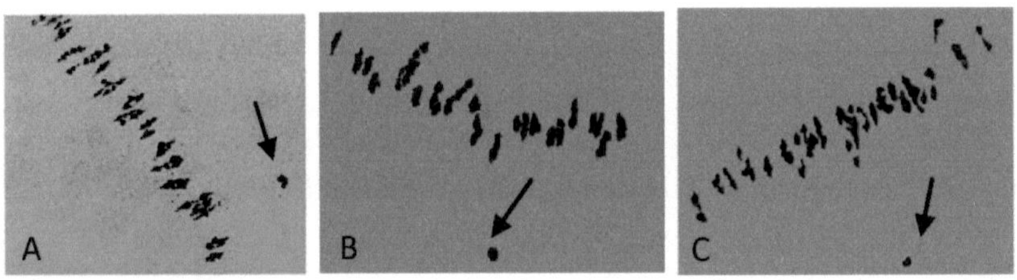

Figure 12. Meiotic configurations in primary monosomics in cotton *G. hirsutum* obtained irradiation of the seeds by thermal neutrons in M_1, M_2 and M_3 generations. Meiotic metaphase I cells showing 25 bivalents and 1 univalent in plant (A) 1474/28_{10}-1 ; (B) 359/9; (C) 368/4_1. The arrows point to the univalents. Note that the background of figures was cleaned using Adobe Photoshop CSS extended version 12.

cotton plant 1063/6_3-13 had semisterile pollen due to different number of unpaired univalents (from 2 to 28) in different PMCs. Desynapsis level was estimated as intermediate. Other six desynaptic plants were characterized with weak desynapsis level and formed from 2 to 14 univalents. As a result, 17 primary monosomics were isolated from the progenies of 7 desynaptic plants and one unexamined plant from the desynaptic plant progeny (Table 4).

All the initial desynaptic plants differed by their number of unpaired chromosomes (from 2 to 28 univalents). Disruptions in unpaired chromosome disjunction led to a random univalent distribution between the cell division poles, forming numerous tetrads with micronuclei (to 13.42±0.87%), lowering of meiotic index (to 75.07±1.11% in 356/8 desynaptic plant), and pollen fertility reduction to semisterility (61.35±2.43%). Meiotic index is a normal tetrad percentage and an indicator of meiotic stability, which proposed by Love [49] for evaluation of meiosis in wheat. We observed that pollen fertility was varied among the flowers on the same plant (from 2.61±1.27% to 91.81±1.18% in 179/2 desynaptic plant; Table 4).

Material	Mo	Chromosome number	Total number of cells	Chromosome associations			Pollen fertility	
				Number of univalents	Frequency of chromosome associations (in average per cell) univalents	bivalents	Total number of pollen grains	Fertility, (%)
$1609/6_6$-DPP		52	60	2-12	4.77±0.48	23.62±0.24	656	70.12±1.79
$1609/6_6$-22	Mo55	51	22	1-3	1.45±0.18	24.77±0.09	466	93.99±1.10
$1609/6_6$-4	Mo69	51	33	1	1.00±0.00	25.00±0.00	499	98.27±0.58
$1063/6_3$-13-DPP		52	42	2-28	14.33±0.9	18.83±0.45	405	65.68±2.36
$1063/6_3$-13_3	Mo70	51	25	1-3	1.08±0.08	24.96±0.04	639	95.15±0.85
$1063/6_3$-13_4	Mo71	51	24	1	1.00±0.00	25.00±0.00	352	96.02±1.04
$1063/6_3$-13_5	Mo72	51	21	1	1.00±0.00	25.00±0.00	632	96.87±0.69
$1063/6_3$-13_6	Mo73	51	30	1-3	1.47±0.15	24.77±0.08	612	98.53±0.49
$1570/14_9$-3-DPP		52	42	2-8	2.43±0.31	24.79±0.15	440	94.09±1.12
$1570/14_9$-3_{18}	Mo78	51	18	1	1.00±0.00	25.00±0.00	-	-
$1570/14_9$-13-DPP		52	15	2-6	2.67±0.46	24.67±0.23	467	95.29±0.98
$1570/14_9$-13_7	Mo85	51	16	1	1.00±0.00	25.00±0.00	984	97.97±0.45
179/2-DPP		52	32	2-8	2.50±0.37	24.75±0.19	157-537	2.61±1.27-91.81±1.18
$179/2_{12}$	Mo87	51	20	1	1.00±0.00	25.00±0.00	217-693	40.09±3.33-92.93±0.97
356/8-DPP		52	18	2	1.67±0.18	25.17±0.09	401	61.35±2.43
$356/8_5$	Mo58	51	33	1-3	1.12±0.08	24.94±0.04	685	81.02±1.50
$356/8_6$	Mo59	51	24	1	1.00±0.00	25.00±0.00	222-1292	2.25±1.00-70.12±1.27
$356/8_7$	Mo60	51	22	1	1.00±0.00	25.00±0.00	307	38.44±2.78
$356/8_8$-unknown kariotype		-	-	-	-	-	452	53.98±2.34
$356/8_8$-14	Mo79	51	22	1	1.00±0.00	25.00±0.00	666	92.94±0.99
$356/8_8$-15	Mo80	51	20	1	1.00±0.00	25.00±0.00	447	99.78±0.22
$356/8_8$-5	Mo84	51	39	1-3	1.41±0.13	24.79±0.07	322	98.14±0.75
$356/8_8$-2	Mo91	51	19	1-3	1.11±0.11	24.95±0.05	65-726	53.85±6.18-89.81±1.12
$1067/9_3$-2_6-DPP		52	10	2-14	7.80±1.38	22.10±0.69	-	-
$1067/9_3$-2_{22}	Mo89	51	44	1-3	1.09±0.06	24.95±0.03	1145	97.64±0.45

Table 4. Chromosome pairing at metaphase I observed in PMCs and pollen fertility in the cotton desynaptic parental (DPPs) and their monosomics (Mo) progenies. Bold faced rows are parental desynaptic plants.

One unique desynaptic plant-356/8 (row number/plant number in M_1 generation in field) was observed from the desynaptic progenies studies. This plant produced monosomics in high frequency with a small size of univalents and strong phenotypic differences, suggesting monosomy for different chromosomes of cotton genome. In previous we identified two new monosomics (Mo30 and Mo67) using progeny of translocation plants [33].

Meiotic metaphase I analysis of 94 cotton primary monosomics showed modal chromosome pairing with 25 bivalents and univalent in 38 plants. Fifty monosomic plants were characterized with the presence of additional univalents side by side bivalents. Thus, in 34 monosomics, the formation of three univalents in some PMCs was observed due to lack of pairing of single pair of chromosomes. Three monosomics formed five univalents in some PMCs suggesting the absence of pairing in two chromosome pairs. Another five monosomics were characterized with the presence of unpaired chromosomes in 20 – 30% PMCs. In 8 chromosome deficient plants, a strong desynaptic effect was detected as they formed from 3 to 11 univalents in 40 – 60% PMCs studied. None of the studied PMCs in the monosomic plant Mo52 revealed normal chromosome pairing because it characterized with the presence of 3 to 15 univalents. The variation in the number of univalents could be explained by different expression of synaptic genes in different cells [44]. Later, disomic desynaptic plants were found in the progeny of two plants, which produced up to 52 univalents in PMCs. This finding confirmed our hypothesis of independent parallel mutations in desynaptic genes of original plants.

Some of monosomic plants showed (Mo6, Mo7, Mo19, Mo30, Mo56, Mo61, and Mo62) univalents, bivalents and trivalents (from 0.04 ± 0.04 to 0.12 ± 0.06 in average per cell) formed at metaphase-I of meiosis. Those results suggested association of univalent with two homeologous chromosomes. Such trivalents formed by pairing of homologous chromosomes were also found in other monosomic plants [50]. Moreover, two of them (Mo56 and Mo61) were also characterized with additional univalents. The other 12 cotton primary monosomics showed quadrivalent associations with different frequencies suggesting heterozygosity for their translocation. Analysis of the sizes of monosomes revealed medium univalent size in 44 monosomics (Fig. 13 C, D); whereas there were 22 monosomics with large univalents (Fig. 13 A, B). The number of monosomics having small univalents was slightly higher (27); moreover, among these, 6 monosomics with very small univalents were detected (Fig. 13 E, F). Therefore, according to a preliminary assignment of monosomes considered on the basis of their sizes to the subgenomes, 22 large monosomes can be assigned to the A_t-genome and 27 monosomes of small sizes to the D_t-genome.

It is known that only three chromosome pairs of G. hirsutum have long arms that are two or three times the length of the short arms [51]. Monosomes of medium sizes demand special translocation tests with subgenome and chromosome number assignment of the translocated chromosomes. The analysis of subgenome assignment of unidentified monosomes of medium sizes showed the A_t subgenome location [52] and significant deviation from the expected 1:1 ratio of the A_t-subgenome monosome number to the D_t-subgenome ones. This observation implied that preferential loss of the A_t-subgenome chromosome was caused by specific genetic regulation system of chromosome disjunction and was not due to size of monosomes [52]. In

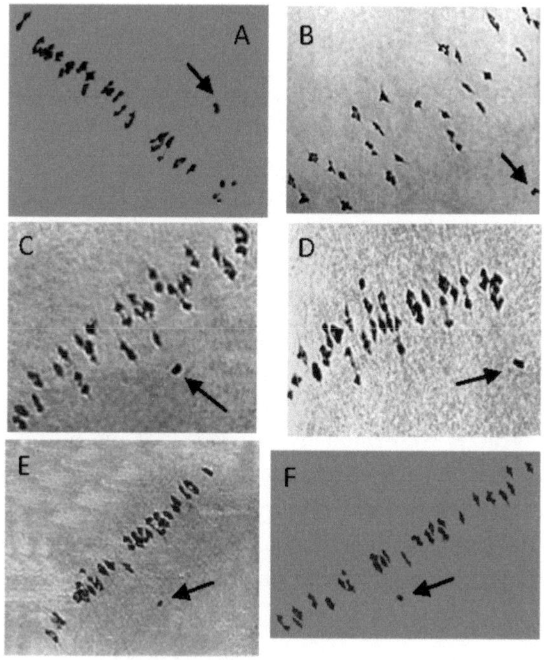

Figure 13. Meiotic configurations in monosomic lines in cotton *G. hirsutum*. Meiotic metaphase I cells showing 25 bivalents and 1 univalent in (A) Mo13 and (B) Mo16 (large univalent size); (C) Mo11 and (d) Mo4 (medium univalent size); (E) Mo80 and (F) Mo89 (small univalent size). The arrows point to the univalents. Note that the background of figures was cleaned using Adobe Photoshop CSS extended version 12.

our experiments, we detected a nearly 2 : 1 ratio of the A_t-to the D_t-subgenome monosomes for all that monosomes of medium sizes to be from A_t-genome. The ratio observed us is not significantly different from the ratio given by Myles and Endrizzi [52]. This confirms a greater tolerance of G. hirsutum to loss of the large A_t-genome chromosome than the small D_t-genome chromosomes.

Analysis of the tetrads was carried out for 87 primary monosomics of our collection. Most of the monosomics (73 or 83.91%) had high meiotic index (more than 90%) than that of the control plants (95.11±0.46%). That indicates regular univalent chromosome disjunction. Fourteen of the monosomics (16.09%) were characterized with lowering of meiotic index from 89.33% (Mo74) to 68.32% (Mo4). Moreover, 10 of the monosomics had a smaller reduction of meiotic index (to 80%) compared others two monosomics (Mo4 and Mo16). These monosomics were induced in M_1 generation by pollen gamma-irradiation in doses of 20 and 25 Gy, leading to strong meiotic index reduction (to 68.32±1.10% and 76.07±0.93%, respectively). We also observe an increase of percentage of tetrads with micronuclei (to 6.87±0.60% and 21.56±0.90% respectively) in comparison with the control line (1.42±0.25%).Two other monosomics (Mo88 and Mo90), selected from M_3 generation treated by thermal neutrons and pollen with gamma-rays were characterized with different meiotic index in various buds. Variation limits were also observed for the number of tetrads with micronuclei.

Meiotic index decrease in 6 monosomics (Mo16, Mo28, Mo52, Mo74, Mo88 and Mo90) could be explained because of the presence of a additional univalents at meiotic metaphase I. In contrast, meiotic index decrease in 4 monosomics (Mo8, Mo21, Mo23 and Mo57) was connected with simultaneous translocation heterozygosity that led to chromosome disjunction disturbances and the production of tetrads with micronuclei. However, meiotic index decrease in 3 monosomics with the modal chromosome pairing (Mo4, Mo34 and Mo37) and increase of number of tetrads with micronuclei In Mo4 (to 6.87±0.60%) directly demonstrated disturbances in monosome disjunction and imbalanced gamete formation. Therefore, the low frequency of tetrads with micronuclei in cotton monosomic argues for stability of monosomes, which seldom undergo irregular division (misdivision) of univalent centromeres [43]. This is confirmed by the fact that we found only 9 monotelodisomics and one isochromosome in more than 1000 cytologically examined plants of the progeny of various monosomics from our cytogenetical collection. These results are in contrast with earlier data on the degree of chromosome lagging in wheat monosomics, where the frequency of tetrads with micronuclei varied from 34.1 to 65.2% [53].

Pollen fertility after acetocarmine staining was studied in 93 primary cotton monosomics, isolated mainly from different types of irradiation. High pollen fertility was detected only in 30 plants with chromosome deficiencies that pointed out probable early haplo-deficient microspore abortion prior to mature pollen stage. Remaining monosomics were characterized with pollen fertility decrease. Thus, 17 monosomics had small lowering of pollen fertility (to 70%), 11 – semisterile pollen (to 40%) and 15 – strong pollen fertility reduction (to 5%) (Fig. 14). Pollen sterility was established in 6 monosomics (Mo5, Mo7, Mo10, Mo44, Mo45 and Mo47) derived from M_1 generation after irradiation of pollen and in two monosomics (Mo57 and Mo74) isolated after thermal neutron seed irradiation. Monosomics Mo5 and Mo44 did not produce any seeds from self-pollination and intercrossing that suggest their complete sterility. In 11 monosomics pollen fertility was varied among different flowers on the same plant; moreover, the variation limits were strongly differed. Reproduced monosomics from the 3 other families (Mo22, Mo39 and Mo46) also had pollen fertility variation in different flowers on the same plant from semisterile or low to reduced pollen fertility.

The reproduction of the monosomic plants was studied in the self-pollination and outcrossed progenies under the field and greenhouse conditions. Comparative analysis of the cotton monosomics produced both in the field and greenhouse revealed distinct morphological differences in comparison with disomic sibs. As a result, monosomics were reproduced in 18 generations under field condition. However, we did not analyze most of the progenies and determine exact transmission frequency in the field due to limited space, time and cost. Thirteen of 18 reproduced later under greenhouse condition whereas five monosomics (Mo22, Mo36, Mo39, Mo46 and Mo53) plants did not produce daughter monosomics.

The progenies of 81 different monosomics were studied in the greenhouse. All monosomic families strongly differed in number of plants studied, and in only 18 families were all

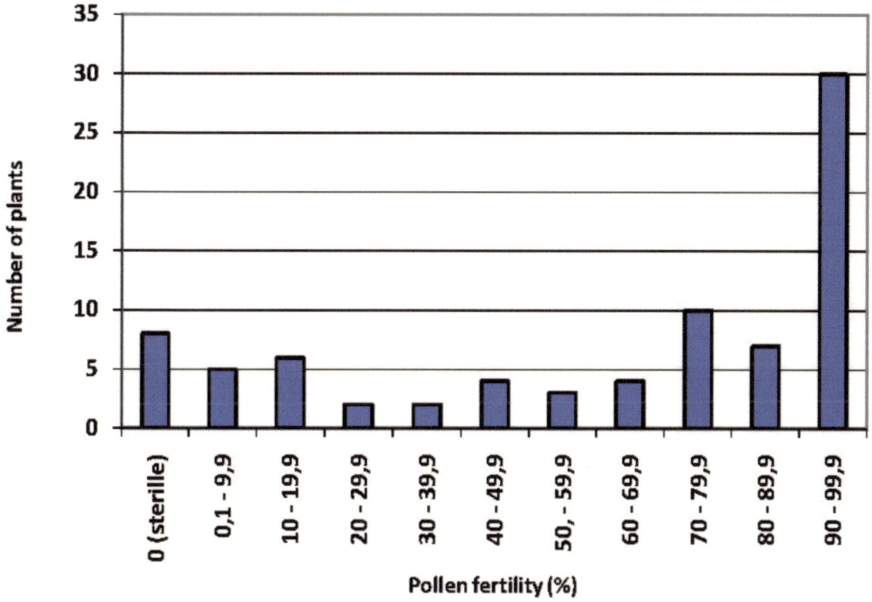

Note: the remaining 11 monosomics were not included in the histogram due to their varied pollen fertility level in different flowers.

Figure 14. Percentage distribution of pollen fertility for 82 cotton monosomic plants.

progenies cytologically examined for monosome transmission rate (Table 5). This demonstrated a large variation in transmission rate from high (44.44% in Mo16 and Mo84) to very low (1.79% in Mo34). The highest transmission rate (from 30.43% in Mo72 to 44.44% in Mo16 and Mo84) was observed in 12 monosomic plants (Mo16, Mo31, Mo58, Mo59, Mo62, Mo66, Mo71, Mo72, Mo77, Mo82, Mo84 and Mo90). Results suggested frequent transmission of haplo-deficient gametes. On the other hand, 12 other monosomics (Mo3, Mo4, Mo9, Mo15, Mo34, Mo35, Mo40, Mo41, Mo56, Mo61, Mo67 and Mo85) had the lowest transmission rate (from 1.79% in Mo34 to 9.38% in Mo67) due to rare *n-1* gamete transmission that demanded to use a large population for their recovery. The remaining 26 monosomic plants were transmitted with medium range of frequency (from 14.29% in Mo10 and Mo74 to 29.41% in Mo11). Significant variability in transmission rates could be explained by differences in the viability of haplo-deficient gametes involving specific chromosomes. Theoretically, after selfing monosomics must produce progenies with *2n*, *2n-1* and *2n-2* chromosome number in the ratio 1:2:1, but, in fact, cotton nullisomic gametes with *2n-2* are nonviable whereas *n* and *n-1* gametes form in unequal frequencies because of lower haplo-deficient gamete viability and their incompetitiveness in comparison with normal gametes. Thus, all the differences in detected transmission rates involve deficiencies in various chromosomes of the cotton genome. Nevertheless, transmission rate similarities in some monosomes in our collection could indicate identities that should be explored.

Mo	Total no. of plants	No. of studied plants	Discomics (26II)	Monotelodisomics (25II+1t)	Monosomics (25II+1I)	Trans-mission (%)	No. of progenies
			Transmission of monosomes studied in outcrossed progenies				
(Mo1)*	6	6	5	0	1	16.67	1
(Mo2)	6	6	5	1	1	16.67	1
Mo3	29	24	23	0	1	4.17	3
Mo4	45	29	27	0	2	6.9	2
(Mo10)	7	7	6	0	1	14.29	2
Mo11	52	34	24	0	10	29.41	4
Mo13	27	21	18	0	3	14.29	3
Mo15	44	42	41	0	1	2.38	5
(Mo28)	5	5	4	0	1	20.00	1
Mo34	64	56	54	1	1	1,79	3
Mo41	15	14	13	0	1	7,14	2
Mo56	26	26	24	0	2	7.69	4
Mo63	19	13	11	0	2	15.38	2
(Mo74)	12	7	6	0	1	14.29	1
			Transmission of monosomes studied in selfed progenies				
Mo7	29	19	14	0	5	26.32	2
Mo9	48	34	32	0	2	5.88	3
Mo16	22	18	10	0	8	44.44	3
Mo17	33	31	24	0	6	19.35	9
Mo19	38	31	24	1	6	19.35	4
(Mo27)	9	9	7	0	2	22.22	2
Mo31	25	25	16	0	9	36.00	5
Mo35	24	23	21	0	2	8.70	3
Mo38	17	17	14	0	3	17.65	2
Mo40	33	33	32	0	1	3.03	2
Mo42	30	25	21	0	4	16.00	2
(Mo48)	11	11	9	0	2	18.19	3
Mo50	37	26	20	0	6	23.07	3
(Mo58)	5	5	3	0	2	40.00	1
Mo59	22	22	13	0	9	40,91	1

http://dx.doi.org/10.5772/58589

Mo	Total no. of plants	No. of studied plants	Discomics (26II)	Monotelodisomics (25II+1t)	Monosomics (25II+1I)	Trans-mission (%)	No. of progenies
Mo60	16	14	10	0	4	28.57	3
Mo61	41	18	16	1	1	5.56	3
Mo62	61	24	17	0	11	35.48	3
Mo66	31	31	20	0	11	35.48	3
Mo67	40	35	32	0	3	9.38	4
Mo69	18	18	13	0	5	27.78	2
Mo70	18	18	15	0	3	16.67	3
Mo71	20	20	13	0	7	35.00	2
Mo72	23	23	16	0	7	30.43	2
Mo73	28	24	18	0	6	25.00	2
Mo75	35	15	11	0	4	26.67	3
Mo76	31	18	14	0	4	22.22	4
(Mo77)	22	10	6	0	4	40.00	1
Mo79	31	22	16	0	6	27.27	3
Mo80	48	20	17	0	3	15.00	3
Mo81	21	12	9	0	3	25.00	2
(Mo82)	17	11	7	0	4	36.36	2
Mo84	31	18	10	0	8	44.44	2
Mo85	48	26	25	0	1	3.85	2
Mo89	47	21	17	0	4	19.05	3
Mo90	16	16	11	0	5	31.25	1

*Families shown in parenthesis are too small to provide a very informative assessment.

Table 5. Transmission of the monosomes in the progenies of cotton monosomics (Mo) under greenhouse condition

In cytogenetic analysis, 30 out of 52 cotton monosomic lines showed modal chromosome pairing with 25 bivalents plus one univalent at metaphase-1 of meiosis. The remaining 20 monosomic lines were characterized by the presence of additional univalents in PMCs; moreover, three lines (Mo10, Mo11 and Mo39) had highest frequencies of such univalents (from 1.21±0.10 to 1.33±0.08 in average per cell, respectively). The line Mo4 was characterized by the presence of rare trivalents (0.12±0.06 in average per cell) that suggested pairing of the monosomic chromosome with homoeologous chromosome. Appearance of additional univalents in the monosomic lines was seen previously in cotton. Homozygotization of daughter monosomic genotype led to meiosis stabilization and absence of additional univalents in subsequent generations.

Monosomic lines were also distinguished by sizes of the univalents. Thus, 8 lines were characterized with univalents of large sizes, 29 monosomic lines had univalents of medium sizes, 11-had small univalents. The remaining 4 monosomic lines had extremely small univalents that suggested a different sub-genome origin and genetic non-uniformity. In three monosomic lines (Mo1, Mo9 and Mo46), the sizes of univalents differed various in the parental and daughter monosomics, underlining the possibility of univalent shifts in progeny.

Analysis of tetrads of microspores showed a high meiotic index in the majority of the monosomic lines with the exception of the line Mo84 which varied in both meiotic index (from 49.90±1.12% to 95.48±0.27%) and tetrads with micronuclei (from 12.44±0.74 to 0.53±0.10%) in different buds. The meiotic index variation led to variation in pollen fertility (from 65.14±1.45% to 94.46±0.36%) within individual flowers of the same plant. It should be noted that lower meiotic index was recorded in wheat monosomic lines and a high percentage of tetrads with micronuclei confirmed that univalents frequently lagged during chromosome disjunction [54].

Pollen fertility analysis of cotton monosomic lines after acetocarmine staining showed high pollen fertility in the majority of the lines. Only line Mo10 was characterized with strong lowering of the character (to 19.35±2.37%) that suggested its partial sterility of chromosome deficient pollen. Six other lines (Mo22, Mo34, Mo39, Mo46, Mo84 and Mo89) showed variation in pollen fertility in different flowers within the same monosomic plants. In the three parental monosomics (Mo22, Mo39 and Mo46) variation in pollen fertility among different flowers within the same plants was also observed (13.43-91.37%; 2.53-34.21%; 2.10-92.46%, respectively). The ranges of variation in pollen fertility were wider in two monosomics (Mo22 and Mo46). A similar effect detected in daughter monosomics, confirmed the genetic determination of such variation and suggested possible chromosome localization of the gene(s) for male gametophyte viability in the deficient chromosomes. It is known that the majority of cotton chromosome deficiencies are not transmissible via pollen due to non-functionality of chromatin-deficient pollen [54]. Besides, Kakani et al. [19] reported that gene(s) responsible for pollen spine development were located on long arm of chromosome 12 using the advanced technique of confocal laser scanning microscopy and substitution lines.

A study of the morphology of cotton monosomic plants revealed the specific influence of monosomy on many characters that were differentiated them from disomic sibs. Such characters were thin stem, feeble leafing, small leaves, short internodes, crooked sympodia, small flowers and bolls, as well as deformed and obligospermous bolls. At the same time, 4 monosomic lines (Mo35, Mo36, Mo40 and Mo50) looked like disomic sibs. Although the majority of the monosomic lines had a compact bush, 10 lines (Mo3, Mo7, Mo11, Mo31, Mo35, Mo39, Mo60, Mo69, Mo73 and Mo89) were characterized by a scattered bush. Two lines (Mo7 and Mo56) differed by having a crooked sympodia and 3 other lines (Mo75, Mo76 and Mo82) had elongated internodes. In 3 lines (Mo13, Mo34 and Mo66), a dense stem pubescence was observed whereas leaf pubescence was feeble (Figure 15). Three monosomic lines (Mo16, Mo31 and Mo48) had difference in leaf sizes within the same plant

http://dx.doi.org/10.5772/58589

and two other lines (Mo9 and Mo76) had leaf folding in the area of the main rib or lobe division, respectively.

Four monosomic lines (Mo4, Mo10, Mo46 and Mo67) differed by having feeble budding and flowering (to 10-15 flowers during the summer) whereas three other lines (Mo22, Mo39 and Mo56) had strong budding and flowering (to 40-60 flowers during the summer) but low seed and boll set (from 10,10±0,78 to 20,71±0,52 per one boll). Many monosomic lines were characterized by small flowers and bracts; however, 6 lines (Mo4, Mo10, Mo16, Mo34, Mo46 and Mo48) were distinguished by a strong reduction in flower sizes (from 38mm to 48mm). Taken together, 7 monosomic lines (Mo9, Mo31, Mo39, Mo71, Mo72, Mo73 and Mo76) had large bracts (to 65x67mm for Mo9) and 5 monosomics (Mo4, Mo10, Mo34, Mo46 and Mo80) had small bracts (to 25x21mm for Mo10). Some chromosome deficient lines (Mo31, Mo72 and Mo76) differed by having a large number of bract teeth (from 14 to 18) whereas other lines had small number of bract teeth (Mo4, Mo10, Mo19, Mo34, Mo46 and Mo80) (from 8 to 12) (Figure 16). In the Mo39 line additional bracts were present, in the Mo17 the bracts were asymmetrical and in the Mo27 the bracts were deformed with feebly expressed teeth.

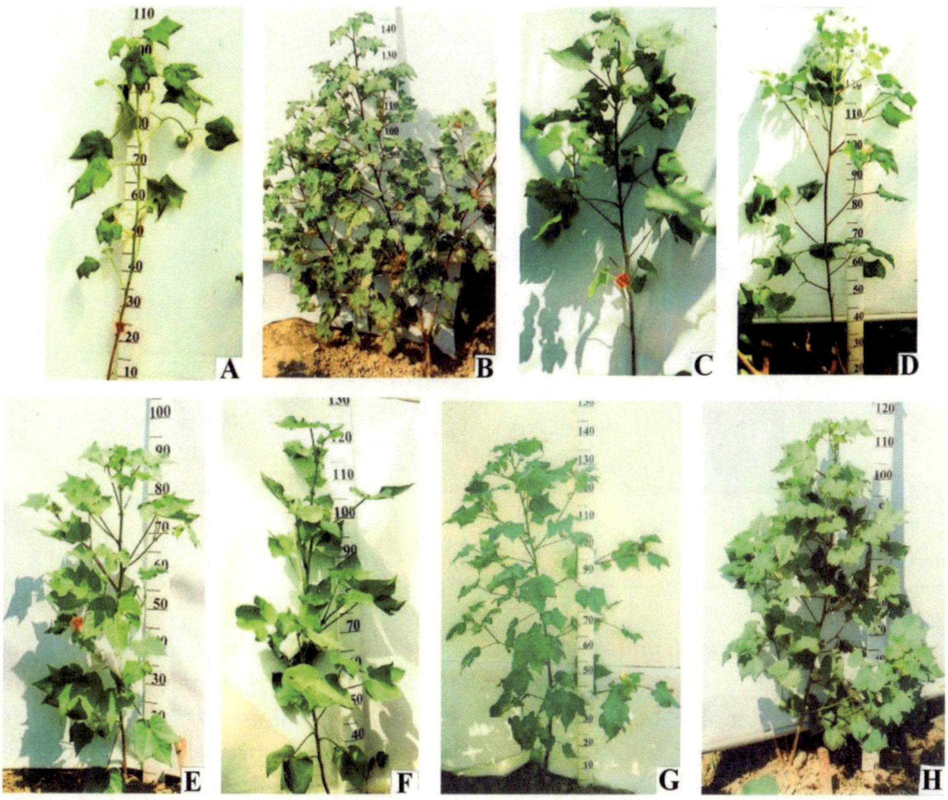

Figure 15. Some examples of morphology of cotton monosomic lines: (A) Mo11; (B) Mo31; (C) Mo50; (D) Mo76; (E) Mo81; (F) Mo82; (G) Mo89; (H) Mo90.

The most variability was observed for the character "presence/absence of nectarines" where in 15 monosomic lines not all bracts had nectarines, and Mo66 lacked any external nectarines. Nectarines of different sizes within a single flower were presented in 6 monosomic lines (Mo9, Mo27, Mo31, Mo39, Mo84 and Mo89) (Figure 17).

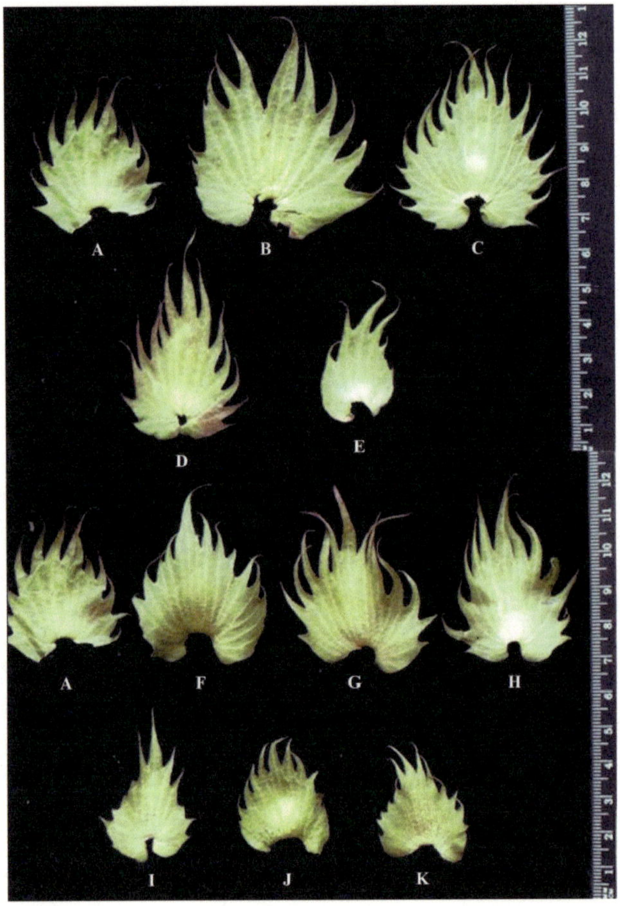

Figure 16. The bracts in the different cotton monosomic lines : (A) parental line L-458; (B) Mo39; (C) Mo72; (D) Mo31; (E) Mo66; (F) Mo84; (G) Mo89; (H) Mo81; (I) Mo88; (J) Mo4; (K) Mo92.

Monosomy had an influence on the stigma structure and sizes in a flower. Thus, there were shorter stigmata in 3 lines (Mo17, Mo19 and Mo28) and a broad "reverting" stigma in Mo39. A new phenotypic marker for cotton monosomy – "reduced" stigma was detected in Mo62. Analysis of Mo62 progeny revealed the presence of reduced stigma only in monosomic cytotypes whereas disomic ones had normal stigma as did the control (Figure 18). This trait it makes possible to distinguish cytotypes within the progeny without cytological analysis. However, stigma reduction rate was varied in different flowers within the same plant: a little reduction stigma (to 7-9 mm); medium reduction (stigma to 2-6 mm), and strong reduction

http://dx.doi.org/10.5772/58589

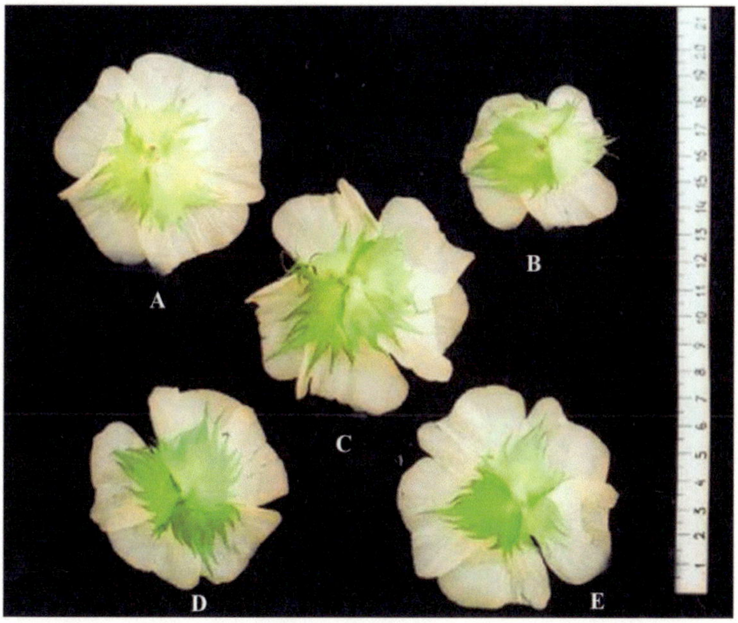

Figure 17. Outside view of nectaries in some cotton monosomics: (A) parental line L-458; (B) Mo13; (C) Mo39; (D) Mo71; (E) Mo72.

(stigma to 1 mm). Moreover, as a rule, strongly reduced stigmas were located inside the staminate column. Besides flowers with reduced stigma, there were flowers in which the stigma was closed inside the stylar tissue. A dependence of stigma reduction rates related to the seasons of a year was also established.

All daughter monosomics of Mo62 were fertile both as male and female but had lower seed number per a boll (22.30±1.83) and lower seed set (76.90±2.47 %) in comparison with the parental line L-458 (34.40±0.62 and 89.81±1.55, respectively). A monosome of *G. hirsutum* with a strong reduction of stigma but still fertile, has not been described. Thus the monosome in Mo62 for the chromosome of cotton genome could be new.

The most important changes due to monosomy concerned sizes and shapes of bolls as majority of them formed smaller round bolls almost ranging from spherical to elongated bolls with beaks or without beaks compared to control plants. Many of the bolls of monosomics were ribbed or deformed due to a number of abortive ovules and immature seeds (Figure 19). As a result, the number of seeds per boll and seed set were lower in all monosomic lines (from 9.50±1.62 in Mo13 to 32.61±3.99 % in Mo76) in comparison with the parental line (34.40±0.62 and 89.81±1.55, respectively). Mo4 was characterized with variation of boll sizes within the same monosomic plant and also the fruit occurred in clusters. Flowers and fruit clusters were also observed in Mo19. Mo66 was distinguished by a large broad beak at the top of an ovoid boll (Figure 19 D). Thus, it was shown that an individual chromosome deficiency had a specific influence in plant morphology and that some of them had unique marker characters. However, the clear similarity both morphological and cytogenetic features in some monosomics of our

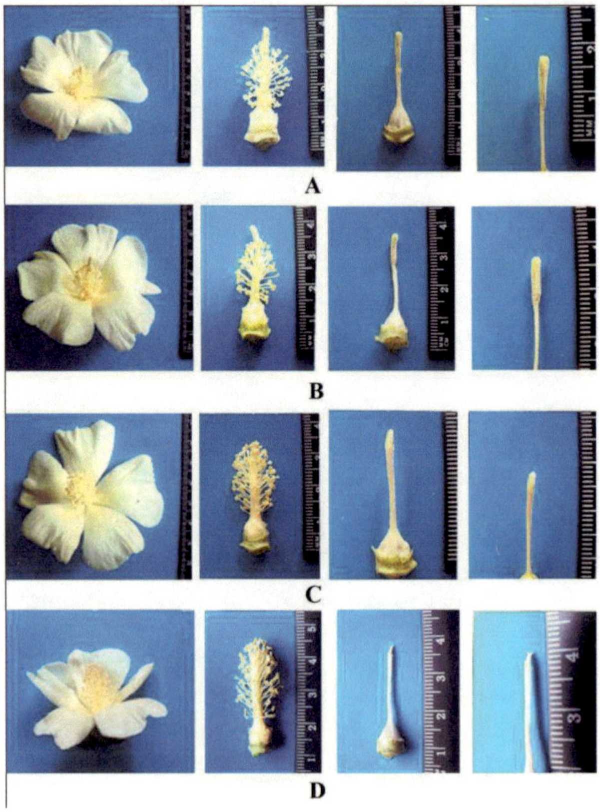

Figure 18. The flowers of the different cytotypes from progeny the monosomic line Mo62: (A) parental line-L-458; (B) disomic cytotype with normal stigma; (C) monosomic cytotype with medium reduction of the stigma; (D) monosomic cytotype with strong reduction of the stigma.

collection suggested probable redundancy for the same monosomic chromosomes among the plants.

Many small chromosomes presence in karyotype analysis of tetraploid cotton *G. hirsutum* and absence of distinctive morphological markers for the chromosomes make it impossible to distinguish and identify chromosomes in karyologic analysis. Therefore, we identified monosomes to be specific chromosomes of the cotton genome using the known translocation test on hybrids of monosomics with translocation lines from the Uzbek Cytogenetic Collection (Table 6). Analysis of hybrid chromosome pairing was used to reveal monosomic translocation F_1 hybrids and to study "critical configurations". The recently developed 28 translocation lines (Tr1-Tr28) from our collection were used for monosome identification according to the method described previously [6].

Eleven monosomics (Mo3, Mo10, Mo11, Mo19, Mo27, Mo39, Mo48, Mo53, Mo56, Mo73 and Mo85) were associated with the chromosomes of seven translocation lines (Tr1, Tr3, Tr5, Tr8, Tr11, Tr12 and Tr16) as chromosome pairing of 24 bivalents plus one trivalent was observed

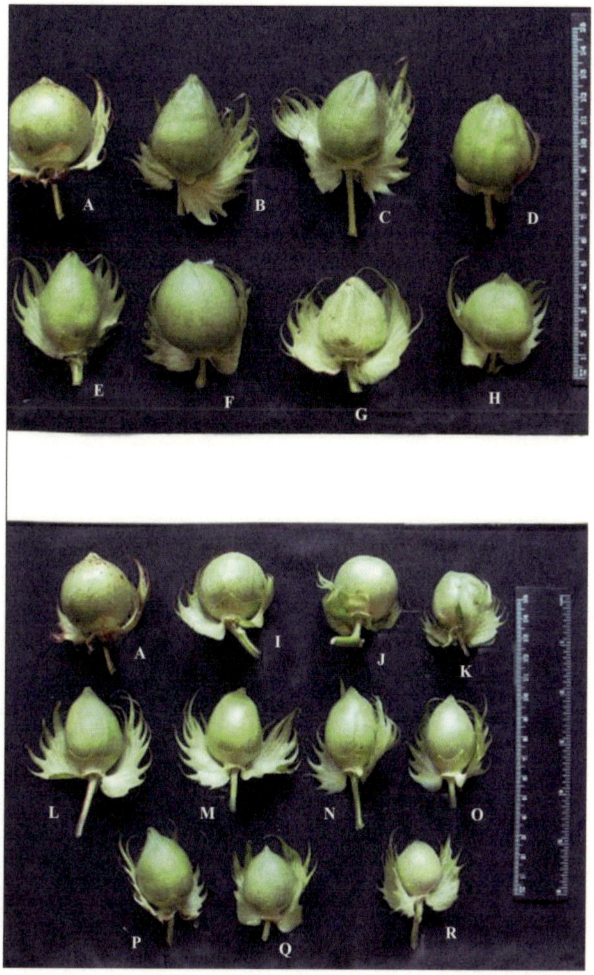

Figure 19. The bolls of the different cotton monosomic lines: (A) parental line L-458; (B to H) – Mo72; Mo31; Mo66; Mo60; Mo50; Mo39; Mo16 and (I to R) Mo80; Mo4; Mo92; Mo89; Mo81; Mo76; Mo62; Mo75; Mo87; Mo88.

in PMCs of the F_1 monosomic hybrid plants (Fig. 20). We also identified four monosome pairs (Mo10 and Mo73; Mo39 and Mo56; Mo48 and Mo53; Mo11 and Mo19) that were associated with the translocation lines Tr3, Tr5, Tr12 and Tr16, respectively (Table5). Thus, three of the above-mentioned monosome pairs (Mo10 and Mo73, Mo39 and Mo56, Mo11 and Mo19) involved the same chromosomes with the each pair. In future analyses, hybrids from crosses of the monosomics and other translocation lines, involving the same chromosomes, will confirm our interpretation about the missing chromosome or chromosome segment and identification of the monosomic line. However, there is evidence for monosomes Mo48 and Mo53 that nonhomologous as the chromosomes from two different sub-genomes all involved with translocation line Tr12.

Monosomics	Translocation lines							Total number of crosses tested
	Tr1	Tr3	Tr5	Tr8	Tr11	Tr12	Tr16	
Mo3			-		+	-		4
Mo7			-	-		-	-	7
Mo10		+	-	-				3
Mo11	-	-	-	-	-	-	+	14
Mo13	-					-	-	13
Mo19		-	-				+	5
Mo27			-	+				5
Mo31	-	-	-	-	-	-	-	25
Mo35				-				3
Mo36								3
Mo38	-		-	-				9
Mo39			+	-				6
Mo41					-			1
Mo48						+		4
Mo50	-	-	-	-		-		19
Mo53				-		+		2
Mo56			+	-		-	-	8
Mo60			-	-			-	9
Mo62	-		-					6
Mo66	-	-	-	-	-	-	-	12
Mo67	-							2
Mo69	-		-	-	-	-	-	21
Mo70		-	-		-	-	-	11
Mo71	-	-			-	-	-	12
Mo72	-	-						9
Mo73	-	+	-	-	-	-	-	14
Mo75	-	-	-	-	-		-	18
Mo76	-			-				9
Mo77								6
Mo79	-		-	-			-	10
Mo80			-		-			4
Mo81	-		-		-	-	-	12
Mo84								1
Mo85	+					-		4
Mo89							-	5

Note:+associated,-independent

Table 6. Cytological test for indentification of the monosomes with the help of translocation lines.

We had isolated 4 monosomics (Mo70 – Mo73) from the progeny of the same desynaptic plant and proposed possible monosomy for different nonhomologous chromosomes of the cotton genome. Indirect confirmation was available with the detection of monosome Mo73 homology and one of the chromosomes involved into interchanges in the line Tr3 whereas the other three monosomes from the progeny of the same desynaptic plant (Mo70, Mo71 and Mo72) did not has any chromosomes in common in the Tr3 interchange. Another monosome (Mo85), isolated from the other desynaptic progeny, showed homology with a chromosome involved in an interchange with Tr1. This test revealed that the chromosomes of Tr1 were rarely involved in translocations. Translocation line Tr1 had common chromosomes only with two lines – Tr2 and Tr20 with multiple interchanges [41]. This verified our assumption that new or rare monosomes would occur in progenies of desynaptic forms of cotton [33].

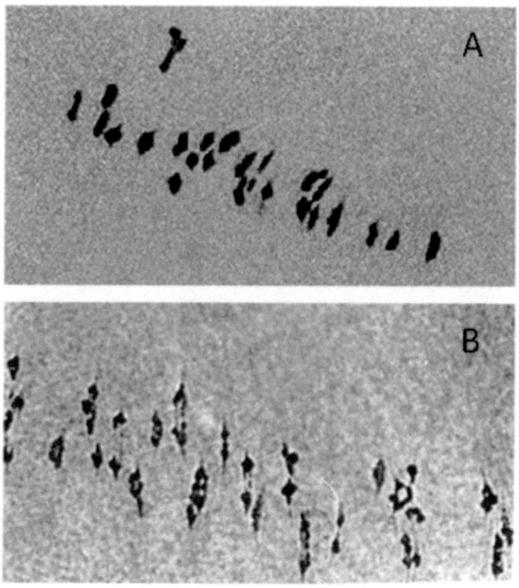

Figure 20. "Critical configurations" of the chromosomes at the meiotic metaphase I cells showing 24 bivalents and 1 trivalent in cotton F_1 plants from crosses the monosomics x translocation lines: (A) Mo19 xTr16; (B) Mo85 x Tr1. The arrows point to the univalents. Note that the background of figures was cleaned using Adobe Photoshop CSS extended version 12.

Translocation tests involving other 24 monosomic lines have not yet revealed any homology of the monosomes and the chromosomes involved in interchanges because they showed detections of chromosome pairing with 23 bivalents plus one univalent plus one quadrivalent (Figure 21). However they did demonstrate the differences in the studying level of the lines as well as depended on transmission rates of the monosomics in hybrid progenies. There is an evidence of the comparative rareness of other monosomes from our collection.

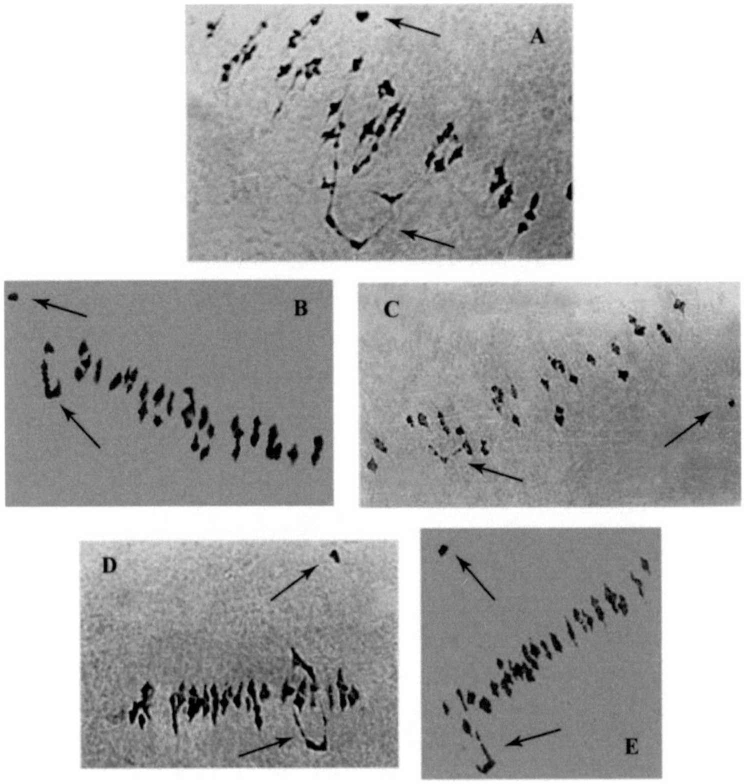

Figure 21. "Critical configurations" of the chromosomes at the meiotic metaphase I cells showing 23 bivalents and 1 univalent and one hexavalent (A) and 23 bivalents and 1 univalent and one quadrivalent (B-E) in cotton F_1 plants from crosses the monosomics x translocation lines: (A) Mo13 xTr2; (B) Mo56 x Tr6, (C) Mo75 xTr16; (D) Mo77 x Tr21; (E) Mo77 x Tr25. The arrows point to the univalents, quadrivalents and hexavalent. Note that the background of figures was cleaned using Adobe Photoshop CSS extended version 12.

6. Monotelodisomics, monoisodisomics and haploids in cotton *G. hirsutum* L.

Other type of chromatin deficiency namely monotelodisimics are characterized with absence of a chromosome arms. As a result 25 normal bivalents and one heteromorphic bivalent with arm deficiency formed in meiosis. There are 11 monotelodisomics following pollen and seed irradiation and 9 from different monosomic progenies in our collection at present time. Misdivision of a chromosome via centromere region followed by irradiation produced telocentric chromosome formation. Centromere inactivation caused loss of a chromosome arm. Telosome pair was detected as two different size univalents with various frequencies in the monotelodisomics (to 1.85±0.15 in average per cell). A high frequency of heteromorphic bivalents (to 0.95±0.05 in average per cell) was registered in monotelodisomics (Figure 22). Among the plants with arm deficiencies three had also a translocation.

http://dx.doi.org/10.5772/58589

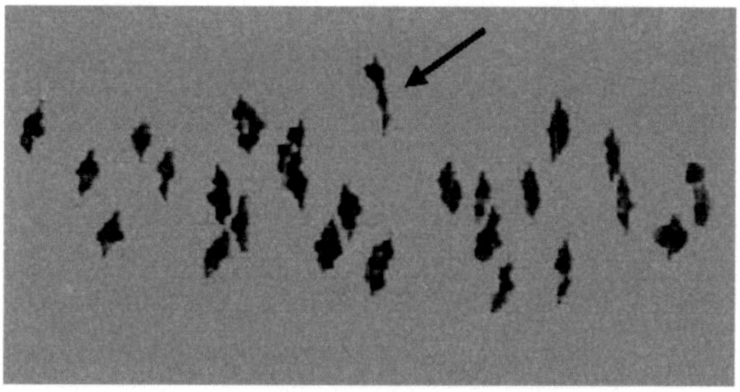

Figure 22. Meiotic configurations in monotelodisomic plant in cotton *G. hirsutum*. Meiotic metaphase I cells showing 25 normal bivalents and 1 heteromorphic bivalent with arm deficiency in plant M_1-1608/2. The arrow point out to the heteromorphic bivalent. Note that the background of figures was cleaned using Adobe Photoshop CSS extended version 12.

Monotelodisomics with the translocation had a telocentric chromosome as univalent in the majority of PMCs. As it is known, telocentrics for short arms are less often paired with normal homologous chromosomes [55]. Meiotic index was high (from 81.86±0.85 to 99.56±0.16), but the pollen fertility reduced in the monotelodisomics.

Isochromosome formation was also connected with damaging action of radiation to centromere chromosome regions. As a result of centromere inactivation instable telocentric formed its arm developed on 180^0, gave an isochromosome. Three monoisodisomics our collection were differed with isochromosome pairing at metaphase I of meiosis. If one of them had heteromorphic in most PMS (to 0.96±0.04) in other plants the isochromosome was often as univalent (to 0.91±0.22 an average on PMS). In spite of high Mi (to 98.55±0.25) in two monoisodicomics pollen fertility was reduced.

Deficiencies for one chromosome arm occurred in the progenies of 9 monosomics. Thus, in four monosomic progenies (Mo2, Mo19, Mo34 and Mo61) that differed with respect to monosome transmission rates, monotelodisomics were produced due to univalent instability and resulted in misdivision. In the progenies of Mo6, Mo21, Mo22, Mo49, Mo54 and Mo68 daugher monosomics failed to produce, but monotelodisimics (from the progenies of Mo6, Mo21, Mo22, Mo49 and Mo68) and a monoisodisomic plant (from the progeny of Mo54) were detected. The results suggested an irregular univalent chromosome centromere misdivision in the parental monosomics that led to a single chromosome arm missing and formed either telocentric or isochromosome in the case of an arm doubling. Our results demonstrated the rather rare occurrence of telo-and isochromosomes in the monosomic progenies studied, which showed univalent misdivision to be rare.

Haploid plants of cotton are characterized by presence of 26 univalent chromosomes and by significant decrease in vigour and fertility, size of lives, bolls and flowers. Our collection includes four haploid plants. One haploid was obtained by irradiation of the seeds by fast neutrons (1005/22), other two (1579/6 and $171/4_{17}$) – by pollen irradiation in M_1 and M_2 generations and one – from monosomic progeny ($175/4_{18}$-57). Meiosis was studied in the microsporocytes of the haploid plants 1005/22. Among 44 studied PMCs at metaphase I only five cells had open bivalents (to 0.14±0.06 on average per cells) (Figure 23 A). Others PMCs were characterized by presence of 26 univalents (Figure 23 B, C). As results, the range of polyads observed in PMCs.

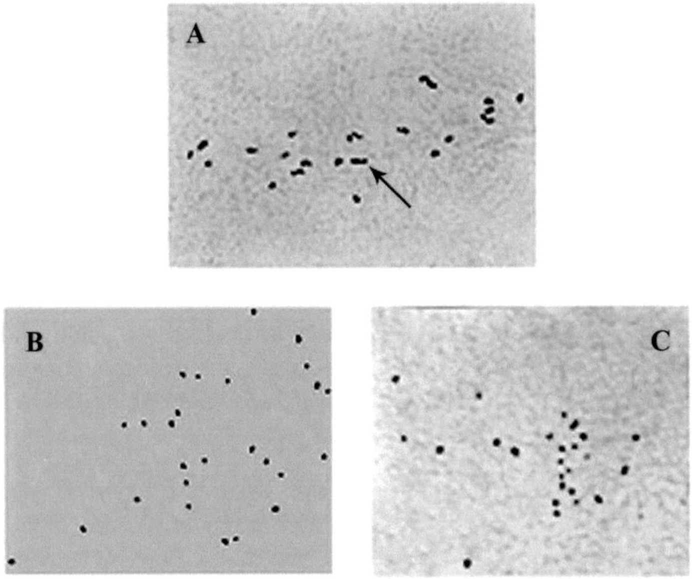

Figure 23. Meiotic configurations in haploid plant $171/4_{17}$ in cotton *G. hirsutum*. Meiotic metaphase I cells showing (A) 25 univalent and 1 bivalent; (B-C) 26 univalent. The arrow point out to the bivalent. Note that the background of figures was cleaned using Adobe Photoshop CSS extended version 12.

All the 26 chromosomes remained as univalents in other two haploid plants (1579/6 and $175/4_{18}$-57). Most abnormal haploid plant (1579/6) had low habit and a thin stem, compact bush, and scarce foliage. It was completely sterile. Its prominent feature was the complete absence of chromosome pairing. In all PMCs, meiosis studies revealed 26 univalents, scattered throughout the cells. Analysis of sporads revealed a significant decrease in meiotic index (to 18.97±1.31%), an increase in the number of tetrads with micronuclei (to 12.01±1.09%), and formation of abundant monads, dyads, triads, and polyads. The complete absence of chromosome pairing resulted in the formation of imbalanced and abortive gametes and pollen sterility. Haploid plant $171/4_{17}$ had rare open bivalents and one trivalent in several PMCs. Some PMSs of the two haploid had 26 bivalents. Non-disjunction during premeiotic mitosis could give rise to such a diploid cell.

Analysis of sporads revealed a significant decrease in meiotic index (to 13.12±0.92%), the decrease in the number of tetrads with micronuclei (to 3.02±0.46%), and formation of abundant pentads (16.51±0.01%), hexads (22.33±1.13%), heptads (17.17±1.02%) and oktads (10.46±0.83%) (Figure 24). In three years few bolls were obtained on this haploid plant (Figure 25).

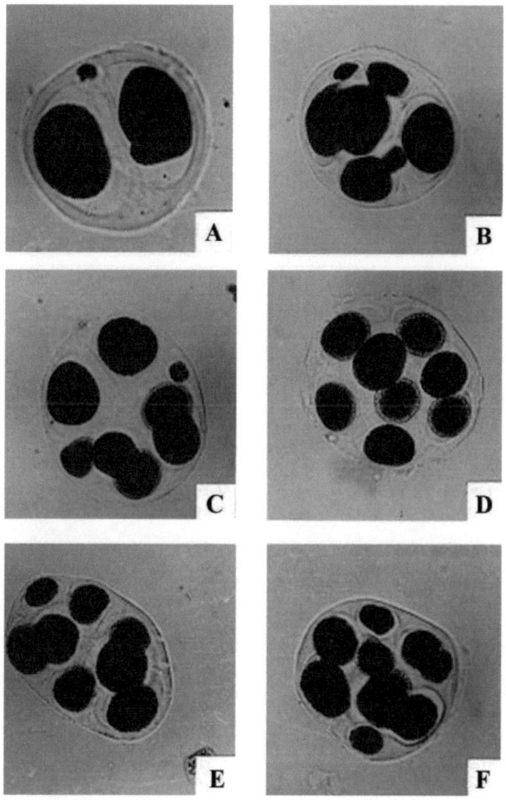

Figure 24. Meiosis in haploid plant $171/4_{17}$ in cotton *G. hirsutum*. Abnormal sporads: (A) diad with micronuclei; (B) pentad with two micronucleis; (C) heksad with two micronucleis; (D and E)-oktads; (F) abnormal poliad.

Different mechanisms are proposed to explain the emergence of haploids during pollen irradiation. One of them suggests that haploids result from female parthenogenesis induced by pseudofertilization with irradiated pollen. According to another mechanism, fertilization occurs before zygotization, but the damaged paternal genome is eliminated early in development [56]. Some authors believe that haploids of *G. hirsutum* are completely sterile, wheareas haploids *G. barbadense* are fertile and produce seeds after pollination with normal pollen [57]. Moreover, a line of the latter species is known that frequently produced haploids of the androgenous and matroclinous types.

7. Storage and propagation cytogenetical collection of cotton

Seeds Cytogenetical Collection of cotton maintained under room conditions (20-25^0 C). There is no facility available for cold storage of seeds. They are placed in to parchment paper bags. Each bag has catalogue number and year of collection. Bags are stored in special metal boxes (30 x 11 cm) and boxes are placed in wooden-cases. Monosomic and translocation plants and of their hybrids are grown at the greenhouse conditions in soil. All data collected are stored as a hard copy catalogue book that is being conversed to electronic format.

8. Location, maintenance and funding

The Cytogenetical Collection of cotton currently stored in the National University of Uzbekictan at Tashkent. It is funded by Committee for Coordination of Science and Technology Development (CCSTD) under the Cabinet Ministry of Uzbekistan.

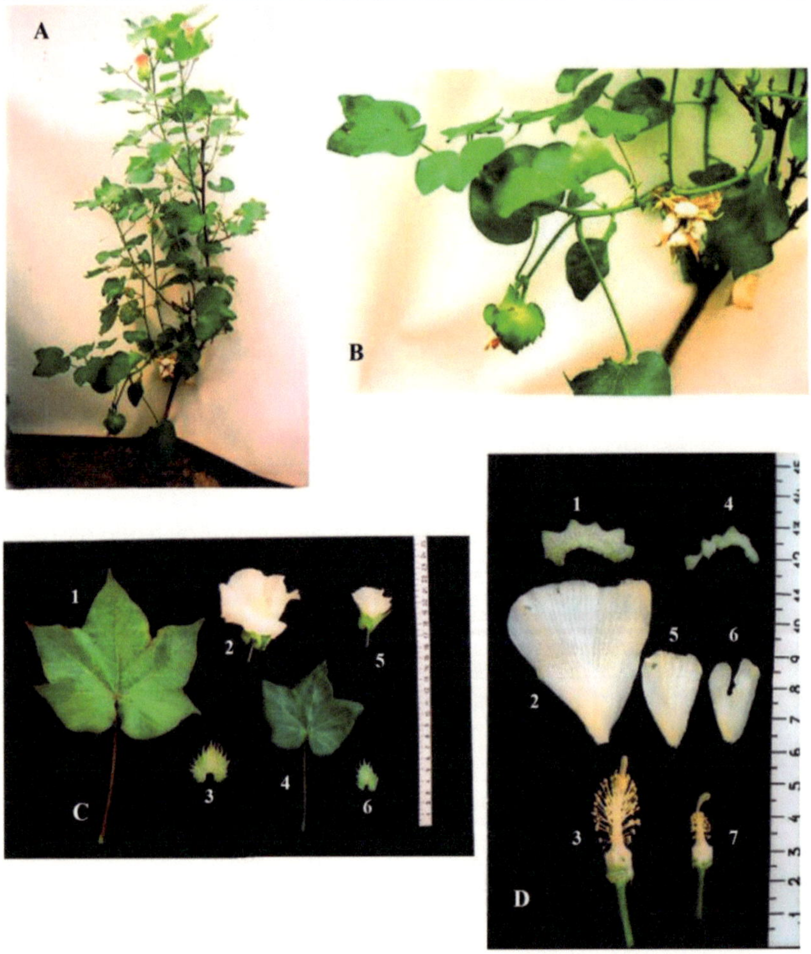

Figure 25. Haploid plant $171/4_{17}$ in cotton *G. hirsutum* obtained in M_2 after pollen irradiation. (A) haploid plant; (B) fertile branch with two bolls; (C) leaf, flower and bract in parental line L-458 (1-3) and haploid plant (4-6); (D) cup, petal and staminate column in parental line L-458 (1-3) and haploid plant (4-7).

http://dx.doi.org/10.5772/58589

9. Conclusions

In conclusion we studied new Cotton Cytogenetic Collection adapted to the Central Asian condition in contrast Cytogenetic Collection from USA using different types of seed and pollen irradiation. We propose the presence of unique cotton aberrations involved chromosomes for absent chromosomes in American collection. The results suggested a detection of "reduced" stigma as a useful phenotypic marker for cotton monosomics which makes it possible to distinguish different cytotypes without cytological analyses. The results demonstrated of new unique desynaptic cotton plants in which progeny produced monosomics with high frequency. We observed the very occurrence of univalents misdivision probably owing to monosome stability in the unique genetic background. Our cotton monosomic lines are unique and should be a valuable cytogenetic tool not only for chromosome assignment of new marker genes and genome enrichment with new chromosome deficient plant, but also for a development of new cotton chromosome substitution lines and germplasm introgression.

Alternatively, the creation of chromosome substitution lines through crossing of each of the new monosomics with *G.barbadense* genotype (Pima 3-79) is in progress. This will serve as a foundation to apply molecular marker (e g., SSPs) for the identification of our monosomics in hybrids with chromosome substitutions for a given monosome. At the same time, our monosomic cotton lines with initial cytogenetic characteristics, which developed using single genome background, should be useful germplasm for cotton researchers to use as material for future breeding genetic, cytogenetic and molecular-genetic investigation of cotton genome.

In future we plan to identify the chromosome deficiencies by molecular markers (SSR) to map of cotton genome. Also we will continue identification monosomic lines of our cytogenetic collection using a well-defined tester-set of translocation lines of the USA Cytogenetic Collection, kindly provided by Dr. D.M. Stelly, Texas A&M University, USA, under USDA germplasm exchange program.

Acknowledgements

This work was partially supported by research grants 38/96, 28/98, 26/2000, F.4.15 and F-5-31 from Committee for Coordination of Science and Technology Development (CCSTD) of the Republik of Uzbekistah. We thank Dr. Svetlana Polyarush and Artyom Maknyov for their help in design of the chapter.

Author details

Marina Sanamyan, Julia Petlyakova, Emma Rakhmatullina and Elnora Sharipova

National University of Uzbekistan, Department of Biology and Soil, Cotton Genetics Laboratory, Uzbekistan

References

[1] Brown MS. Identification of the chromosomes of *Gossypium hirsutum L.* by means of translocations Journal Heredity 1980; 71 (4) 266 – 274.

[2] Endrizzi JE., Turcotte E.L., Kohel R.J. Genetics, cytology and evolution of *Gossypium* Advantes Genetics 1985; (23) 271-375.

[3] Ray DT., Endrizzi JE. A tester-set of translocations in *Gossypium hirsutum L.* Journal Heredity 1982; (73) 429-433.

[4] Ray DT. Metaphase I configurations of the reciprocal translocations in a cytogenetic tester set of *Gossypium hirsutum L.* Journal Heredity 1984; 75 (5) 371-377.

[5] Brown MS., Endrizzi JE. The origin, fertility and transmission of monosomic in *Gossypium* American Journal Botany 1964; 51 (1) 108-115.

[6] Endrizzi JE., Brown MS. Identification of monosomes for six chromosomes in *Gossypium hirsutum* American Journal Botany 1964; 51 (2) 117-120.

[7] Galen DF., Endrizzi JE. Induction of monosomes and mutations in cotton by gamma irradiation of pollen Journal Heredity 1968; 59 (6) 343-346.

[8] Endrizzi JE., Ramsay G. Monosomes and telosomes for 18 of the 26 chromosomes of *Gossypium hirsutum* Canadian Journal Genetics Cytology 1979; 21 (4) 531-536.

[9] Endrizzi JE., Ramsay G. Identification of ten chromosome deficiencies of cotton. Cytological identification of eight chromosomes and genetic analysis of chromosome deficiencies and marker genes Journal Heredity 1980; 71 (1) 45-48.

[10] Edwards GA., Brown MS., Niles GA., Naqi SA. Monosomics of cotton Crop Science 1980; 20 (4) 527-528.

[11] Stelly DM. Interfacing cytogenetics with the cotton genome mapping effort: conference proceedings, conference proceedings, January 10-14, 1993, Beltwide Cotton Conference 1993, New Orleans, Louisiana, 1993 1545-1550.

[12] Ji Y., Raska DA., Mc Knight TD., Islam-Faridi MN., Crane CF., Zwick MS., Hanson RE., Price HJ., Stelly DM. Use of meiotic FISH for identification of a new monosome in *Gossypium hirsutum L.* Genome 1997; 40 34-40.

[13] Raska DA., Stelly DM., Islam-Faridi MN., Woods ME. Identification of a new monosome in cotton: chromosome 21: conference proceedings, 2005, New Orleans, USA, 2005.

[14] Stelly DM. Localization of the Le_2 locus of cotton (*Gossypium hirsutum L.*) Journal Heredity 1990; 81 (3) 193-197.

[15] Endrizzi JE., Ray DT. Monosomic and monotelodisomic analysis of 34 mutant loci in cotton Journal Heredity 1991; 82 53-57.

http://dx.doi.org/10.5772/58589

[16] Endrizzi JE., Ray DT. Mapping of the cl_1, R_1, yg_1 and Dw loci in the long arm of chromosome 16 of cotton Journal Heredity 1992; 83 1-5.

[17] Samora PJ., Stelly DM., Kohel RJ. Localization and mapping of the Le_1 and Gl_2 loci of cotton (*Gossypium hirsutum L.*) Journal Heredity 1994; 85 (2) 152-157.

[18] Saha S., Stelly DM. Chromosomal location of Phosphoglucomutase 7 locus in *Gossypium hirsutum* Journal Heredity 1994; 85 (1) 35-39.

[19] Kakani A., Saha S., Sapra VT., Zipf A., Stelly DM. Genetic mechanism and chromosomal location of pollen-specific gene (s) in *Gossypium* Crop Science 1999; 39 668-673.

[20] Kohel RJ., Yu J., Park Y.-H., Lazo GR. Molecular mapping and characterization of traits controlling fiber quality in cotton Euphytica 2001; 121 163-172.

[21] Kohel RJ., Stelly DM., Yu J. Tests of six cotton (*Gossypium hirsutum L.*) mutants for association with aneuploids Journal Heredity 2002; 93 (2) 130 – 132.

[22] Karaca M., Saha S., Jenkins JN., Zipf A., Kohel R., Stelly DM. Simple sequence repeat (SSR) markers linked to the Ligon Lintless (Li_1) mutant in cotton Journal Heredity 2002; 93 (3) 221 – 224.

[23] Mei M., Syed NH., Gao W., Thaxton PM., Smith CW., Stelly DM., Chen ZJ. Genetic mapping and QTL analysis of fiber-related traits in cotton (*Gossypium*) Theoretical Applied Genetics 2004; 108 280 – 291.

[24] Abdurakhmonov I.Y., Buriev Z.T., Saha S., Pepper A.E., Musaev J.A., Almatov A., Shermatov S.E., Kushanov F.N., Mavlonov G.T., Reddy U.K., Yu. J.Z.Yu., Jenkins J.N., Kohel R.J., Abdukarimov A. Microsatellite markers associated with lint percentage trait in cotton, *Gossypium hirsutum* Euphitica 2007; 156 141-156.

[25] Liu S., Saha S., Stelly DM., Burr B., Cantrell RG. Chromosomal assignment of microsatellite loci in cotton Journal Heredity 2000; 91 (4) 326-332.

[26] Lacape JM., Nguyen TB., Thibivillers S., Bojinov B., Courtols B., Cantrell RG., Burr B., Hau B. A combined RFLP-SSR-AFLP map of tetraploid cotton based on a *Gossypium hirsutum x Gossypium barbadense* backcross population Genome 2003; 46 612-626.

[27] Stelly DM., Saha S., Raska DA., Jenkins JN., McCarty JC., Gutierrez OA. Registration of 17 Upland (*Gossypium hirsutum*) cotton germplasm lines disomic for different *G. barbadense* chromosome or arm substitutions Crop Science 2005; 45 2663-2665.

[28] Saha S., Wu J., Jenkins JN., McCarty JC., Gutierrez OA., Stelly DM., Percy RG., Raska DA. Effect of chromosome substitutions from *Gossypium barbadense L.* 3-79 into *G.hirsutum L.* TM-1 on agronomic and fiber traits Journal Cotton Science 2004; 8 162-169.

[29] Saha S., Raska DA., Stelly DM. Upland (*Gossypium hirsutum*) x Hawaiian cotton (*G. tomentosum* Nutt. Ex Seem.) F1 hybrid hypoaneuploid chromosome substitution series Journal Cotton Science 2006; 10 263-272.

[30] Sanamyan MF, Musaev DA Detection and cytological study of the aneuploid and euploid plants with translocations of chromosomes in cotton *Gossypium hirsutum* L. Genetika 1990; 26 (3) 506-515 [In Russian].

[31] Sanamyan MF, Musaev DA Production and cytogenetic study of the homozygous translocation stocks of cotton. Genetika 1992; 28 75-82 [In Russian].

[32] Sanamyan MF, Musaev DA Cytological and morphological peculiarities of the new translocated lines of cotton. Dokl. Akad. Nauk Republ. Uzbek. 1995; 11-12:63-65 [In Russian].

[33] Sanamyan MF, Petlyakova JE, Musaev DA The development and a cytogenetic study of monosomics of *Gossypium hirsutum* L. Biologia Plantarum 2000, 43 193-197.

[34] Sanamyan MF., Petlyakova JE., Rakhmatullina EM., Sharipova EA. Development of cotton (*Gossypium hirsutum* L.) cytogenetic collection: conference July 30-August 3, 2001 Conf. Genetic collections, isogenic and alloplasmic lines. Novosibirsk, 47-51.

[35] Sanamyan MF, Petlyakova JE. Cytogenetic analysis of cotton monosomics. Biologia Plantarum 2002; 45 367-373.

[36] Sanamyan M.F., Petlyakova JE, Rakhmatullina EM, Sharipova EA. Development and use of radiation-induced chromosomal translocations and primary monosomics of cotton (*G. hirsutum* L.): conference proceedings, 3-6 June, 2002, III ICGI workshop. China, Cotton Sci, 14 (Suppl.) 79-80.

[37] Sanamyan MF, Rakhmatullina EM. Cytogenetic analysis of translocations in cotton. Plant Breeding 2003 122 511-516.

[38] Sanamyan MF. Evaluation of the effect of pollen irradiation on karyotype variability in M_1 cotton plants. Russian Journal of Genetics. 2003a; 39 (7) 791-798.

[39] Sanamyan MF. Evaluation of the effect of pollen irradiation on karyotype variability in M_2 cotton plants. Russian Journal of Genetics. 2003b; 39 (8) 909-916.

[40] Sanamyan MF., Petlyakova JE, Rakhmatullina EM, Sharipova EA. Origin and cytogenetics of new cytogenetic stocks of cotton G.hirsutum L.): conference proceedings, October 10-13, 2004, ICGI-2004 Workshop. India, Hyderabad Andhra Pradesh, 99-100.

[41] Sanamyan MF. Cytogenetics of translocant and monosomic plants of cotton *Gossypium hirsutum* L.", of dokt. Thesis, National University of Uzbekistan, Tashkent, Uzbekistan; 2006.

[42] Sanamyan MF., Petlyakova JE., Sharipova EA., Abdurakhmonov IY. Morphological characteristics and identification of new monosomic stocks for cotton (*Gossypium hirsutum* L.) *Advances in Bioscience and Biotechnology* 2010; 1 372-383.

[43] Sanamyan MF., Petlyakova JE., Sharipova EA., Abdurakhmonov IY. Cytogenetic characteristics of new monosomic stocks of cotton (*Gossypium hirsutum* L.) 2011; *Genetics Research International* 2011; ID 273642, 12 pages.

[44] Bogdanov Yu.f., Grishaeva T.M., Kolomiets O.L., Fedorova Yu.S. Cytogenetic regularities in synapsis of meiotic chromosomes in animals and plants Genetica 1996; 32 (11) 1474-1493. [In Russian].

[45] Sjodin J. Induced translocations in *Vicia faba L.* Hereditas 1971; 68 (1) 1-33.

[46] Burnham C.R., White F.H., Livers R. Chromosomal interchanges in barley Cytologia 1954; 19 191-202.

[47] Burnham C.R. Tester – set of translocations Maise Genet. Coop. News 1954; 28 59-60.

[48] Brown MS. The identification of A and D genome chromosomes in translocations in *Gossypium hirsutum* by means of species crosses Texas Journal Science 1967; 19 423.

[49] Love RM. Varietal differences in meiotic chromosome behavior of Brazilian wheat Agronomy Journal 1951; 43 72-76.

[50] Khush G.S. Cytogenetics of aneuploids. New York and London: Academic Press, 1973.

[51] Menzel M.Y., Brown M.S. Genetic lengths and break points in twelve chromosomes of *Gossypium hirsutum* involved in ten reciprocal translocations Genetics 1978; 88 (3) 541-558.

[52] Myles E.L., Endrizzi J.E. Aneuploids induced by deficiencies of chromosome 9 and analysis of the time of nondisjunction in cotton Genome1989; 32 12-18.

[53] Morrison J.W., Unrau J. Frequency of micronuclei in pollen quartets of common wheat monosomics Canadian Journal of Botany 1952; 30 371-378.

[54] Endrizzi J.E., Turcotte E.L., Kohel R.J. Qualitative genetics, cytology and cytogenetics // Cotton.-Madison, Wisconsin: American Society of Agronomy, 1984.-P. 81-129.

[55] Endrizzi J.E., Bray R. Cytogenetics of disomics, monotelo-and monoisodisomics and ml_1st_1 mutants of chromosome 4 of cotton Genetics 1980; 9 979-988.

[56] Snape J.W., Parker B.B., Simpson E., Ainsworth C.C., Payne P.I., Law C.N. The use of irradiated pollen for differential gene transfer in wheat (*T. aestivum*) Theoretical Applied Genetics 1983; 65 (2) 103-112.

[57] Endrizzi J.E. Use of haploids in *Gossypium barbad*ense L. as a source of aneuploids Current Science 1966; (2) 34-35.

Chapter 11

Cotton Germplasm Collection of Uzbekistan

Ibrokhim Y. Abdurakhmonov, Alisher Abdullaev, Zabardast Buriev, Shukhrat Shermatov, Fahriddin N. Kushanov, Abdusalom Makamov, Umid Shapulatov, Sharof S. Egamberdiev, Ilkhom B. Salakhutdinov, Mirzakamol Ayubov, Mukhtor Darmanov, Azoda T. Adylova, Sofiya M. Rizaeva, Fayzulla Abdullaev, Shadman Namazov, Malohat Khalikova, Hakimjon Saydaliev, Viktor A. Avtonomov, Marina Snamyan, Tillaboy K. Duiesenov, Jura Musaev, Abdumavlyan A. Abdullaev and Abdusattor Abdukarimov

Additional information is available at the end of the chapter

http://dx.doi.org/10.5772/58590

1. Introduction

Uzbekistan, the northernmost cotton growing country, is the sixth largest cotton producer and the second largest cotton exporter in the world [1] with annual production of 0.85-1.0 million metric tons of fibre valued at ~US$0.9 to 1.2 billion [1; 2]. Cotton is grown in ~30% of all lands available for crop cultivation in the country. Uzbekistan's cotton lint fibre yield was close to the world average of 753 kg/ha in 2010/11 [4] and was estimated at 804 kg/ha in 2012/13 and 812 kg/ha in 2013/14 [1; 5].

Cotton farming is affected by commonly observed cotton pathogens and pests, as well as major environmental stress factors (salinity, drought, heat, etc.) that greatly impacts the quality and yield characteristics of cotton cultivars. Therefore, the major objectives of the cotton breeding programs of Uzbekistan are the improvement of cotton fibre quality, lint yield, agronomic productivity, maturity,and resistance to various diseases, pests and abiotic stresses. During the past century of cotton production Uzbekistan prioritized and promoted cotton research and farming methods that resulted in increased cotton farming expertise, and the breeding of highly adapted, very-early maturing cotton cultivars suitable to be grown in the northern latitudes and arid zones [6; 7; 8]. This led to the development of a large number of cotton germplasm resources, which are being preserved and maintained for cotton genetics and breeding research that target current and future needs of the cotton improvement for different soil-climatic regions of Uzbekistan [1; 2; 3; 8].

Aspects of Uzbekistan cotton germplasm resources including the content, distribution, descriptions, characterizations, utilization, genetic and molecular diversity, maintenance, and ongoing and prospective research previously have been highlighted in several documents [2; 3; 7; 8; 9; 10]. In this chapter, we provide a detailed inventory of the Uzbekistan cotton germplasm collection, review previous reports and add updated information including the development and characterization of novel germplasm resources.

2. History and development of Uzbekistan cotton collection

The past century of cotton production in Uzbekistan has developed well-established cotton research programs and distinguished cotton scientists who initiated and devoted themselves to collecting important materials for cotton research. As highlighted in previous reports [3; 8] the cotton germplasm collection initiative was began by Drs. N. I. Vavilov and F. M. Mauer in 1930 in the former Soviet Union. Subsequently, Uzbekistan cotton germplasm founder and leader Dr. A. Abdullaev and his group expanded this initiative and established a collection of Uzbekistan germplasm materials through the (1) coordination of scientific efforts of continuous selection of cultivated cotton varieties, (2) continuation of collecting and preserving wild cotton species and landraces from centres of origin during many scientific expeditions, and (3) germplasm exchange worldwide.

According to Abdullaev et al. [8], several expeditions to Central Asia, Afghanistan, China, India, Turkey, Iran, Korea and Japan to obtain germplasm were made during 1920-1930, Dr. N. I. Vavilov, P. M. Jukovsky and Dr. F. M. Mauer, and in 1950s Dr. D. V. Ter-Avanesyan. In later periods from 1974 to 1998, Dr. A. Abdullaev visited to Mexico, Peru, China, India and Sri-Lanka, Australia and Pakistan and obtained germplasm. These historic scientific expeditions enriched Uzbekistan collection with Old World (Afro-Asian and Indian) diploid cottons (*G. herbaceum* and *G. arboreum*), and a number of wild, exotic and cultivated tetraploid and diploid cottons around the world [8].

The Uzbekistan collection has been periodically enriched as a result of germplasm exchanges with collections worldwide. In the most recent exchanges within the framework of USDA-Uzbekistan Cooperation programs, approximately ~ 1000 *G. hirsutum* exotic and varietal accessions were exchanged with the US cotton germplasm collection [11; 12]. Annually, 100-120 cotton accessions from the collection of Uzbek Research Institute of Cotton Breeding and Seed Production (UzSRICBSP) are exchanged with world centres. During the period of 2001-2003, the Institute received 990 accessions from and sent 260 cotton accessions to the US cotton germplasm collection [7].

3. Content of Uzbekistan cotton germplasm collection

3.1. Main collections

The main cotton germplasm collections are being historically preserved at the research centres and institutions of the Academy of Sciences of Uzbekistan (ASUz), Ministry of Agriculture and Water Resources of Uzbekistan (MAWR), and the biology department of the National University (NU) of Uzbekistan. Table 1 summarizes and highlights the general content and description of cotton germplasm resources of these main collections. These collections maintain cultivars, wild and primitive, predomesticated landraces, hybrids breeding and genetic stocks, cytogenetic and mutant lines of widely cultivated allotetraploids(*G. hirsutum* and *G. barbadense*) representing the primary gene pool, and two cultivated Asian diploids (*G. herbaceum* and *G. arboreum*) representing the secondary gene pool. Although some redundancy of accessions maintained by collections could be possible and is a subject for future comparative inventory work, each collection has its own specificities and has been formed according to distinctive research efforts conducted by the scientists of these institutions for past decades.

Germplasm type	*G. hirsutum*	*G. barbadense*	*G. arboreum*	*G. herbaceum*	Other species	Total
Institute of Genetics and Plant Experimental Biology (IG&PEB), Academy of Sciences of Uzbekistan (ASUz)						
Cultivar/Line	3735	827	736	338		5636
Wild landraces	402	6	25	11	45	489
Hybrids	321	84	30	20	187	642
Unclassified	445	53	66	178		742
Total	4903	970	857	547	232	7509
Uzbek Scientific Research Institute of Cotton Breeding and Seed Production (UzSRICBSP), Ministry of Agriculture and Water Resources (MAWR), Republic of Uzbekistan						
Cultivar/Line	6597	908	200	161	28	7894
Wild landraces	568	27	38	21	101	755
Hybrids	1200	645	232	162	58	2297
Unclassified	722	648	155	294	35	1854
Total	9087	2228	625	638	222	12800
Uzbek Research Institute of Plant Industry (UzRIPI), Ministry of Agriculture and Water Resources (MAWR), Republic of Uzbekistan						
Cultivar/Line	2105	64	44	55	314	2582
Wild landraces	846	8	25	43	99	1021
Mutants	1	1	-	-	-	2
Hybrids	76	152	-	-	19	247
Unclassified	1414	482	74	9	240	2219
Total	4442	707	143	107	672	6071

Germplasm type	*G. hirsutum*	*G. barbadense*	*G. arboreum*	*G. herbaceum*	Other species	Total
			National University of Uzbekistan (NUUz)			
Genetic stocks of inbred and RI lines	771	-	-	-	-	771
			Cytogenetic stocks/Mutants			
Primary monosomics	94	-	-	-	-	94
Tertiary monosomics	22	-	-	-	-	22
Monotelodisomics	20	-	-	-	-	20
Monoisodisomics	4	-	-	-	-	4
Haploids	4	-	-	-	-	4
Disynaptics	31	-	-	-	-	31
Translocations	235	-	-	-	-	235
						0
Total	1181	0	0	0	0	1181
			Centre of Genomics and Bioinformatics, ASUz, MAWR, and "UzCottonIndustry" association			
			Mapping panels			
Association mapping individuals	986	286	-	-	-	1272
Nested association mapping cross combination	20	-	-	-	-	20
			Chromosome substitution line hybrids			
F_1 to F_4 generation families	260	-	-	-	-	260
CSUZ-RILs individuals	301	-	-	-	-	301
			Transformed lines			
Tissue culture derived (T_{1-6})	1444					1444
Hybrids (F_{1-6} and BC_{1-5}) with local cultivars	1852					1852
			MAS-derived germplasm			
MAS – F_{1-2} and BC_{2-4} families	51				14	65
MAS gene pyramiding families	24					24
Total	4938	286	0	0	14	5238
Grand total	24571	4190	1623	1292	937	32580

Table 1. Summary of the content of Uzbekistan cotton germplasm collections

Cotton germplasm collection of the Institute of Genetics and Plant Experimental Biology (IG&PEB) of the ASUz, founded and headed by academician and Prof. Abdumavlyan Abdullaev, preserves a total of 7,500 cotton accessions. The collection specifically aims to gather, maintain, and study wild cotton species, primitive, pre-domesticated landraces and domesticated genotypes from entire *Gossypium* genus. The IG&PEB cotton germplasm collection, also referred to as "wild collection", was formed as a result of scientific expeditions to the centres of origin of *Gossypium* species and a 50 years of research efforts by IG&PEB scientists and research programs. IG&PEB cotton collection maintains more than 40 wild A-to G and K-genome *Gossypium* species [2; 3; 8] and targets the study of the taxonomy, phylogeny, evolution, hybridization compatibility, and introgression of wild germplasm for breeding purposes, all of which make the collection unique compared to others. The detailed description, content, geographic coverage and history of *G. hirsutum* and *G. barbadense* germplasm development in Uzbekistan were discussed by Abdullaev et al., 2013, where authors report the representation of 4 continents, ~33 geographic regions and ~103 countries by the IG&PEB collection [8].There are a large number di-and tri-genomic hybrids and their diploid and allotetraploid progenies recovered from tedious sexual crosses within and/or between wild, primitive and domesticated genotypes within different gene pools [13; 14; Dr. Rizaeva, personal communication]. Some of examples such as tri-genomic hybrids were highlighted in previous reports [14; 15].

MAWR has two distinctive cotton collections: one is preserved at the UzSRICBSP, another is in the Uzbek Research Institute of Plant Industry (UzRIPI), which was a Central Asian branch of All Union scientific-research institute after N.I. Vavilov. The UzSRICBSP collection preserves more than 12,000 cotton accessions from primary and secondary gene pools and refereed to as "breeding" germplasm resources that resulted from continuous breeding and selection efforts of the institute's scientists as well as cotton germplasm exchange efforts [16]. Geographically, this collection represents 107 countries of origin for cotton accessions [7]. The uniqueness of UzSRICBSP collection is its wide representation and coverage of cultivar germplasm developed and collected over the past century from worldwide breeding efforts. This collection also maintains synthetic tetraploid, pentaploid and octoploid hybrids [7; 16]. There are small differences in germplasm accession numbers reported here (Table 1) and by Ibragimov et al. [7]. However, our inventory is based on the latest information obtained from this collection (Dr. H. Saydaliev, a germplasm curator of the UzSRICBSP, personal communication).

The UzRIPI cotton collection has contents similar to those of the IG&PEB collection and preserves a total of over 6,000 accessions (Table 1) from primary and secondary gene pools as well as accessions of other gene pools of wild species. Among all the collections, UzRIPI cotton collection is the richest resource for primitive, and pre-domesticated landrace stocks for all *Gossypium* gene pools in the country. However, there is a need to conduct comparative re-inventory between UzRIPI and IG&PEB collection to identify the distinctive versus redundant germplasm accessions. Because UZRIPI was the Central Asian branch of All Union scientific-research institute after N.I. Vavilov some level of redundancies to Russian VIR collection is expected that requires future study.

The NU collection is tasked with maintaining of a total about 1200 germplasm resources that include 771 genetic stocks and recombinant inbred lines, formed during study of key cotton traits and mutations [3; 17; 18]. Additionally, the NU collection has a unique set of over 400 cytogenetics stocks primarily derived from radio-mutagenesis of a single genotype of *G.*

hirsutum line L-458 [19; 20]. Readers can find detailed description of Uzbekistan's cytogenetic cotton collection in this book.

3.2. Novel resources

Efforts focused on genetic mapping of important traits, application of marker-assisted breeding as an aid for contemporary breeding, and the development of cotton tissue culture-based transgenomics programs and their integration into conventional cotton improvement efforts have resulted in the creation and collection of novel germplasm resources in Uzbekistan. These novel germplasm resources were developed in the past decade by scientists of Centre of Genomics and Bioinformatics (CGB), ASUz, MAWR, and "UzcottonIndustry association" within the framework of international collaborations and government funding [1; 21; 22]. The CGB collection with over 5,000 germplasm resources (Table 1) includes (i) panels of association mapping and nested-association mapping populations [22; 23; 24], (ii) hybrids and recombinant inbred lines ($F_{1\text{-}4}$) derived from the combination of sexual top crosses between 9 commercialized Uzbek cotton cultivars and 16 different chromosome substituted lines (CS-B) [25; 26; 27; 28; 29], (iii) germplasm resources developed through marker-assisted selection (MAS) programs that bear novel quantitative trait loci (QTL) loci mobilized from unique donors to the genetic background of commercial Uzbek cotton cultivars via molecular markers, and (iv) tissue culture-derived, genetically modified (GM) germplasm and their hybrids to local cultivars that bear RNA interference (RNAi), synthetic hairpin oligonucleotides, anti-sense, or overexpression genetic constructs for *de novo* characterized genes and sequence signatures in the CGB laboratories [1; 22; 30; 31; 32].

It is noteworthy to mention that association mapping individuals (Table 1) were selected from the IG&PEB collection and re-grown at the Mexico Winter Nursery of USDA-ARS by Drs. Russel Kohel and John Yu, (cotton germplasm Unit of USDA-ARS at College Station,Texas) for phenotypic evaluations and seed increase. Increased seeds grown at the Mexican environment kindly were sent back to Uzbekistan by Dr. Richard Percy (USDA cotton germplasm curator) and currently backed-up at the CGB and IG&PEB collections. Additionally, chromosome substituted (CS-B) lines were received within the frame of USDA-Uzbekistan Cooperation Programs, kindly provided by Dr. David Stelly (Texas A&M University), Dr. Sukumar Saha and Dr. Johnie Jenkins, USDA-ARS, Starkville, Mississippi, and now are preserved in both CGB and IGPEB collections. CGB scientists in collaboration with USDA partners are developing CS-B specific chromosome substituted recombinant inbred lines (CSRILs) in the background of important Uzbekistan cultivars. Further, development of cotton tissue culture and trangenomics efforts [21], and the mobilization of useful genetic constructs into commercialized cultivars has created novel germplasm resources, useful for cotton improvement and helpful to address many problems associated with improving and boosting yield and quality [1; 22; 32].

4. Storage, maintenance and funding

The above-mentioned main collections and novel germplasm resources are stored and maintained in each institution and managed separately by its scientists. The IG&PEB, UzS-RICBSP, and NU collections are stored under room temperature conditions (20-25°C) and there is no facility available for cold storage of germplasm accessions [3; 8]. In contrast, UzRIPI [33] and CGB collections are stored in short term (under+4°C) cold room facilities that were established as a result of government and international funding (in the case of UzRIPI, [33]. No long term cold storage (-20 or-80 °C) facilities, requiring attention and investment, are available for any of the germplasm collections in Uzbekistan, as highlighted by Campbell et al. [3] and Abdullaev et al. [8].

Germplasm accession seeds are preserved according to commonly practised procedures used over the decades of germplasm maintenance efforts in each collection. For instance, according to previous reports [8] germplasm seeds are ginned and put into paper bags with a label of catalogue number, accession name, year of collection and origin. Paper bags also contain *"the weight of seeds (50 g or 100 g individual or total pick respectively"*) and *"bags are stored in special metal boxes (30 x 11 cm) and boxes are placed in wooden-cases"* [8]. Other collections follow similar storage procedure with some modifications in types of storage boxes and variations in labelling of bags. Since 2003, after the reconstruction of the building for germplasm resources at UZRIPI, cotton germplasm seed have been stored in plastic containers [33].

Consequently, germplasm resources, in particular those without short term cold room facility, are scheduled for seed renewal every 8-10 years under forced self-pollination in the open field conditions [3]. Each organization has its own, but very similar protocols, schemes of planting, growing and evaluating germplasm (see [8] for detailed protocol for IG&PEB cotton collection), government research grants and field extension stations with up to 8-10 staff working on germplasm maintenance. During a seed renewal year, accessions of re-grown germplasm are phenotypically evaluated for major agronomic and morpho-biological and fibre quality traits [3; 8].

Germplasm evaluation records from each collection are maintained as a hard copy catalogue book that contains all descriptions about accessions (origin, year, collector, collected sites, seed renewal, etc), and data from the past 50 years of evaluations [e.g. 34] In UzRIPI, there is a "Unified Council for Mutual Economic Assistance (COMECON) list of descriptors for the species *Gossypium L* [35]. IG&PEB has started using modified "Cotton descriptor" of International Plant Genetic Resource Institution [see below for detail description; 3; 8]. Moreover, data records on germplasm accession characteristics and description are being currently entered into electronic Microsoft database formats (personal communications with germplasm heads of all collections). All cotton collections also have their own greenhouse facilities to vegetatively maintain [7; 8] wild and primitive accessions, unique multi-genomic hybrids, mutants, and cytogenetics stocks as well as transformed and somatically regenerated lines.

As reported by Campbell et al. [3], all germplasm related activities and maintenance of the Uzbekistan cotton collections are funded by the Committee for Coordination of Science and Technology Development under the Cabinet of Ministry of Uzbekistan, MAWR, and ASUz where funds are given as competitive research and "a unique facility" maintenance grants. Moreover, each institution receives international grants for projects that utilize the germplasm resources, and therefore, budget funding for germplasm related works [3].

5. Sharing and exchange

As highlighted in the recent reports by Campbell et al. [3] and Abdullaev et al. [8], all existing cotton germplasm resources, deposited and preserved in the country, are available for cotton researchers, breeders, and students who are conducting the cotton research. Written requests should be addressed to the directors of institutions, and should describe the purpose of the germplasm usage and specify the amount of seeds requested. Directors of institutions, with approval and on the responsibility of germplasm curators, grant the distribution of requested germplasm. If a specific germplasm with commercial interest is requested, a bi-lateral agreements are sought defining the condition of sharing that varies according institutions' internal regulations. All granted requests are registered in the germplasm exchange book of the collection.

Previously, germplasm requested by foreign institutions were officially sent under a standard "research purposes only" Material Transfer Agreement (MTA) and accompanied by proper phytosanitary certificates upon approval of the National Coordinator of Plant Genetic Resources (PGR) of Uzbekistan and responsible offices at the MAWR. Presently, any genetic and biological material sharing is granted by approval of Committee for Coordination of Science and Technology Development under the Cabinet of Ministry of Uzbekistan with "a research purpose only" MTA.

6. Characterization and utilization of the collection

Detailed evaluation, characterization, and cataloguing of germplasm accessions in the collections are very important to the utility of the collections by the local and world cotton research community interested in using 'candidate' accessions for breeding purposes. As mentioned above, during the periodic renewal of seed of germplasm accessions to maintain the collection, accessions are evaluated and characterized for the major characteristics and traits useful for both biodiversity estimates and cotton improvement. Each collection has its independent programs and objectives toward this goal; therefore, there was a need to develop a unified germplasm evaluation methodology and descriptors [11; 12].

http://dx.doi.org/10.5772/58590

6.1. Cotton germplasm descriptor and database

In UzRIPI, there is a computerized "CAC-DB" database for plant germplasm resources developed for Central Asian and Transcaucasian countries using Microsoft FoxPro [36; 37]. In this database, the principle information systems of the International Centre for Agricultural Research in the Dry Areas (ICARDA) and the N.I. Vavilov Research Institute of Plant Industry (VIR) is used. Major characteristics for the entire cotton collection of the UZRIPI as well as UzSRICBSP have been described in an electronic catalogue in Microsoft Excel (Dr. Fyzulla Abdullaev, germplasm specialist of the UzSRICBSP, personal communication).

Within the framwork of USDA-Uzbekistan cooperation programs, CGB scientists in collaboration with IG&PEB colleagues and cotton germplasm Unit staff worked on updating the cotton cataloguing system. Scientists suggested the use of a modified version of the "Descriptor for Cotton" which was originally developed and approved by IPGRI in 1985 (http://www/ipgri/cgiar.org). After considering recommendations from more recent descriptors for plant germplasm resources (e.g., Descriptor for Groundnuts-1992; and Descriptor for Pistachio-2002) and consulting with IG&PEB germplasm curator and leaders (Dr. Abdumavlyan Abdullaev and Dr. Sofiya Rizaeva), some modifications were introduced to the "Descriptor for Cotton-1985" of IPGRI. In the modified descriptors, two categories: "characterization and preliminary evaluation" and "further characterization and evaluation" were combined into one category "characterization and evaluation" because of the lack of preliminary information for accessions that were brought from abroad to the IG&PEB collection. New sub-categories, such as 1) cotton boll size, and 2) natural leaf defoliation properties were introduced; in "Susceptibility to biotic stresses" diseases and disease sources, specific to Uzbekistan, were introduced. At present, about 1,000 Upland germplasm accessions have been characterized for main agronomic, fibre quality properties and molecular diversity [12; 23; 24] using the modified "Descriptor for Cotton-1985" [Table 2; 8].

Further, ~1000 *G. hirsutum* cotton accessions were selected from IG&PEB cotton collection and evaluated for major morphological, agronomic and fibre quality traits in the Uzbekistan and Mexican growing environments in collaboration with Germplasm Unit of USDA-ARS at College Station, Texas, USA [12; 23; 24; 38]. Data from the evaluations was collected according to above mentioned descriptor. Consequently, pc-GRIN software package (used in creating US plant germplasm database) and Microsoft Access software packages were used to develop initial basic electronic database of IG&PEB collection. This initial database contains most of information about accessions and morphological trait data, including fibre quality and yield properties as well as molecular-genetic data for each accession (such as in microsatellite marker genotypes, molecular diversity, etc.). There is ongoing effort to expand this database through adding additional germplasm accessions from periodic germplasm seed renewal evaluations. There is a need to apply the same procedure for all existing collections and coordinate future joint efforts toward this goal.

No	Trait	Characteristic or short description	Value	Notes
1	SCIENTIFIC NAME	Latin name		Name of genus, species, subspecies etc. (ex.: *Gossypium hirsutum spp. mexicanum*)
2	ACCESSION NAME	Name of line or cultivar		Ex.: TM-1, 3-79
3	ACCESSION NUMBER	Number of accession in collection catalogue		Ex.: 1, 2, 3...
4	ORIGIN	Place of sample origin		Collection, author/scientist, country etc.
5	YEAR	Year of acceptance to collection		YYYY
6	RENEWAL	Last time of seeds renewal		DD.MM.YYYY
7	HOMOGENIETY	Not uniform	0	Homogeneity of cotton germplasm population
		Uniform	1	
8	GROW HABIT	Prostrate	3	Growth of habit (Bush shape)
		Compact	5	
		Erect	7	
9	ANTOCYAN	Weak	0	Colour of the plant in general
		Middle	1	
		Strong	2	
		Not became brown	3	
10	STEM HAIRINESS	Naked	1	Hairiness of the plant stem
		Very weak	2	
		Weak	3	
		Middle	5	
		Strong	7	
11	LEAF HAIRINES	As above		Hairiness of the leaves
12	LEAFSHP	Palmate(normal)	1	Leaf shape
		Semi-digitate(semi-okra)	2	
		Digitate(okra)	3	
		Lanceolate(super okra)	4	
13	LOBE NUMB		Numeric	Number of leaf lobe
14	EMERGENCE		Numeric	Days to emergence of cotton seedlings
15	SEEDENERGY %		Numeric	The energy required for seed germination
16	SEEDTERM %	Seed energy in thermostat (%)	Numeric	The energy required for seed germination in thermostat
17	BRHGHT (HS)		Numeric	Height of the first fruit branch in cm.
18	BRANCHTYPE	Branching Type		Distance of first sympodial fruit branch from first fruit brunch in cm
		0-5 cm	1	
		5-10 cm	2	
		10-15 cm	3	
		15-20 cm	4	
19	HIEGHT (cm)		Numeric	Plant height in cm.

No	Trait	Characteristic or short description	Value	Notes
20	MONO		Numeric	Number of monopodia
21	SYMP		Numeric	Number of sympodia
22	STEAMNODE		Numeric	Number of total stem nodes
23	PETAL colour	White	1	Petal colour
		Cream	2	
		Light yellow	3	
		Yellow	4	
		Lavender	5	
		Red	6	
		bicolour	7	
24	PEATAL SPOT	absent	1	Petal spot
		present	9	
25	POLLEN colour	White	1	Pollen colour
		Cream	2	
		Yellow	3	
		Purple	4	
26	PHOTO	Not photoperiodic	0	Sensitivity to day/night length
		Slightly photoperiodic	1	
		Photoperiodic	2	
		Strictly photoperiodic	3	
27	FLOWERING		Numeric	Days to 50% of plants flowering
28	OPENING		Numeric	Days to 50% of bolls opening
29	BOLL SH	Round	1	Boll shape
		Oval	2	
		Conical	3	
30	BOLL OPEN	Normal	1	Level of Boll opening
		Intermediate	2	
		Strom-proof	3	
31	BOLL NUM		Numeric	Number of boll
32	BOLL WEIGHT	Boll weight (g)	Numeric	Average weight in grams of a 10 boll sample
33	LOCULES NUM		Numeric	Locules per boll
34	SEED WEIGHT		Numeric	Weight of 100 seeds in grams (could be applied to cultivated plants only)
35	SEED FUZZ	Fuzzy	1	Fuzz grade (amount of fuzz on seeds)
		Sparse fuzz	2	
		Naked seed	3	
36	FUZZ colour	White	1	Fuzz colour
		Green	2	
		Grey	3	
		Brown (Tan)	4	
37	LINT colour	White	1	Lint colour

No	Trait	Characteristic or short description	Value	Notes
		Cream	2	
		Light brown	3	
		Brown	4	
		Green	5	
38	fibre LENGHT		Numeric	fibre length in millimeter
39	T0	fibre strength (g/tex)	Numeric	The fibre strength of a bundle of fibres measured on a Stelometre with the jaws holding the fibre bundle tightly apprised. Measured in grams force per tex.
40	MIC	Micronaire	Numeric	The fitness of the sample taken from the ginned lint measured by the Micronaire and expressed in standard curvilinear micronaire units
41	UI%		Numeric	fibre maturity in %
42	YELLOWNESS	fibre yellowness	Numeric	Hunter's B value, a measure of increasing yellowness of the cotton, taken with a Nickerson-Hunter colourimeter
43	REFLECT	Reflectance (RD)	Numeric	A measure of the percentage of reflectance on a Nickerson-Hunter colourimeter. The higher the value the lighter the cotton.
44	LINT	Lint (yield) percentage	Numeric	The weight of lint ginned from sample of seed cotton expressed as percentage of the weight of seed cotton
45	LINT INDEX		Numeric	The weight of lint from 100 seed in gram
46	ELO	The percentage of fibre elongation	Numeric	The percentage of elongation at break of the centre 1/8 each of the fibre bundle measured for T1 strength on the Stelometer
47	CGRD		Numeric	colour grade of fibre
48	AREA	Area of seed in %	Numeric	Seed covered area with fibre
49	DISEASE RES	Highly Resistant (≥86% -100%)	1	Percentage of plants Resistant to pests/ insects or phytopathogen (fungi, bacteria, virus etc.)
		Resistant (≥76%-85%)	2	
		Moderate (≥51%-75%)	3	
		Susceptible (≥31%-50%)	4	
		Highly susceptible (1%-30%)	5	
50	ENVRES	Special resistance to environmental conditions	As above	Resistance to salt, drought, low water, temperature etc.

Table 2. The descriptor developed for Uzbek cotton germplasm collection (Source: from Abdullaev et al., 2013)

6.2. Germplasm characterization and utilization

Cotton germplasm Units of each collection work extensively on characterization of their own germplasm resources within the framework of various projects. IG&PEB cotton germplasm Unit scientists, as mentioned above, investigate the evolution, taxonomy, phylogeny, hybridization compatibility, usage and introgression of wild germplasm. On the basis of investigations of the gene pools from IG&PEB collection, Abdullaev et al. [39] updated the Mauer taxonomy system for *Gossypium* L. and highlighted new species discovered at the end of XX century in their updated taxonomy, which was unknown for Mauer [40]. Researchers also have created hybridization compatibility schemes and identified phylogenetic relations between different cotton species [41]. Accordingly, the IG&PEB collection has developed a number of hybrids within and between different gene pools and cotton species. Cotton species and gene pools preserved in IG&PEB collection were studied for morphological and anatomical characteristics in detail and an "Atlas of *Gossypium* L. genus" has been published [41].

Being a breeding collection of cultivated cottons in Uzbekistan, the UzSRICBSP researchers mainly use their collection to study genetics of various agronomic traits and disease resistance aspects of germplasm accessions during the variety development process [7; 16]. The NU collection, in particular the genetic stocks and cytogenetic stocks has been characterized in detail for the genetic traits [17] and cytogenetic aberrations [19; 20; 42]. The unique cytogenetic collection preserved at the NU also is being characterized using molecular markers and identification of chromosome specificities of the monosomics is in progress (Dr. Marina Sanamyan, personal communication).

Cotton germplasm resources were the foundation to develop highly adapted, disease resistant and superior agronomic quality cotton cultivars for Uzbekistan that were highlighted in a number of past reports [2; 3; 6; 8; 10]. In particular, forecasting the benefit of utilization of wild cotton germplasm accessions in conventional breeding of cotton in early 1960s by germplasm leaders, Drs. F. Mauer and A. Abdullaev [3; 8; 43] boosted the new variety development in Uzbekistan that provided timely responses to cotton production problems in the country. Over the past several decades, Uzbekistan breeders have developed more than 200 new cotton cultivars highly adapted [7] to the different soil-climatic regions of Uzbekistan, with high resistance characteristics to the major cotton diseases and pests, having high-yield and better fibre qualities [6; 7; 8; 44]. It is noteworthy to highlight here that the major accomplishment of Uzbekistan cotton breeders for the past century of efforts was the development of very early-maturing and productive cotton cultivars with 105-120 days of vegetation period, which made cotton growing suitable and profitable in the northern latitudes like Uzbekistan. This was only possible because of the existence and efficient exploitation of cotton germplasm resources that should be highlighted and valued as Uzbekistan's cotton breeders greatest commitment.

Further, as highlighted in recent reports [3; 8; 21] with the advances in cotton sciences and the development and application of modern molecular genetics tools and approaches for plant germplasm analysis [45], initial efforts by Uzbekistan scientist to characterize a selected global set of ~1000 *Gossypium hirsutum* L. accessions from Uzbekistan cotton germplasm at molecular level have occured. This global set represented 37 cotton growing countries and 8 breeding ecotypes as well as wild landrace stocks. Using this selected set of global Upland germplasm resources, molecular genetic diversity, population diversification and strata, and the extent of linkage disequilibrium (LD) for the cotton genome were characterized [10; 11; 12; 23; 24].

Efforts also identified several SSR markers associated with main fibre quality traits along with donor accessions, bearing "golden" QTLs useful for MAS programs [23; 24]. As a result, a successful MAS program has been established in Uzbekistan that facilitated to mobilize novel haplotypes of important fibre quality QTLs from donor accessions preserved in cotton germplasm collection to commercial cultivars. In that fibre trait-associated DNA markers were used as a tool to manipulate the transfer of QTLs during a genetic hybridization [38; 46; 47].

The MAS program, extensively utilized during past decade in Uzbekistan that involved several donor (germplasm accessions) and recipient (commercial cultivars) germplasm not only improved and developed novel MAS cultivars through mobilization of novel untapped loci but also created novel germplasm resources useful for cotton breeders and future cotton breeding [Table 1; 10; 38; 46; 47]. Several first generation MAS-derived cultivars were developed and submitted for State Variety Testing Committee of Uzbekistan for future commercialization that are being field-trailed for improved agronomic and fibre qualities across the Uzbekistan regions. Moreover, as a ongoing effort, Uzbekistan researchers initiated a gene-pyramiding approach to combine major fibre quality traits into single genotype of several commercial Upland cotton cultivars of Uzbekistan using these effective molecular markers as a breeding tool and donor genotypes from cotton germplasm collections [38; 46; 47].

As a continuation of efforts to characterize cotton germplasm resources at the molecular level, about 300 *G. barbadense* (so called extra long staple fibre Pima cotton) accessions with wide geographic origin covering 17 countries worldwide were recently genotyped with SSR markers to estimate molecular diversity, phylogeny, population structure, and linkage disequilibrium level. These Pima cotton accessions were exchanged with USDA-ARS at Shafter, California, evaluated for major agronomic, morphological and fibre quality traits in the Uzbekistan or/and CA growing environments, and used for molecular mapping of fibre quality traits useful for MAS programs [8; Abdullaev et al., 2014 unpublished]

Use of cotton germplasm resources and their characterization at the molecular level further helped us to select the most diverse *G. hirsutum* accessions to create nested association mapping (NAM) panel. The creation of NAM populations is efficient approach to enhance power [48] of association mapping in cotton [10; 49]. Currently, a panel of 4000 $F_{2:3}$ generation NAM population individuals has been developed from genetic crosses between 20 most diverse *G. hirsutum* accessions and Uzbek cultivar Namangan-77, a genetic standard for *G. hirsutum.* NAM population individuals are also being genotyped with a large number of SSR markers and evaluated for major agronomic characteristics in different environments of Uzbekistan to conduct fine association mapping studies [22; Abdurakhmonov et al., 2014, unpublished].

Currently, genotyping of additional cotton germplasm accessions from major collections using widely available SSR markers is in progress that will help to characterize and organize the entire cotton germplasm resources of Uzbekistan. In perspective, we also aim to apply novel molecular tools such as SNP platforms and genotyping-by-sequencing (GBS) technologies to

http://dx.doi.org/10.5772/58590

better characterize the selected cotton germplasm resources, AM and NAM panels that require additional funding, coordinated efforts and international collaborations.

7. Conclusion

Due to the importance of cotton production for the country and the historic expertise on cotton farming and production developed during the past century, Uzbekistan has prioritized and promoted the breeding programs, leading to a collection of one of the richest cotton germplasm resources in the world. Developed and maintained by several leading cotton research institutions in Uzbekistan, cotton germplasm collections preserve over 25,000 major cotton germplasm accessions of *Gossypium* species, wild, primitive, pre-domesticated landraces stocks, cultivar and breeding lines, mutants, genetic and cytogenetic stocks, and various types of within and between cotton gene pool hybrids. These resources were collected from the centres of origins of *Gossypium* species during scientific expeditions and through germplasm exchange with world germplasm centres, and developed by scientists and breeders of Uzbekistan for the past century. Consequently, these germplasm resources were the basis for the development of Uzbekistan's main commercial cultivars with early maturity and high productivity, making cotton profitable in the northernmost cotton growing country. This greatest achievement and commitment of cotton breeders timely responded and solved many past and current problems of cotton production as well as it will help to sustain the cotton production in Uzbekistan in the future.

Although each cotton collection has its own specific goals and objectives for preserved materials, there is a huge need for conducting joint re-inventory for clarification of redundancies between some of collections. There is a need for building short-term and long term cold storage rooms for all collections available in the country to better preserve the collection for future generations and cotton production. Moreover, although initial efforts have been made, coordinated efforts are needed to create a unified electronic database to systematize the germplasm records for all collections that will help for better utilization of the accessions in the breeding programs.

There are over 5,000 novel germplasm resources that were developed for past decade of collaborative efforts on molecular genetic characterization of cotton germplasm resources and establishment of modern MAS and GM programs. The modern cotton genomics and bioinformatics programs in combination with conventional cotton breeding efforts will further enhance the characterization and utilization as well as efficient documentation and systematization of the germplasm resources in Uzbekistan.

Acknowledgements

We thank the Uzbekistan government for continual funding support for cotton germplasm collections and research. We acknowledge the Office of International Research Programs

(OIRP) of the United States Department of Agriculture (USDA) and USA partner laboratories for the financial support of cotton germplasm related works through project P120/P120a.

Author details

Ibrokhim Y. Abdurakhmonov[1], Alisher Abdullaev[1], Zabardast Buriev[1], Shukhrat Shermatov[1], Fahriddin N. Kushanov[1], Abdusalom Makamov[1], Umid Shapulatov[1], Sharof S. Egamberdiev[1], Ilkhom B. Salakhutdinov[1], Mirzakamol Ayubov[1], Mukhtor Darmanov[1], Azoda T. Adylova[1], Sofiya M. Rizaeva[2], Fayzulla Abdullaev[2,4], Shadman Namazov[3], Malohat Khalikova[3], Hakimjon Saydaliev[3], Viktor A. Avtonomov[3], Marina Snamyan[4], Tillaboy K. Duiesenov[5], Jura Musaev[4], Abdumavlyan A. Abdullaev[2] and Abdusattor Abdukarimov[1]

1 Centre of Genomics and Bioinformatics, Academy of Sciences of Uzbekistan, Ministry of Agriculture and Water Resources of Uzbekistan, and " UzCottonIndustry" association, Tashkent, Uzbekistan

2 Cotton Germplasm Unit, Institute of Genetics and Plant Experimental Biology, Academy of Sciences of Uzbekistan, Tashkent, Uzbekistan

3 Uzbek Scientific Research Institute of Cotton Breeding and Seed Production, Ministry of Agriculture and Water Resources of Uzbekistan, Tashkent, Uzbekistan

4 Department of Biology, National University of Uzbekistan, Uzbekistan

5 Uzbek Research Institute of Plant Industry, Ministry of Agriculture and Water Resources, Uzbekistan

References

[1] Abdurakhmonov IY. Role of genomic studies in boosting yield. In: Overcoming of no-growth in yield, Papers presented in fifth technical seminar, 72nd Plenary meeting of International Cotton Advisory Board (ICAC), Cartagena: Columbia; September 29-October 4, 2013, (Available at: https://www.icac.org/cotton_info/publications/tech_seminar/pub_tech_seminar/tis2013; verified on February 10, 2014).

[2] Abdurakhmonov IY. Exploiting genetic diversity. In: Ethridge D (eds): Plenary Presentations and Papers: Proceedings of World Cotton Research Conference-4; Sept 10-14, 2007, Lubbock, TX USA.

[3] Campbell BT, Saha S, Percy R, Frelichowski J, Jenkins JN, Park W, Mayee CD, Gotmare V, Dessauw D, Gband M, Du X, Jia Y, Constable G, Dillon S, Abdurakhmonov IY *et al.* Status of global cotton germplasm resources. Crop Sci 2010; 50: 1161-1179.

[4] Cotton Fact Sheet, ICAC. 2011. (available at http://www.icac.org/econ_stats/country_fact_sheets/fact_sheet_uzbekistan_2011.pdf, verified on February 10, 2014).

[5] Cotton: World Statistics. 2009. Bulletin of International Cotton Advisory Committee (ICAC). Washington D.C., USA.

[6] Abdukarimov A, Djataev S, Abdurakhmonov IY. Cotton Research in Uzbekistan: Elite varieties and future of cotton breeding: Proceedings of WCRC-3, 2003, South Africa.

[7] Ibragimov PS, Avtonomov VA, Amanturdiev AB, Namazov SE, Zaurov DE, Molnar TJ, Eisenman SW, Orton TJ, Funk CR, Percival J, Edward A. Uzbek Scientific Research Institute of Cotton Breeding and Seed Production: Breeding and germplasm resources. J. Cotton Sci 2008; 12:62-72.

[8] Abdullaev A, Abdullaev AA, Salakhutdinov, Rizaeva S, Kuryazov Z, Ernazarova D, Abdurakhmonov IY. Cotton germplasm collection of Uzbekistan. In: Egamberdieva D, Abdurakhmonov I (eds). Cotton Research in Uzbekistan. Asian and Australasian Journal of Plant Science and Biotechnology 7 (Special Issue 2) 2013; 1-15.

[9] Chen ZJ, Scheffler BE, Dennis E, Triplett BA, Zhang T, Guo W *et al*. Toward sequencing cotton (*Gossypium*) genomes. *Plant Physiol.* 2007; 145:1303-1310.

[10] Abdurakhmonov IY, Buriev ZT, Shermatov SE, Abdullaev AA, Urmonov HU, Kushanov FN, Egamberdiev SS, Shapulatov UM, Abdukarimov AA, Sukumar S, Jenkins JN, Kohel RJ, Yu JZ, Pepper AE, Kumpatala SP, Ulloa M. Genetic diversity of *Gossypium* genus.: M. Caliskan (eds). Plant Genetic Diversity. Croatia: Intech; 2012a p313-338.

[11] Abdurakhmonov IY, Abdullaev A. Rizaeva S, Buriev Z, Adylova A, Abdukarimov A, Saha S, Kohel R, Yu J, Pepper A. Evaluation of G. hirsutum exotic accessions from Uzbek cotton germplasm collection for further molecular mapping purposes: Cotton Beltwide conference: Proceedings, 2004, San Antonio, Texas, USA.

[12] Abdurakhmonov IY, Buriev ZT, Salakhuddinov IB, Rizaeva SM, Adylova AT, Shermatov SE, Abdukarimov A, Kohel RJ, Yu JZ, Pepper AE, Saha S, Jenkins JN. Characterization of *G. hirsutum* wild and variety accessions from Uzbek Cotton Germplasm collection for morphological and fibre quality traits and database development: Cotton Beltwide Conference, Jan. 3-6, 2006, San Antonio, Texas, USA.

[13] Rizaeva SM. Interspecific hybridization of cotton and development of new cotton donor accessions (in the example of New World cottons). PhD thesis. Institute of Plant Experimental Biology of the Academy of Sciences of Uzbekistan, 1996.

[14] Rizaeva SM, Abdullaev AA, Klyat VP, Arslonov DM, Kuryazov ZB. Creation of donors with naturally early leaf defoliation. Uzbek Biol. Journal 2001; 4:65-70.

[15] Abdurakhmonov IY, Abdullaev AA, Saha S, Buriev ZT, Arslanov D, Kuryazov Z, Mavlonov GT, Rizaeva SM, Reddy UK, Jenkins JN, Abdullaev A, Abdukarimov A.

Simple sequence repeat marker associated with a natural leaf defoliation trait in tetraploid cotton. Journal of Heredity 2005; 96:644-653.

[16] Saydaliev H. World cotton germplasm collection of Uzbek Research Institute of Cotton Breeding and Seed Production. Uzbek biology Journal 2006; *4:79-82 (in Russian).*

[17] Musaev JA, Abzalov MF, Almatov A, Sanamyan MF, Gubanova N, Nadjimov U. Cotton genetics and genetic collection of isogenic, monosomic and translocation lines. Bulletins SCST of the republic of Uzbekistan 1997; 28–39.

[18] Abdurakhmonov IY, Buriev ZT, Saha S, Pepper AE, Musaev JA, Almatov A, Shermatov SE, Kushanov FN, Mavlonov GT, Reddy UK, Yu JZ, Jenkins JN, Kohel RJ, Abdukarimov A. Microsatellite markers associated with lint percentage trait in cotton, *Gossypium hirsutum*. Euphytica 2007; 156: 141-156.

[19] Sanamyan MF, Petlyakova JE, Sharipova EA, Abdurakhmonov IY. Morphological characteristics and identification of new monosomic stocks for cotton (*Gossypium hirsutum* L.). Advances in Bioscience and Biotechnology 2010; 1: 372-383.

[20] Sanamyan MF, Petlyakova JE, Sharipova EA, Abdurakhmonov IY. 2011. Cytogenetic Characteristics of New Monosomic Stocks of Cotton (*Gossypium hirsutum* L.). Genetics Research International 2011; (2011): 27364.

[21] Abdurakhmonov IY, Buriev Z, Shermatov S, Abdullaev A, Kushanov F, Abdukarimov A, Saha S, Jenkins J, Yu J, Kohel R, Percy R, Ulloa U, Stelly D, Pepper A. Cotton genomics and transgenomics in Uzbekistan: Proceedings of the International Cotton Genome Initiative, 2012b, Conference.

[22] Abdurakhmonov IY, Shapulatov UM, Shermatov SE, Buriev ZT, Abdullaev AA, Kushanov FN, Egamberdiev SS, Salahutdinov IB, Ubaydullaeva HA, Makamov AH, Darmanov MM, Ayubov MS, Norov TM, Tulanov AA, Mavlonov GT, Abdukarimov A. Achievements and perspectives of cotton "omics" in Uzbekistan: Proceedings of the International Cotton conference Bremen, March 19-21, 2014, Bremen, Germany.

[23] Abdurakhmonov IY, Kohel RJ, Yu JZ, Pepper AE, Abdullaev AA, Kushanov FN, Salakhutdinov IB, Buriev ZT, Saha S, Scheffler BE, Jenkins JN, Abdukarimov A. Molecular diversity and association mapping of fibre quality traits in exotic *G. hirsutum* L. germplasm. Genomics 2008; 92:478-87.

[24] Abdurakhmonov IY, Saha S, Jenkins JN, Buriev ZT, Shermatov SE, Scheffler BE, Pepper AE, Yu JZ, Kohel RJ, Abdukarimov A. Linkage disequilibrium based association mapping of fibre quality traits in *G. hirsutum* L. variety germplasm. Genetica 2009; 136:401-17.

[25] Stelly D, Saha S, Raska D, Jenkins J, McCarty J, Gutierrez O. Registration of 17 Upland (*Gossypium hirsutum*) germplasm lines disomic for different *G. barbadense* chromosome or arm substitutions. Crop Science 2005; 45: 6:2663-2665.

[26] Saha S, Wu J, Jenkins J, McCarty J, Stelly D, Percy R, Raska D, and Gutierrez O. Effect of chromosome substitutions from *Gossypium barbadense* L. 3-79 into *G. hirsutum* L. TM-1 on agronomic and fibre traits. Journal of Cotton Science 2004; 8:162-169.

[27] Saha S, Stelly DM, Raska DA, Wu J, Jenkins JN, McCarty JC, Makamov A, Gotmare V, Abdurakhmonov IY, Campbell BT. Chromosome substitution lines: concept, development and utilization in the genetic improvement of Upland cotton, Plant Breeding, Ibrokhim Y. Abdurakhmonov (Ed.), Croatia: InTech; 2012.

[28] Jenkins J, Wu J, McCarty J, Saha S, Gutierrez O, Hayes R, Stelly D. Genetic effects of thirteen *Gossypium barbadense* L. chromosome substitution lines with Upland cotton cultivars: I. Yield and yield component. Crop Science 2006; 46:1169-1178.

[29] Jenkins J, Wu J, McCarty J, Saha S, Gutierrez O, Hayes R, Stelly D. Genetic effects of thirteen Gossypium barbadense L. chromosome substitution lines in topcrosses with Upland cotton cultivars: II fibre quality traits. Crop Science 2007; 47:561-570.

[30] Abdurakhmonov IY, Buriev ZT, Logan-Young CJ, Abdukarimov A, Pepper AE. Duplication, divergence and persistence in the phytochrome photoreceptor gene family of cottons (*Gossypium* spp.). BMC Plant Biol 2010; 10:119.

[31] Abdukarimov A, Abdurakhmonov IY, Buriev ZT, Bozorov TA. Small interfering RNA (siRNA) for knocking down gene expression in plant cells. Uzbekistan patent IAP 04300. Official bulletins of State Patents #2-6, 2011.

[32] Abdurakhmonov IY, Buriev ZT, Saha S, Jenkins JN, Abdukarimov A, Pepper AE. Cotton PHYA1 RNAi enhances major fibre quality and agronomic traits of cotton (*Gossypium hirsutum* L). Nature Communications 2013; 5: 3062.

[33] Mavlyanova RF, Abdullaev FKh, Khodjiev P, Zaurov DE, Molhar TJ, Goffreda JC, Orton TJ, Funk CR. Plant Genetic Resources and Scientific Activities of the Uzbek Scientific Research Institute of Plant Industry. J Hort Science 2005; 40 (1):10-14.

[34] Muratov UH, Tadjibaev T, Alikhodjaev SS, Munasov K. Catalog of cotton cultivars. Tashkent: University Press; 1992. (in Russian).

[35] Lemishev N, Atlanov A, Podolnaya L, Korneychuk B. Unified Council for Mutual Economic Assistance (COMECON) list of descriptors for the species Gossypium L. Leningrad: VIR; 1989.

[36] Abdullaev FK. Information Technology Use for Documentation of Genepool in Uzbekistan.Genetic Resources of Cultivated Plants in XXI Century: Current Status, Problems, Perspectives: Abstracts of II Vavilov International Conference.-26-30 November 2007. St.Petersburg. pg. 669-670. (in Russian).

[37] Abdullaev FK. Management of Plant Genetic Resources by the Information Technology Base. Soil-Water Journal. 2013, 2: 2 (2).

[38] Abdurakhmonov IY. Understanding and utilization of molecular diversity in cotton genome: TWAS Prize 2010 lecture, 22nd General meeting of TWAS, November 20-23, 2011, Trieste, Italy.

[39] Abdullaev A, Klyat VP, Rizaeva SM, Abdullaev AA, Abdurakhmonov IY. Cotton germplasm collection and an updated taxonomy of *Gossypium* L. 4th World Cotton Research Conference: Abstracts of World Cotton Research Conference-4; Sept 10-14, 2007, Lubbock, TX USA.

[40] Mauer FM. Origin and taxonomy of cotton. In Cotton. Academy of Sciences of USSR: Tashkent; 1954. (in Russian).

[41] Abdullaev AA, Dariev AC, Omelchenko MV, Klyat VP, Rizaeva CM, Saydaliev H, Khalikova MB.. Atlas of *Gossypium L.* genus. Tashkent: Fan; 2010.

[42] Sanamyan MF, Rakhmatullina EM. Cytogenetic analysis of translocations in cotton. Plant Breed 2003; 122 (6): 511–516.

[43] Abdullaev, AA, Klyat VP, Rizaeva SM. Cotton introduction in Uzbekistan-history and perspectives of using of plant introduction: problems and perspectives: Proceedings of 4th National scientific-applied conference; July 3-4, 2009; Tashkent Uzbekistan. (in Russian).

[44] Nematov SH, Batalov AM, Sultanov AA, Nematov IH. Development of Productive Cotton Cultivars with Increased fibre Quality for Bukhara Region of Uzbekistan. In: Egamberdieva D, Abdurakhmonov I (eds). Cotton Research in Uzbekistan; Asian and Australasian Journal of Plant Science and Biotechnology 7 (Special Issue 2) 2013; 16-18.

[45] Abdurakhmonov IY, Abdukarimov A. Application of association mapping to understanding the genetic diversity of plant germplasm resources. International Journal of Plant Genomics 2008; 574927.

[46] Abdurakhmonov IY, Buriev ZT, Shermatov SE *et al.* Marker-assisted selection for complex fibre traits in cotton: 5th World Cotton Research Conference, Special session of ICGI, November 7-12, 2011a, Mumbai, India.

[47] Abdurakhmonov IY, Buriev ZT, Shermatov SE, Kushanov FN, Makamov A, Shopulatov U, Turaev O, Norov T, Akhmedov Ch, Mirzaakhmedov M, Abdukarimov A. Utilization of natural diversity in Upland cotton (G. *hirsutum*) germplasm collection for pyramiding genes via marker-assisted selection program: Presentation in 5th Asian Cotton Research and Development Network conference, February, 2011b, Lahore, Pakistan.

[48] Stich B, Melchinger AE. An Introduction to Association Mapping in Plants. CAB Reviews: Perspectives in Agriculture, Veterinary Science, Nutrition and Natural Resources 2010; 5:1-9.

[49] Kumpatla SP, Buyyarapu R, Abdurakhmonov IY, Mammadov JA. In: Ibrokhim IY (eds). Genomics-assisted plant breeding in the 21st Century: Technological Advances and Progress. Plant Breeding, Croatia: InTech; 2012.